MASTER
MEDICINE

Medical Biochemistry

Commissioning Editor: Timothy Horne
Project Development Manager: Barbara Simmons
Project Manager: Nancy Arnott
Designer: George Ajayi

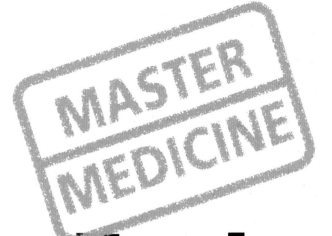

Medical Biochemistry

A core text with self-assessment

ALEXANDER C. BROWNIE

PhD DSc FRSE
Formerly Consultant in Biochemistry,
University of Dundee;
SUNY Distinguished Teaching Professor Emeritus,
Senior Curriculum Advisor, School of Medicine,
University at Buffalo, NY, USA

JOHN C. KERNOHAN

MA PhD
Formerly Senior Lecturer, Department of Biochemistry,
University of Dundee, UK

ELSEVIER
CHURCHILL
LIVINGSTONE

EDINBURGH   LONDON   NEW YORK   OXFORD   PHILADELPHIA   ST LOUIS   SYDNEY   TORONTO 2005

ELSEVIER
CHURCHILL
LIVINGSTONE

First edition   1999
Second edition   2005

ISBN   0443100152

British Library Cataloguing in Publication Data
A catalogue record for this book is available from the British Library

Library of Congress Cataloging in Publication Data
A catalog record for this book is available from the Library of Congress

Notice
Medical knowledge is constantly changing. Standard safety precautions must be followed, but as new research and clinical experience broaden our knowledge, changes in treatment and drug therapy may become necessary or appropriate. Readers are advised to check the most current product information provided by the manufacturer of each drug to be administered to verify the recommended dose, the method and duration of administration, and contraindications. It is the responsibility of the practitioner, relying on experience and knowledge of the patient, to determine dosages and the best treatment for each individual patient. Neither the Publisher nor the authors assumes any liability for any injury and/or damage to persons or property arising from this publication.
The Publisher

ELSEVIER   your source for books,
journals and multimedia
in the health sciences
www.elsevierhealth.com

Working together to grow
libraries in developing countries

www.elsevier.com | www.bookaid.org | www.sabre.org

ELSEVIER   BOOK AID
International   Sabre Foundation

The
publisher's
policy is to use
**paper manufactured
from sustainable forests**

Printed in China

Preface

Biochemistry and medicine

Most biochemists will tell you that the enormous strides that have been made in advancing medical knowledge have been largely the result of the development of methods that allow us to examine physiological and pathological processes at the molecular level. In fact, almost every branch of clinical medicine research is carried out using the latest molecular biology techniques. The fact that the newspapers report these advances on an almost daily basis and terms such as 'recombinant DNA', 'cloning' and 'proteonics' are printed without explanation is surely reason enough why medical graduates must be better informed than the lay public.

Surely the parents of a child with a metabolic disorder (diabetes affects millions in the UK alone!) should expect their general practitioner to know enough about intermediary metabolism that they can explain the diagnostic techniques available and the biochemical basis of treatment regimens.

You need to understand the background to the screening of newborn infants for inborn errors of metabolism, which is carried out routinely in most technically advanced countries. Interpretation of the data requires knowledge of basic aspects of metabolism and biochemical genetics.

Given the major role that (bad) diet plays in the extraordinarily high incidence of coronary heart disease in the UK (the rate is not low in North America or in Northern Europe), it is surely unacceptable for medical students not to understand basic aspects of lipoprotein metabolism. Similarly, it is imperative that our medical graduates appreciate the mechanisms that are involved in the beneficial actions of vitamins in important periods of life such as pregnancy and growth and development.

If you have a patient who may have had a heart attack, you need to know about the enzyme assays that support the diagnosis and when you may need to request more specific tests.

Table 1 is a (incomplete) list of clinical biochemical studies carried out on patients in hospital and on outpatients and the core biochemistry related to these tests.

The fact that a biochemistry laboratory of high or moderate sophistication is present in every hospital re-emphasises the importance of this discipline. Now all one need do is get on with the task of studying biochemistry.

Table 1 Some clinical biochemical studies and the related biochemistry

Clinical biochemistry	Core biochemistry
Blood glucose	Carbohydrate metabolism and its control
Blood urea	Amino acid catabolism; the urea cycle; liver function
Serum cholesterol	Lipid and lipoprotein metabolism
Serum fatty acids	Lipid and lipoprotein metabolism
Serum albumin	Protein synthesis; liver function; nutrition
Prothrombin time	Blood coagulation, protein synthesis
Lactate dehydrogenase	Enzyme kinetics; electrophoresis; enzyme assay
Creatine kinase	Enzyme kinetics; electrophoresis
DNA analysis	DNA structure and DNA replication
Serum thyroxine and thyroid-stimulating hormone	Endocrine system
Phenylalanine	Amino acid catabolism; inheritance of disease
Ketone bodies	Ketogenesis; starvation; diabetes mellitus
Serum uric acid	Purine nucleotide metabolism
Serum calcium	Control of calcium metabolism; parathyroid hormone; vitamin D and calcium
Serum bilirubin	Haem degradation; liver function
Liver function tests	Enzyme assays; liver metabolism
Plasma and urinary creatinine	One-carbon metabolism; muscle creatine metabolism
Haemoglobin A_{1c}	Glucose homeostasis; diabetes mellitus

Acknowledgements

Both authors have been teaching general biochemistry to medical, dental and science students for many years. During this time we have had many colleagues whose input to jointly taught courses have impacted on our teaching and therefore this text. A.C.B. wishes to express his indebtedness to the late Dr John F. Moran, University at Buffalo, and Dr Steven Simasko, College of Veterinary Medicine, Washington State, with whom he taught metabolism and endocrinology in Buffalo and who influenced the treatment of these topics in the first edition. Likewise, Dr Josephine Alfano, University at Buffalo, reviewed the chapter on the endocrine system.

The authors thank their colleagues at the University of Dundee, Professor Michael J. Rennie and Michael Stark, who provided material on protein turnover and biochemical genetics, respectively. Dr Roger Booth reviewed Chapters 1–11 in the first edition.

An important contribution to the writing of the second edition was the careful review of chapters in the first edition by colleagues of A.C.B. in Buffalo. The authors are greatly indebted to Professors Murray Ettinger, Mark O'Brian, Richard Erbe, Michael Duffy, and Mulchand Patel of the School of Medicine and Biomedical Sciences, University at Buffalo, for their critiques and insightful suggestions.

We thank Barbara Simmons at Elsevier for her guidance in producing this second edition.

Lastly, we acknowledge the support of our wives, Willy Brownie-Bakhuizen and Kathy Kernohan, who once more tolerated our commitment to many hours of work on the text when we were supposed to be retired.

Contents

Using this book

Philosophy of this book

Both the General Medical Council in Great Britain and the Licensing Committee on Medical Education in the United States have recommended significant changes in the medical curriculum. Phase 1 of such a new curriculum emphasises integration, a system approach and the presentation of core knowledge. The teaching of a core biochemistry course to medical or dental students represents a major challenge. The problem that we face in designing biochemistry courses is that it is difficult to identify *anything* that is not core. This applies especially in the rapidly developing area of molecular biology and the fact-rich area of metabolism. However, almost every day newspapers tell the public about latest findings that affect the quality of health care delivery and this book will help you develop a base of knowledge upon which you can build.

Layout of the book

This book covers General and Applied Biochemistry. Some of our colleagues have provided us with the learning objectives for their lectures and we have designed the book to conform to these. Since this is a text primarily directed at medical students, we have included brief 'clinical notes' in order to demonstrate the applications of core biochemistry knowledge to clinical practice. With a more generous page allowance we could have included many more.

We recognise that self-assessment by our students is the key to them dealing with the intensity of the medical curriculum and have prepared many exercises that complement the various chapters in this core text. We have completely reorganised the Multiple Choice Questions in the book and have adopted the *Single Best Answer* approach that experts in evaluation have shown to be best for evaluating students' understanding of a discipline. Stems are now longer, especially in the applied biochemistry areas, and problem-solving is encouraged wherever possible. Because of this decision we have over a hundred new questions in the book.

Studying biochemistry

Core knowledge essential for students in the life sciences has not become easier, but because of the application of the tools of modern molecular biology we can now describe the systems in a clearer fashion. How should students deal with the knowledge explosion in a core course? Our advice is as follows:

- Make sure to take basic courses in chemistry, biology, mathematics and physics prior to entry into medical school.
- Read the appropriate section of this core text *before* attending lectures. If detailed lecture notes are part of the course, read them in advance as well. If necessary, read relevant material in one of the many excellent comprehensive texts available.
- Try to be *honest* and admit when there are areas or points that you find confusing. The key is not to delay in filling these gaps in your understanding. Often you can clear up problems by talking to a colleague but, failing that, talk to a teacher or teaching assistant. Students who fail miserably and who have not asked for help do not impress anyone!
- You will find that many new terms will be introduced in your biochemistry lectures. Be consistent in listing these terms along with their definition. Prepare a *glossary* by making use of this text and others. Writing down definitions and descriptions will help fix the information in your memory.
- During the course, prepare a list of headings of the various subsections of the material well spaced out on sheets of paper. Closer to examination time take these sheets and fill in as much of the gaps as you can. Comparison with your lecture notes will establish two things: (a) what you know well and (b) what you need to study. In this way you avoid reading through your entire course notes or course book again and again. This is a diagnostic approach to gauging your knowledge.
- Your aim should be to arrive at the examination hall *knowing* what you know. You are there simply to let the teachers know *what* you know. You need to engage in *regular and extensive self-assessment*. Each chapter in this book ends with a series of self-assessment questions. Try them after you have reviewed the material in the chapter. Make sure you use any self-assessment exercises that your teachers have prepared; they may be easy to access through your

university computer network. You need to get used to the type of questions your teachers tend to ask.

Examination techniques

There is a lot of variation in exam formats used in the different universities. Since medical classes are usually large, easily scored multiple choice questions (MCQs) are frequently used, but it is also useful to develop skills in answering short essay questions. Here are some hints that apply to MCQs:

1. MCQs need particular attention since a single word can change the answer dramatically.
2. **Read the stem more than once**.
3. Although the MCQs in this book are all of the *single best answer* type, many teachers use MCQs where there can be any number of correct answers so you need to make decisions **true** or **false** for every option. If you are given no guidance as to the number of true or false statements in an MCQ, in most cases you get credit for all correct answers selected, but you lose points for incorrect ones (negative marking). Make sure you know what system is being used
4. *Read the exam instructions carefully before you start!*
5. Know if the examiners allow for challenges! This is often possible if you receive a copy of the exam or if it is posted.
6. Words in the stem such as *direct* and *indirect* can make terrific differences to the answers. Words such as *all* or *never* are often giveaways that the choice is false but there is no hard and fast rule.

7. Do not spend too much time on tough questions. Go through all of the questions answering those you feel most confident about and then return to the others. If guessing is not punished, make sure you answer every MCQ.
8. If an MCQ has a long clinical vignette as the stem, see if you can arrive at an answer before you look at the options.
9. If your exams are taken at a computer terminal, make sure you practise with sample questions at a terminal; this will improve your chances of success in degree exams.

Here are some hints that apply if you are taking exams with short answers or essays.

1. Make sure to start by sketching out the major points you will cover; if necessary, ask for scrap paper! This helps to organise your answer and will be appreciated by the examiner.
2. Do not fail to illustrate your answers with well-conceived, clear diagrams.
3. Do not drift from the point of the question; examiners get tired and angry reading through a mass of irrelevancy!
4. Ration your time since it is advisable to answer *all* of the required essays.
5. Practise writing answers to questions that appeared in previous years' exams; they are usually provided but, if not, ask for them! Find out if your teacher is willing to give you an opinion on your practice efforts.

1 Molecules in cells and water

Overview

Water is the most abundant molecule in living matter. It has unique physical and chemical properties. It enables or moderates the range of transient and weak molecular interactions involved in biochemical processes. It is also a reactant or product in many biochemical reactions.

1.1 What is biochemistry about?

Learning objective

You should be able to:

- describe the nature of biochemistry.

Biochemistry is the study of the molecular events that correspond to the phenomenon of life. It is concerned with the relationship between the structure and the function of the molecules that occur in living systems. Biochemists believe that it is possible to give an account of physiological observations, such as muscle contraction, gas exchange in the lung and nerve conduction, in terms of the molecules involved and the laws of physics and chemistry. Most of the processes that interest a biochemist occur, or at least start, in cells, so we begin by asking what kinds of molecules we find in cells.

Molecules in cells

Cells contain a great variety of molecules, ranging from enormous polymers containing millions of atoms to small building block and fuel molecules with fewer than 100 atoms. Before we start our study of the molecules

that are the main subject matter of biochemistry (proteins, nucleic acids, polysaccharides, lipids and metabolites), we must consider the most abundant molecule in cells: water.

1.2 The importance of water

Learning objectives

You should be able to:

- describe the unique physical properties of water

- describe the influence of water in weak intermolecular forces such as hydrogen bonds, electrostatic forces and hydrophobic interactions

- give examples of biochemical reactions in which water is (a) a reactant and (b) a product.

Water accounts for about 60% of the body weight of an adult:

- about 63% of body water is within cells
- 37% is extracellular fluid
- about one-quarter of extracellular fluid is blood plasma.

The importance of water in the body is shown by the precision with which the water content of the body is regulated by physiological mechanisms, including thirst and renal function. Deviations of more than 1% or 2% from the normal have adverse effects on our well-being and performance. Uncontrolled water loss from the body, which can occur in diseases such as cholera and untreated diabetes, is life-threatening.

Water is important in biochemistry not only because of its abundance but also because it influences the behaviour of all other molecules of biochemical interest. All biochemical processes occur in, or in contact with, aqueous solution, so we must bear in mind the properties of water if we are to understand how other molecules interact in cells.

Physical properties of water

The molecular formula for water, H_2O, does not reveal what an unusual substance water is. The molecule

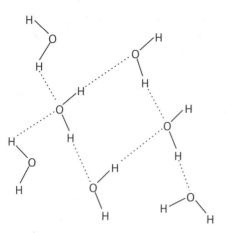

Fig. 1 Cluster of water molecules held together by hydrogen bonds.

contains an oxygen atom making covalent bonds with each of two hydrogen atoms. However, the molecule so formed is highly polar as the 'centre of gravity' of its positive charge does not coincide with its centre of negative charge. This polar nature has a strong influence on its physical properties. Water molecules act as electrostatic dipoles; they attract each other strongly and form clusters (Fig. 1). The clusters formed by water molecules are temporary; molecules are continually leaving one cluster and joining another. Water in the liquid state is highly mobile and has no regular long-range structure.

Polar interactions and hydrogen bonds make water a liquid at temperatures at which all other molecules of a similar size are gases.

Hydrogen bonds

Another important interaction between water molecules that favours cluster formation is the formation of hydrogen bonds. A hydrogen bond is the sharing of two electrons on an oxygen or nitrogen atom with a hydrogen atom carried on another atom, usually oxygen or nitrogen (but not carbon). This bond is weaker and longer than a covalent bond (Fig. 2). The hydrogen bond is about 0.28 nm long compared with a covalent bond length of 0.15 nm. The energy required to break a hydrogen bond is about 20 times lower than that needed to break a covalent bond.

Hydrogen bond formation in water tends to organise water molecules in space. A hydrogen bond is strongest when the hydrogen atom, the oxygen atom to which it

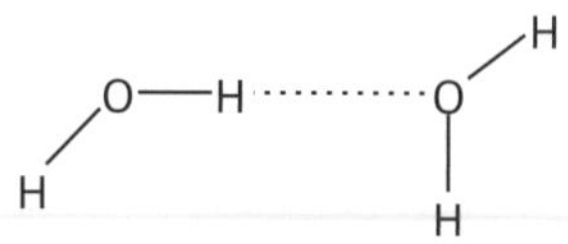

Fig. 2 Hydrogen bond between water molecules.

is covalently bonded and the other atom forming the hydrogen bond are in line. Ice, or solid water, is an array of water molecules held in place by hydrogen bonds; it has a regular long-range structure.

Many molecules of biochemical interest are capable of forming hydrogen bonds. Bonds are formed both within and between molecules, but most hydrogen bonds are formed in competition with the bonds that could be formed with water. Water thus provides a medium in which hydrogen bonds can be rapidly formed and broken.

Although they are weaker than covalent bonds, hydrogen bonds are very important in biochemistry because they are so numerous and because they can be formed and broken so readily. Appropriate spacing of hydrogen bond acceptors and donors provides one mechanism for intermolecular recognition and specific binding.

Solvent and ionising properties of water

Water, being polar, is an excellent solvent for other polar molecules. Molecules such as glucose and the smaller amino acids are polar and are very soluble in water. As a consequence of its polar nature water has a high dielectric constant. This means that it reduces the electrostatic forces between any charged particles it surrounds. Water is thus an excellent solvent for ionic materials. Sodium and chloride ions in a salt crystal attract each other so strongly that the crystal is a highly stable structure in air or in most solvents. In the presence of water, the ions become hydrated (surrounded by a shell of water molecules) and the attractive forces between the ions are greatly reduced. The hydrated ions can readily separate and enter solution.

An *acid* is a molecule that can dissociate to form a hydrogen ion, H^+, and a *base*. Water can promote the dissociation of hydrogen ions from acids in two ways:

- It acts as an acceptor for the hydrogen ion, which should really be represented not as H^+ but as H_3O^+, and even the H_3O^+ is hydrated. H^+ on its own is unstable, so ionisation of acids requires the presence of an ionising solvent such as water.
- If the base is negatively charged, water reduces the attractive force between the base and the departing positively charged hydrogen ion.

For example, the dissociation of acetic acid, a typical weak acid, is promoted in water, where the H^+ produced can be made more stable by hydration:

$$CH_3COOH + H_2O = CH_3COO^- + H_3^+O$$

Hydrogen ions are important in many biochemical processes. They are about 100 times more mobile than any other ions in aqueous solution since water provides

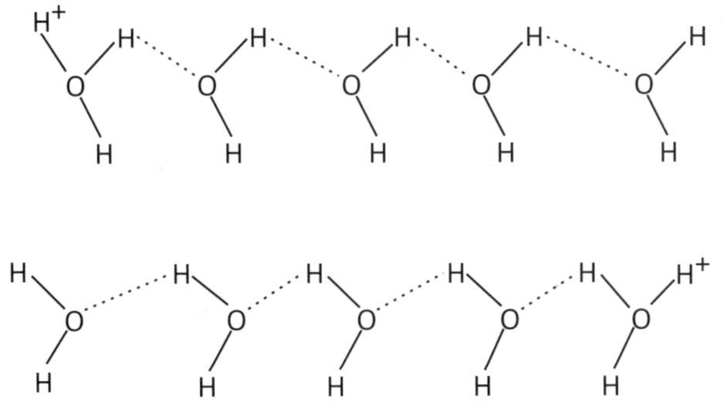

Fig. 3 Mobility of hydrogen ions in water.

a special tunnelling mechanism for their movement. The positive charge representing the hydrogen atom can move through clusters of water molecules with minimal movement of any atoms (Fig. 3).

The concentration of hydrogen ions, [H$^+$], influences many biochemical processes and is controlled in living cells and the fluid surrounding them. It is always quoted in biochemistry as *pH*, where:

$$pH = -\log_{10}[H^+]$$

Strictly speaking, the hydrogen ion activity, not concentration, should be used, but few biochemists make this distinction.

Most molecules of biochemical interest have one or more chemical groupings that can act as acids or bases, groups that can donate or accept a hydrogen ion. Each hydrogen ion lost decreases the charge on the molecule by one unit and each hydrogen ion gained increases the charge. Since dissociation of acids and binding of hydrogen ions by bases are rapid equilibrium processes, the charge on many biochemical molecules varies with the pH of the medium. This usually influences their properties and functions. Some molecules, such as amino acids, can have both positive and negative charges. These molecules are known as *zwitterions*. In most biochemical experiments, pH must be controlled by using buffers.

Water and non-polar molecules

Molecules that are not polar are generally insoluble in water. Water molecules cling to each other, excluding the non-polar molecules, which remain clustered together as solids or immiscible liquids. For example, water is immiscible with liquid hydrocarbons such as hexane and benzene.

Amphipathic molecules and hydrophobic interactions

Many biochemical molecules, long-chain fatty acids and their ions are examples, cannot be classified as simply polar or non-polar. One part of a molecule may be polar and interact readily with water, and is said to be *hydrophilic* or 'water-loving', whereas another part is non-polar and is excluded from water, being *hydrophobic* or 'water-hating'. Such molecules with both a hydrophilic part and a hydrophobic part are said to be *amphipathic*. Water has a powerful influence on such molecules and organises them into biochemically important structures such as:

- membranes (see p. 48)
- folded globular proteins (see p. 21)
- the DNA double helix (see p. 179).

In these structures, hydrophobic parts of molecules associate with other hydrophobic parts to form a core from which water is excluded. The surface of the structure is composed of the hydrophilic parts of the molecules. The surrounding water molecules stabilise the structure.

Water as a reactant

Biochemical reactions often involve water molecules as a reactant or product. Many reactions in metabolism involve the addition or elimination of a water molecule. The polymerisation of building block molecules to make macromolecules such as proteins or nucleic acids involves the elimination of a water molecule and the formation of a covalent bond between the building blocks. Breakdown of the macromolecules, as in digestion, is by *hydrolysis*, the cleavage of the bond between the building blocks with the introduction of a molecule of water. Because it is present in cells at such a high concentration, water drives hydrolysis reactions. The breakdown of biopolymers in aqueous solution is, therefore, energetically favourable, whereas the synthesis of these polymers from their building blocks requires an input of energy.

Self-assessment: questions

Single best answer MCQs

1. Which of the following statements accurately reflects physiological aspects of water?
   a. Water accounts for more than one-half of the mass of the body
   b. Most of the water in the body is outside cells
   c. Most of the extracellular water in the body is in the blood plasma
   d. Water in the body acts as an inert solvent and does not take part in cellular reactions
   e. The water content of the body is so high that changes in its water content are usually well tolerated

2. Identify the correct statement concerning solvent properties of water and its influence on the behaviour of molecules in cells.
   a. Water influences the behaviour of molecules such as long-chain fatty acids even though they are virtually insoluble
   b. Water prevents the ionisation of acids such as acetic acid
   c. Amino acids such as glycine and alanine are almost insoluble in water since they must form zwitterions in solution
   d. In water the attractive electrostatic forces between oppositely charged ions, such as Na^+ and Cl^-, are decreased and the repulsive forces between ions having the same charge are increased
   e. Water is an excellent solvent for non-polar substances such as glucose that have many hydroxyl groups in the molecule

3. From your knowledge of water and hydrogen bonds in cellular processes select the single correct statement from the following.
   a. A water molecule can act as a hydrogen bond donor but not as a hydrogen bond acceptor
   b. Hydrogen bonds occur between water molecules in the liquid state but not in ice
   c. Water molecules can form hydrogen bonds with hydrogen atoms attached by covalent bonds to oxygen and carbon atoms but not to those attached to nitrogen
   d. The occurrence of hydrogen bonds between water molecules gives liquid water a regular three-dimensional structure
   e. Hydrogen bonds, although weak, are numerous and can be made and broken very rapidly

4. Phosphoric acid dissociates in three stages to produce a phosphate ion, according to the following scheme:

   $$H_3PO_4 = H^+ + H_2PO_4^- = H^+ + HPO_4^{2-} = H^+ + PO_4^{3-}$$

   Identify the single correct statement concerning that scheme.
   a. The species $H_2PO_4^-$ is not an acid because it is not a neutral molecule
   b. The species $H_2PO_4^-$ is not a base because it can dissociate a hydrogen ion
   c. The species $H_2PO_4^-$ is not an acid because it can accept a hydrogen ion
   d. The species $H_2PO_4^-$ is both an acid and a base
   e. The species H_3PO_4 is a weaker acid than $H_2PO_4^-$ or HPO_4^{2-}

5. Which of the following statements accurately reflects the influence of water on cellular molecules?
   a. Water has no effect on the structures of macromolecules
   b. Water has no effect on the hydrophobic parts of amphipathic molecules
   c. Water is excluded from cellular membranes so it does not contribute to the stability of their structures
   d. Changes of pH alter the charge carried by proteins and influence their properties
   e. Water hydrates the hydrogen ion so it has a low mobility in aqueous solution

6. Which of the following statements accurately reflects the role of water in biochemical reactions?
   a. Water is a reactant in many reactions involved in the digestion of foodstuffs
   b. Water is present in such high concentration that it has no influence on the equilibrium of cellular reactions
   c. Hydration is the cleavage of a covalent bond with the introduction of the elements of a water molecule
   d. The formation of biological polymers such as proteins and polysaccharides is energetically favoured by the high concentration of water in cells
   e. Water is one of the products of the digestion of foodstuffs

Short essay questions

1. What molecule would you look for first on a planet where you suspected that extraterrestrial life existed? Justify your answer.

2. 'Life is only possible in the presence of liquid water.' Comment on this statement. Also mention any practical applications it might have.

Self-assessment: answers

Single best answer MCQ answers

1. a. **True**. Water accounts for 55–65% of the weight of the body.
   b. **False**. About two-thirds of body water is inside cells.
   c. **False**. About one-quarter of extracellular water circulates as plasma.
   d. **False**. Far from being an inert solvent, water influences interactions between cellular molecules and takes part in many reactions.
   e. **False**. Although the water content of the body is high, it is also precisely regulated and significant changes in water content can be a serious threat to life.

2. a. **True**. Long-chain fatty acids are amphipathic and have polar groups that are hydrophilic.
   b. **False**. Water hydrates H^+ making it more stable. It also promotes dissociation by decreasing the attractive force between H^+ and the acetate ion.
   c. **False**. In water, these amino acids have charged amino and carboxyl groups. Although the molecules have no overall charge they are very polar.
   d. **False**. Water because of its high dielectric constant reduces all electrostatic forces between ions.
   e. **False**. Glucose is very polar.

3. a. **False**. Water can act as both donor and acceptor.
   b. **False**. Ice contains virtually the maximum possible number of hydrogen bonds.
   c. **False**. Hydrogen attached to carbon does not form hydrogen bonds. Hydrogen atoms attached to oxygen and nitrogen generally do.
   d. **False**. Liquid water is composed of temporary irregular clusters of water molecules.
   e. **True**. They are important in most interactions between cellular molecules.

4. a. **False**. Any molecular species from which H^+ can dissociate is an acid.
   b. **False**. Any molecular species that can accept H^+ is a base.
   c. **False**. Any molecular species from which H^+ can dissociate is an acid.

   d. **True**. $H_2PO_4^-$ can act as an acid or a base; it can dissociate or bind H^+.
   e. **False**. H_3PO_4 dissociates more readily than $H_2PO_4^-$; it has more hydrogen atoms and H^+ leaves a neutral molecule more readily than one that has a negative charge.

5. a. **False**. Cellular macromolecules depend on the presence of water for their structures and functions.
   b. **False**. The hydrophobic parts are excluded from the water phase so they tend to cluster together.
   c. **False**. The orientation of amphipathic membrane molecules in the presence of water is a major force for the stability of membrane structure.
   d. **True**. The binding of H^+ to cellular macromolecules, especially proteins, depends on the pH. This changes their charge and the way that they interact.
   e. **False**. Hydrogen-bonded water provides a tunnelling mechanism for hydrogen ion movement, making it very mobile in water.

6. a. **True**. Hydrolysis, the chemical reaction in digestion, requires water.
   b. **False**. The high concentration of water favours hydrolysis.
   c. **False**. This is the definition of hydrolysis. Hydration is the binding of water to other molecules by hydrogen bonds and other weak forces.
   d. **False**. Hydrolysis is favoured by the high concentration of water.
   e. **False**. Digestion consumes water as a reactant. Water is a product of the oxidation of foodstuffs.

Short essay answers

1. Water must surely be the first molecule that is looked for. Any form of life that could exist in the absence of water would be so different from life on earth that it would be impossible to predict what molecular form(s) it would take or which of its molecules to look for. The search for ATP on Mars would not make sense unless investigators already knew that water was present.

2. Most biochemical processes cease or are greatly slowed down in the absence of liquid water. Macromolecules are immobilised in the complete absence of water or in ice, and cannot interact at a sufficient rate with smaller molecules such as nutrients, metabolites and building blocks. The biochemical processes, mostly mediated by microorganisms involved in food spoilage, can be controlled by freezing or by desiccation, the removal of water. Biochemicals often spoil at room temperature. In the laboratory they are generally stored in the refrigerator or deep-freeze, or else in freeze-dried form.

2 Proteins

Overview

Protein molecules have a wide range of functions in living organisms. These functions depend on the ability of proteins to recognise and bind other molecules specifically. Proteins are made up of long chains of amino acids joined by stable peptide bonds. The same set of 20 amino acids is found in all organisms. Part of the structure of each amino acid is common to all and is involved in peptide bond formation. The other part, the side chain, varies from one amino acid to another. The 20 amino acid side chains have a wide range of sizes, shapes and chemical reactivities. Peptide chains contain specific sequences of amino acids and fold to produce three-dimensional structures with sites for binding other molecules. Study of these structures gives many insights into protein function.

2.1 Protein function

Learning objectives

You should be able to:

- give examples of the wide range of protein functions

- explain a common principle underlying most functions of proteins

- define the term: ligand.

Proteins are the first cellular macromolecules to be considered in this book because they are so central to biochemistry. Other macromolecules, while important in some biochemical processes, are generally synthesised, organised, controlled and regulated, packaged and eventually broken down by proteins. It is difficult to think of a biochemical process that does not involve the participation of proteins. The range of protein functions is enormous.

Mechanical functions
Proteins are a major part of the mechanical system of our bodies. Tendons made from collagen, a fibrous protein, are the inelastic ropes that allow our muscles, the protein motors, to move our bones. Bones have some protein content, being made from collagen and a calcium phosphate mineral. The bones are held together at our joints by the fibrous elastic protein elastin.

Energy production
Energy to drive the muscle motors is obtained from metabolic reactions catalysed by enzymes, which are proteins.

Oxygen carriage
Oxygen needed for metabolic reactions that generate energy is carried to our muscles and most other tissues by another protein, haemoglobin.

Regulatory signals
Signal proteins, notably the protein hormone insulin, regulate the concentrations of fuel molecules circulating to our muscles in our blood. Insulin and many other hormones move in our blood between the glands that secrete them and their target cells, where they are detected by protein receptors on the membrane. Once detected, the hormone signal is amplified, combined with other signals and acted upon by further proteins.

Protein synthesis
Proteins are responsible for many aspects of their own synthesis. Nucleic acids, which provide the information for protein synthesis, are synthesised, packaged, regulated and repaired by proteins. Proteins are involved in most stages of ribosome function during protein synthesis

and they are needed to provide the energy for the process.

Proteins bind other molecules specifically

Considering even this incomplete list of protein functions, it is surprising that a common principle can be discerned in all the biochemical functions of proteins. This common principle is that protein molecules are able to recognise and bind other molecules very specifically and with great affinity. This binding of other molecules occurs very rapidly and is often reversible. Many proteins have multiple binding sites, and the binding of one molecule by a protein often influences its ability to bind others.

The molecules that proteins bind are referred to as *ligands*. A ligand is a small molecule or part of a large molecule that can occupy a binding site. Oxygen is a ligand of haemoglobin, substrates and inhibitors are ligands of enzymes and a hormone molecule is the ligand of the receptor molecule with which it interacts.

Examples of ligand binding in protein function

Proteins involved in forming complex structures assemble by ligand binding. For instance, collagen molecules recognise and bind to other collagen molecules in a regular parallel array to form a fibre. This initial assembly is followed by covalent crosslinking to form a more permanent structure and eventually a tendon. Therefore, the ligand for bone collagen molecule is part of another collagen molecule. Collagen molecules that form the matrix of bone have further binding sites where initiation of bone calcification occurs.

Muscle
There are two principal proteins in muscle, *myosin* and *actin*, which each assemble into filaments: the thick and thin filaments, respectively. These filaments slide over each other as the muscle contracts or relaxes. Further binding sites on the proteins allow the filaments to combine with each other and then separate in a cyclical manner when fuelled by ATP and stimulated by calcium ions. This interaction between the filaments enables the muscle to develop tension and to contract. Myosin, therefore, has binding sites for several different ligands: other myosin molecules, actin filaments, ATP and interaction with calcium ions.

Enzymes
These catalytic proteins bind the molecules that participate in the reactions they catalyse, their substrates. This substrate binding often distorts the substrate, making it more reactive. By binding two substrates in an orientation favourable for reaction, the rate of the reaction between them is greatly enhanced. Some enzymes have further binding sites that can be occupied by specific molecules which switch the catalytic activity of the enzyme on or off.

Carriage of oxygen
No molecules composed entirely of amino acids have evolved that are capable of carrying oxygen molecules directly. The haemoglobin which carries oxygen in our blood is formed from a protein, *globin*, which specifically binds an iron-containing organic group, *haem*. Binding of the haem group to globin modifies the properties of haem so that it binds oxygen reversibly, a reaction not possible for haem on its own.

Nucleic acid function
The nucleic acids, particularly DNA, carry genetic information, information on the structures of our proteins. Even in this function, DNA needs the participation of protein molecules. Enzymes copy DNA, so that after cell division each daughter cell contains an accurate copy of the DNA of the original cell. Histone proteins condense the metre length of DNA in each of our cells so that it fits within a cell nucleus with a maximum dimension of perhaps ten millionths of a metre. Other proteins control which parts of the DNA are used to provide information in any particular cell, so that, for example, muscle cells make muscle proteins and liver cells make liver proteins. These functions require proteins that can recognise and bind nucleic acids, either to all DNA for its replication and packaging or to specific parts of the total DNA when controlling its use to direct protein synthesis.

2.2 Amino acids

Learning objectives

You should be able to:

- define and explain the following terms: amino acid, amino acid side chain, peptide bond, polypeptide chain, amino acid residue, N-terminal, C-terminal
- draw a general structure for (a) an amino acid and (b) a peptide bond.

If we are to understand how proteins are able to recognise and bind to other molecules we must learn about the structure of proteins. Proteins are polymers of

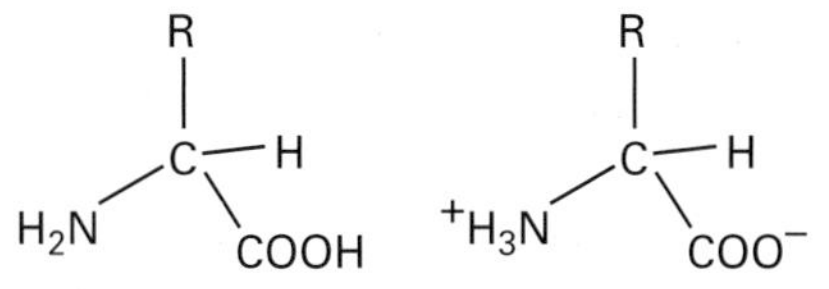

Fig. 4 General structure of an amino acid. Amino acids are often shown as uncharged molecules (left). In solutions with pH near neutrality, as in most physiological situations, the representation with charged amino and carboxyl groups (right) is more accurate.

amino acids. The general structure of an amino acid is shown in Figure 4. Four groups are attached by covalent bonds to a single carbon atom, the alpha carbon. Two of these groups, an amino group and an acidic carboxyl group, give their name to this class of compound and are also involved in forming the *peptide bonds* that join the amino acids into long polypeptide chains. The other two groups attached to the alpha carbon are a hydrogen atom, present in all amino acids, and a variable group, the so-called *side chain*. It is the side chain that distinguishes one amino acid from another. All proteins in animals, plants, bacteria and viruses are synthesised from the same set of 20 amino acids. The side chains of these 20 amino acids contain a limited range of chemical groups. In the few cases, proteins contain an amino acid that is not a member of this set and the protein is synthesised as a precursor protein. A side chain in the precursor protein is then chemically modified to form the unusual amino acid.

Figure 5 shows the structures of the 20 amino acids. They are arranged in groups with similar amino acids together; noting these structural relationships will help you to recognise and distinguish the amino acids. As the figure shows, the type of side chain alters the character and properties of the amino acids. This results in certain amino acids playing particular roles in protein function; for example, the disulphide bond formed by two cysteine residues is often used to hold a protein in a particular folded shape.

L-Amino acids

All of the amino acids except glycine are optically active, or *chiral*, having four different groups attached to the alpha carbon. Each amino acid can exist in two distinct forms, which are mirror images of each other and are not superimposable. Proteins are composed of amino acids of the so-called L series. Amino acids of the D series are very rarely found and never in proteins (they do occur in small peptides in some bacterial cell walls). Glycine has two hydrogen atoms attached to its alpha carbon and exists in only one form.

Figure 5 also shows the two systems of abbreviated names for amino acids that are in common use: an easily learnt three-letter code and a more concise single letter code, which is used for showing long polypeptide sequences. Only the three-letter code will be used in this book.

The peptide bond

Proteins are composed of amino acids joined by peptide bonds. Peptide bond formation involves the elimination of the elements of water between the alpha carboxyl group of one amino acid and the alpha amino group of another (Fig. 6). The dipeptide that is produced has terminal amino and carboxyl groups which (if free) can participate in further peptide bonds to extend the chain. Side chain carboxyl and amino groups, on those amino acids that possess them, are never involved, so polypeptide chains are linear and never branched. The bond formed between the carboxyl carbon and the amino nitrogen is a strong covalent bond that is somewhat shorter than would be expected for a single carbon–nitrogen bond. This is because it has some double bond character (Fig. 7). For this reason, free rotation around the peptide bond is not possible and there are some restrictions on the ways in which a polypeptide chain can be arranged in space.

Another important feature of the peptide bond is the hydrogen-bonding capacity of the atoms around the bond. The oxygen atom attached to the carbon atom of the peptide bond carries a fractional negative charge and is a strong hydrogen bond acceptor. The hydrogen attached to the peptide nitrogen has a fractional positive charge and can form strong hydrogen bonds (Fig. 7). Protein molecules containing many peptide bonds have a great capacity for hydrogen bonding, which must be satisfied. This influences the way in which polypeptide chains fold.

Polypeptide chains typically contain between 50 and 5000 amino acid units. The group of atoms belonging to each amino acid once it is combined in a peptide chain is known as an *amino acid residue*. Many functional proteins contain more than one polypeptide chain.

N-terminal and C-terminal ends

However long a polypeptide chain becomes it will still have an alpha amino group at one end, known as the *N-terminal* end, and an alpha carboxyl group at the other, the *C-terminal* end. Sometimes the N-terminal amino group is not free, but is modified by addition of an acetyl or other group. Similarly, the C-terminal carboxyl group is sometimes modified to its amide. By convention, the sequence of amino acids in a polypeptide

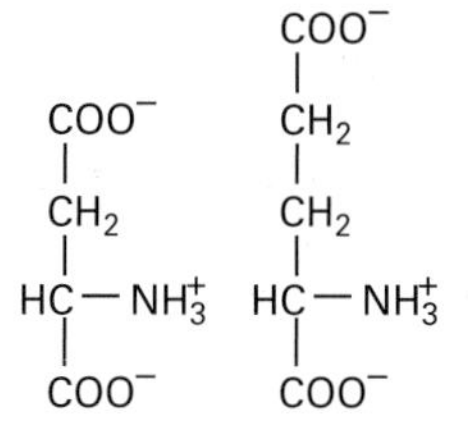

Asp (D)   Glu (E)

Aspartic acid and **glutamic acid** carry acid carboxyl groups on their side chains.

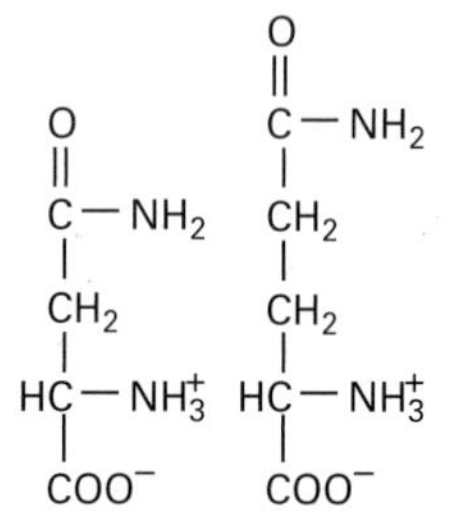

Asn (N)   Gln (Q)

Asparagine and **glutamine** are closely related to aspartic acid and glutamic acid, respectively; the side chain carboxyl groups are modified into uncharged hydrophilic amide groups.

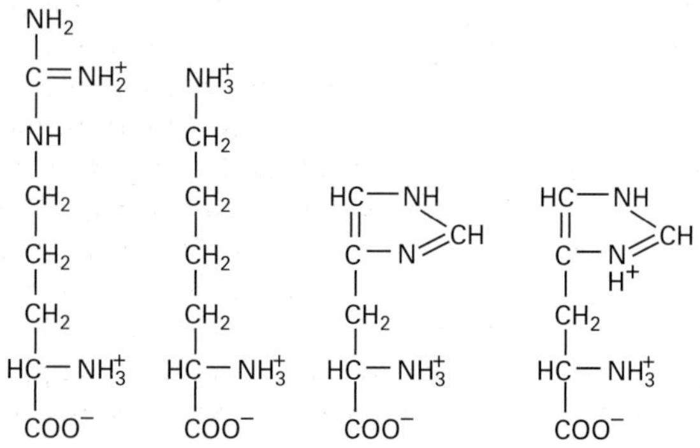

Arg (R)   Lys (K)   His (H)   His (protonated)

Arginine, **lysine** and **histidine** carry basic functional groups. Arginine and lysine side chains usually bind protons under physiological conditions and are positively charged. The imidazole group of histidine can exist in either a positively charged form (protonated) or as an uncharged base. Histidine side chains act as buffers at physiological pH.

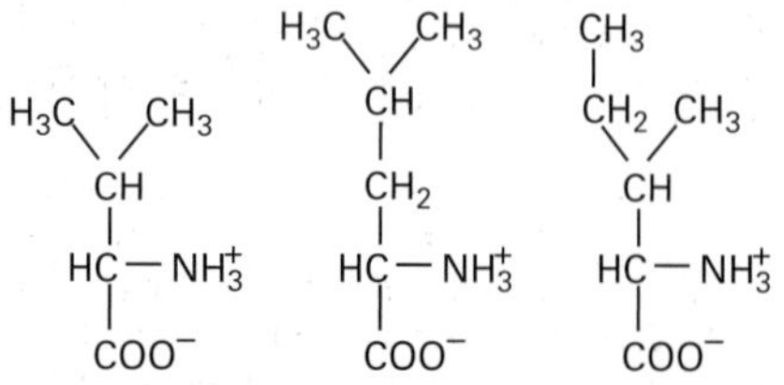

Val (V)   Leu (L)   Ile (I)

Valine, **leucine** and **isoleucine** have branched aliphatic hydrocarbon side chains, which are very hydrophobic.

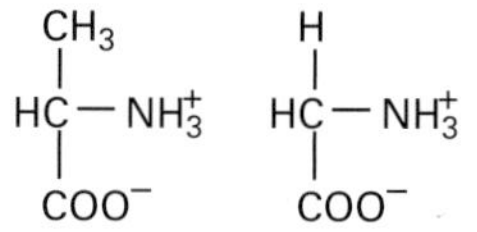

Ala (A)   Gly (G)

Alanine has a methyl group as its side chain; **glycine** has a second hydrogen atom attached do its alpha carbon and can be considered to have no side chain. It is the only amino acid that is not optically active.

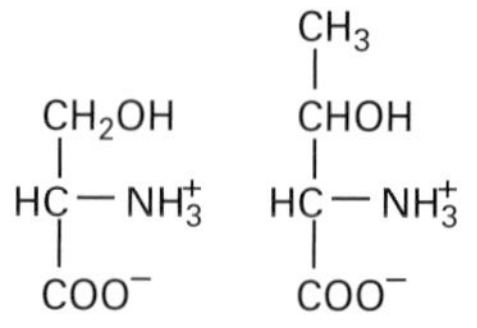

Ser (S)   Thr (T)

Serine and **threonine** have small uncharged side chains containing hydroxyl groups.

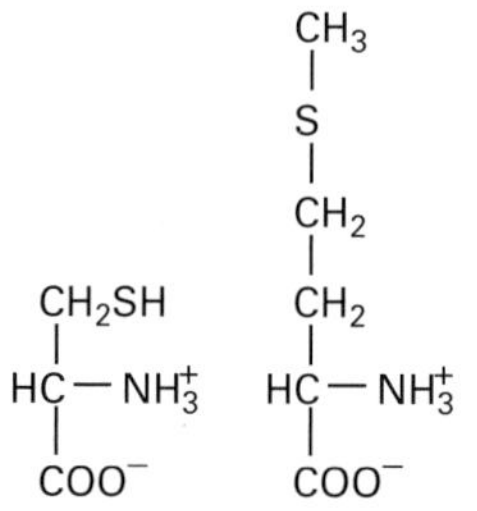

Cys (C)   Met (M)

Cysteine and **methionine** are sulphur-containing amino acids. Cysteine has a thiol or sulphydryl group on its side chain. Two cysteine side chains can react together to form a strong covalent disulphide bond, which is often used to hold different parts of a protein together, both between and within polypeptide chains. Methionine has a methylated sulphur in its side chain.

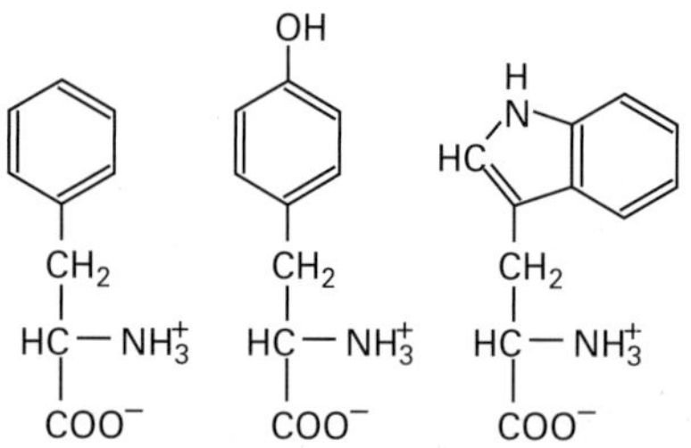

Phe (F)   Tyr (Y)   Trp (W)

Phenylalanine, **tyrosine** and **tryptophan** all have aromatic side chains. Phenylalanine is very hydrophobic, tyrosine less so since its ring carries a phenolic hydroxyl group. Tryptophan, the largest amino acid, has indole, a double aromatic ring containing a nitrogen atom, as its side chain. It is very hydrophobic.

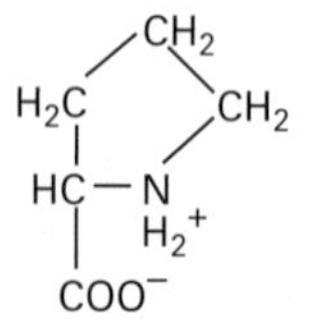

Pro (P)

Proline is the only amino acid to have a secondary amino group, not a primary amino group like all the others. The side chain of proline loops around to make a bond with the amino nitrogen atom, which, therefore, has two covalent bonds to carbon. Striclty speaking proline is an imino acid.

Fig. 5 Structures of the 20 amino acids. These are shown with their ionisable groups in the predominant forms found near pH 7.

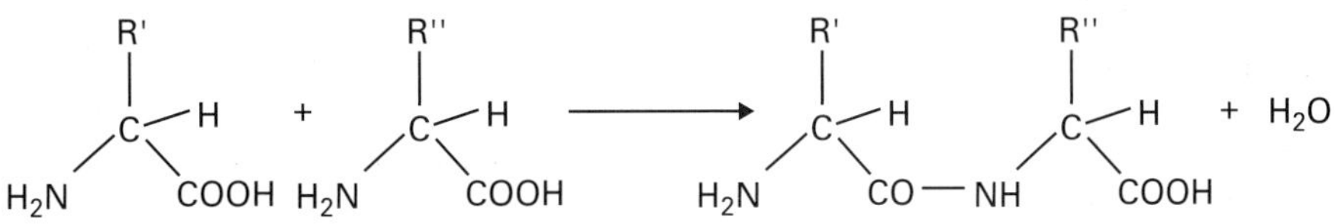

Fig. 6 Peptide bond formation.

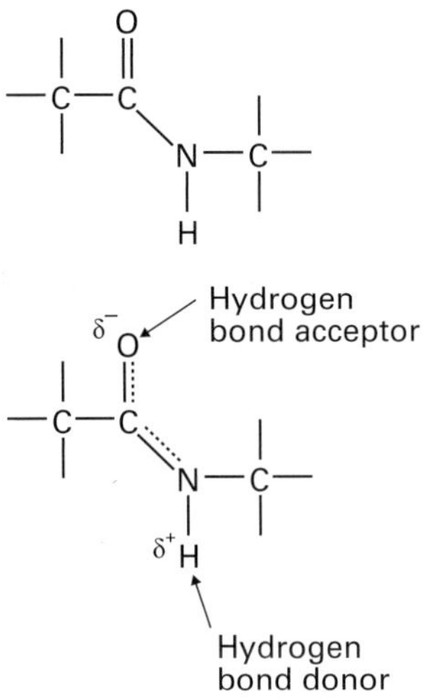

Fig. 7 Nature of the peptide bond. While often shown as the upper form, the properties of the peptide bond indicate that the lower representation is more accurate. The *trans* configuration shown is adopted by almost all peptide bonds in proteins. All six atoms shown are in a single plane. The carbonyl oxygen and the hydrogen on the nitrogen both carry fractional electronic charges and form strong hydrogen bonds. Rotation is allowed around the carbon–carbon bond.

chain is written with the N-terminal on the left. Two amino acids (X and Y) can form two distinct peptides, XY and YX.

2.3 Protein purification and characterisation

Learning objectives

You should be able to:

- give examples of purified proteins that are used therapeutically
- describe the principles of protein electrophoresis
- give examples of the use of protein electrophoresis in clinical investigations.

Proteins occur mixed with other compounds, including other proteins; so one of the first tasks for a biochemist who wishes to study the relationship between structure and function for a single protein is to purify the protein by separating and isolating it from other proteins. Purification is also necessary for proteins used for therapeutic purposes, such as insulin used to treat diabetics and clotting factor VIII used to treat haemophiliacs. Details of the powerful methods that have been developed to purify proteins are beyond the scope of this book, but the principles will be mentioned in outline. The methods depend on differences between the properties of protein molecules, such as:

- ligand binding ability
- size
- solubility
- stability
- electric charge.

A single process can rarely achieve purification of a protein from a complex mixture. Usually it is necessary to combine several purification techniques, each of which removes some of the unwanted components of the mixture while retaining the protein to be purified. Measurement of the amount of the target protein and total protein at the start and finish of each stage shows how successful the stage has been. The ratio of the amount of the target protein to the amount of total protein is known as the *specific activity*. The value of this ratio should increase with each successful stage of purification. Methods for purifying proteins are used empirically. They must be tested experimentally because there is no way of predicting which method will be most successful for any particular protein. The success or otherwise of a particular method cannot necessarily be related to the biochemical activity of the protein that is being purified.

Clinical note:
Plasma fractions for transfusion

Blood donated for transfusion that has not been used within the few weeks it remains useful is not wasted. The proteins from the plasma are fractionated by precipitation with cold ethanol and the separate fractions are used therapeutically to treat such conditions as low plasma volume following burns and surgery, and to give temporary protection against possible infection.

Electrophoresis: separation of proteins by charge

Protein molecules carry electric charge because of their ionised amino acid side chains. The charge depends on the amino acid composition of the protein and also on pH. The charge on each molecule is generally positive at low pH values and falls as the pH increases, reaching zero at a defined pH for each protein, its *isoelectric point*. As the pH rises beyond the isoelectric point, the charge on the protein becomes increasingly negative. Proteins are separated on the basis of their charge by *ion-exchange chromatography*. The chromatography material is a porous hydrophilic material, cellulose is often used, modified chemically to carry charged groups. Ion exchangers are available with either fixed positive or fixed negative charges. When a mixture of proteins flows into the chromatographic column, protein molecules opposite in charge to the charge on the column are bound to the column. Other proteins can be washed through. Changing the pH or increasing the ionic strength of the eluting buffer changes the charge on some of the bound proteins and they will elute. If the pH is gradually changed, a series of different proteins will emerge from the column depending on their isoelectric points.

The techniques of electrophoresis and isoelectric focusing also exploit the differences in charge between different proteins. *Electrophoresis* is the movement of charged molecules in an electric field. Electrophoresis of proteins is usually carried out in buffer solutions supported by a hydrophobic gel that is porous enough to allow protein molecules to penetrate. At the end of the electrophoresis procedure, a specific or a general protein stain is used to locate protein molecules in the gel. The rate at which proteins move through the gel depends on both their charge and their size. Identical molecules will all move at the same rate so that a sample of purified protein will move as a single band. This makes electrophoresis a valuable tool for establishing how many molecular species of protein a given protein preparation contains. *Isoelectric focusing* is a variant of electrophoresis carried out on a gel that has been set up to contain a gradient of pH. A protein molecule introduced to the gel will move in the electric field to a region where the pH matches its isoelectric point. Here it becomes uncharged and moves no further. Electrophoresis is a powerful method for detecting the presence of *isoenzymes*, different molecular forms that have the same catalytic activity. The identification of isoenzymes in plasma is an important diagnostic procedure (see Clinical note, p. 30).

2.4 Protein structure

Learning objectives

You should be able to:

- define the following terms: amino acid composition, amino acid sequence

- explain the four different levels at which protein structure can be described

- describe the general features of the alpha helix and beta sheet as elements of secondary structure

- describe the role of disulphide bonds in some protein structures

- define the following terms: denaturation, protein subunits, domains.

Amino acid composition

A count of the number of times each amino acid occurs in a given protein is known as the amino acid composition of the protein. To determine this, the protein molecule is first broken down into its constituent amino acids by cleavage of the peptide bonds. Although the peptide bond is a strong covalent bond, prolonged heating in acid or alkali hydrolyses it. Proteolytic enzymes may also be used.

Complete hydrolysis is then followed by a chromatographic procedure to separate the amino acids. The amino acid composition of a protein is often the first information that is available about a protein, but this information, of itself, generally does not reveal much about the relationship between the structure and function of the protein. There are a few exceptions. Haemoglobin contains many more histidine residues than the average protein; the histidine side chains act as a buffer at physiological pH, so their presence correlates with the buffering role of haemoglobin in the red cell. One-third of the amino acid residues in collagen, the main structural protein of connective tissue, are glycine and one-quarter are proline or modified proline. These amino acids have a role in collagen fibre formation. With most proteins there is no obvious relationship between amino acid composition and function.

Proteins have varying levels of structure

Proteins often lose their activity if heated; incubation for a few minutes at 60°C to 70°C is sufficient to inactivate many. Exposure to cold dilute acids or bases inactivates the majority of proteins, and high concentrations of urea or solvents such as ethanol also inactivate them. None of these treatments, which are said to denature the protein, would be expected to cleave peptide bonds or any other covalent bonds involved in protein structure. Some higher level of structure, destroyed by denaturation, must be necessary for protein function. The polypeptide chain must be folded in space to assume its functional form.

The structure of proteins can be considered at varying levels of complexity:

- primary: amino acid sequence established by covalent peptide bonds
- secondary: folding of the chains stabilised by hydrogen bonding between residues that are relatively close together
- tertiary: longer range folding stabilised by interactions between side chains; various bonds including hydrogen bonding and covalent bonds may occur
- quaternary: aggregates of more than one protein chain, folded together and held by various types of bond.

The full three-dimensional structures of many proteins have been determined by *X-ray crystallography* and *nuclear magnetic resonance* (NMR) methods. Description of these physical methods is beyond the scope of this book, but their results show that the polypeptide chains in proteins are folded specifically. Many relationships between protein structure and function have been revealed.

Primary structure: amino acid sequence

There appears to be no restriction on the order in which amino acids can be joined in a protein; so, with 20 possibilities at every position in the sequence, there is clearly an enormous number of possible proteins. Information stored in a nucleic acid base sequence directs the machinery of protein synthesis in a cell to make the proteins appropriate for that cell. The primary structure of a protein, the sequence in which amino acids are joined in a protein, makes that protein distinctive and leads to its further levels of structure, or shape, beyond sequence. Small changes in sequence can lead to large changes in properties and functions. Some inherited diseases are known to be caused by a change involving only one amino acid residue, a change that alters or destroys the function of the protein involved.

The amino acid sequences of many proteins have been determined. The methods used were originally chemical but now physical methods of greater sensitivity are used. Protein amino acid sequences can also be deduced from the base sequences of the nucleic acids that direct their synthesis. Proteins carrying out similar functions and proteins having the same function in different species almost always have closely related primary structures. Primary sequences are stored in data bases. This enables predictions about the structure and function of other proteins, often of medical importance, to be made. The interpretation of the X-ray studies on protein crystals to discover the three-dimensional structure of a protein depends on knowledge of the primary structure of the protein.

Secondary structure

The folding of the chain of amino acid residues through hydrogen bonding between residues that are close together in the chain is known as the secondary structure of the protein. Folding patterns such as the *alpha helix*, the *beta sheet* and the *triple helix* (occurring in collagen fibres) are examples of secondary structure. Secondary structure can be identified for most proteins, but the best examples of the importance of this level of structure are seen when we consider the structural proteins, the fibrous proteins that make up the structures in our bodies. Fibre formation by these proteins involves formation of regular secondary structures that extend over long distances.

The alpha helix

In the alpha helix, the backbone of the polypeptide chain is folded into a helix (Fig. 8). Folded in this way, the hydrogen-bonding capacity of the backbone peptide bonds can be completely satisfied within the helix and a stable structure results. For each residue, the amino hydrogen forms a bond to the carbonyl oxygen fourth earlier in the chain and the carbonyl oxygen forms a bond to a later amino hydrogen. Left-handed and right-handed helices are possible but only the latter are found, as they are more stable with L-amino acids. In a right-handed helix the chain rises as we move along it to the right. There are 3.6 residues per turn and the pitch of the helix is 0.54 nm, so each residue adds 0.15 nm to the length of the helix. Structural proteins containing the alpha helix have fibres that can be stretched, especially when wet. The alpha helix is the predominant secondary structure of unstretched keratin, the fibrous protein of hair, skin and nails. Many globular proteins contain short sections of alpha helix separated by sequences folded in other ways. The alpha helix does not involve the amino acid side chains; these project from the helix.

Beta sheets

In beta sheets, polypeptide chains are almost fully extended and run side by side so that hydrogen bonds

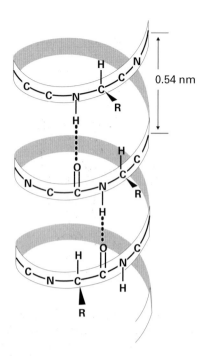

Fig. 8 The alpha helix.

0.54 nm

can be formed between adjacent chains in the sheet (Fig. 9). Stretched keratin can assume the beta sheet structure. Many globular proteins, for example immunoglobulins, contain sections of beta sheet or even barrel-like structures formed from a curved sheet. Peptide chains in a beta sheet may be parallel or antiparallel.

The triple helix and collagen

The triple helix is found principally in collagen, the protein that makes the strong low-elasticity fibres of connective tissue. Three polypeptide chains that are almost fully extended are wound around each other to form a rope-like structure (Fig. 10). Again, much of the stability of the structure results from hydrogen bonds between the backbones of the three chains. For the triple helix to form, it is necessary for each of its component chains to have a glycine residue in every third position in its sequence. Only glycine with a hydrogen atom as its side chain can allow the chains to come close enough to form the structure. The individual chains in the helix

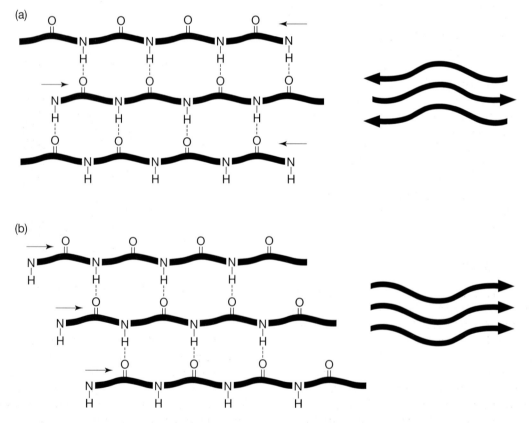

Fig. 9 Beta pleated sheets. Only the hydrogen bonding atoms of the polypeptide backbone are shown. Sheets formed with antiparallel chains (a) are somewhat more stable than those formed from parallel chains (b). Protein structure diagrams, such as Figure 11, show chains in beta sheets as ribbons with arrowheads. Bulky side chains cannot be accommodated on beta sheets composed of parallel chains.

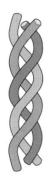

Fig. 10 The collagen triple helix.

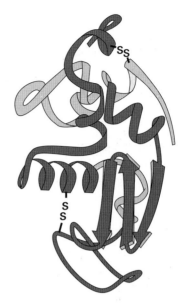

Fig. 11 Tertiary structure of lysozyme. The single polypeptide chain of this small enzyme molecule folds into short sections of alpha helix and a small antiparallel beta pleated sheet, as well as into bends and loops where the chain has no recognisable secondary structure. The structure is stabilised by four disulphide bonds, only two of which are visible in the figure. (Based on Wolf, S.L. (1995) *Cell and Molecular Biology*, Wadsworth.)

are in almost fully extended configurations so fibres composed of collagen molecules combine high strength with low elasticity.

Tertiary structure

Consideration of secondary structure can reveal much about the relationship between the structure of fibrous proteins and the physical properties on which the functions of these proteins depend. When we consider globular proteins, we must describe an even higher level of structure, tertiary structure. Physical studies show that many globular proteins have compact structures; the long polypeptide chains within them must be folded or wound up like a ball of string. Many globular proteins can form crystals; the chains must be folded in the same way in every molecule to give them the identical overall shape needed for them to fit into the crystal. X-ray diffraction studies of protein crystals have led to the determination of the three-dimensional structure of a wide variety of protein molecules. These structures show how the polypeptide chain winds back and forth through the molecule, sometimes in the form of an alpha helix, sometimes forming beta sheets, sometimes in turns and less regular structures (Fig. 11).

Disulphide bonds

Tertiary structures are often stabilised by covalent disulphide bonds. The structures formed by folded polypeptides depend on hydrogen bonds and hydrophobic interactions, so they can be fragile and easily disrupted by changes in temperature or pH. Many proteins, especially those that function outside cells, have their folded structures reinforced by disulphide bonds. These bonds can also hold subunits together. Disulphide bonds are formed when the side chains of two cysteine residues that are close together in the folded structure react together, losing the hydrogen atoms of their sulphydryl (also known as thiol) groups in an oxidation reaction

2 Cysteine   Cystine
—SH + HS— = —S—S— + 2H

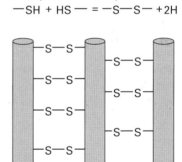

Fig. 12 Disulphide bonds in proteins.

(Fig. 12). Disulphide bonds are strong covalent bonds. They are particularly important in keratin, the fibrous structural protein of hair, skin and nails, where parallel alpha helices are crosslinked by disulphide bonds. Keratin is chemically very resistant because its structure can maintain its integrity even after breakage of some peptide or disulphide bonds. It is greatly weakened by reducing agents, which can convert disulphide bonds into free thiol groups. Chemical depilatories (hair removers) exploit this susceptibility of keratin to chemical reduction, as do industrial processes to remove the bristles from hides in leather production.

Formation of tertiary structure

The tertiary structure that a protein forms is dependent upon its amino acid sequence. Haemoglobin and myoglobin were the first proteins to have their molecular structures described. The relationship between their primary and tertiary structures revealed the general principles of protein tertiary structure. Tertiary structure largely results from the properties of the amino acid side chains. Hydrophobic side chains such as those of phenylalanine, valine, leucine and isoleucine are always found on the inside of the structure, out of contact with the water that surrounds the protein molecule, even in the crystal. Charged groups such as arginine, lysine, histidine, aspartate and glutamate are almost always on the surface of the molecule. There is no empty space within the molecule; the hydrophobic side chains that form much of the core are close-packed. Except on the surface of the molecule, groups capable of forming hydrogen bonds are virtually all in a position to form hydrogen bonds. This is so for both donors and acceptors, on side chains and on the polypeptide backbone. In myoglobin and in each of the four subunits of haemoglobin, about 75% of the residues are involved in the formation of eight short sections of alpha helix. The remaining residues are situated in the connections between the end of one helix and the start of the next. Myoglobin and haemoglobin are atypical globular proteins in that they have a high content of alpha helix and a complete absence of beta sheet.

Denaturation destroys secondary and tertiary structure

While primary structure depends on covalent bonds, which are strong, secondary and tertiary structures are stabilised by a very large number of weak bonds, principally hydrogen bonds, by hydrophobic forces and by the electrostatic forces between charged groups. A few of these weak bonds can be temporarily disrupted without destroying the tertiary structure. Partners in the broken bonds are still close together in space and the bonds can quickly reform. This dependence of structure on a large number of weak bonds gives globular proteins a flexibility and an ability to assume alternative conformations important to their function. However, if too much disruption of the weak stabilising bonds occurs, partners in a broken bond may move too far apart for the bond to be formed again; as a result, the whole structure falls apart.

Primary structure is responsible for specific folding

How do polypeptides achieve the specific folding they need for their function? Anfinsen performed an important experiment, which showed that polypeptides could acquire their secondary and tertiary structures on their own without the involvement of other agents (Fig. 13). He used a purified enzyme, bovine pancreatic ribonuclease (RNAase). This is a relatively small enzyme with only 124 amino acid residues in its single polypeptide chain. Like many enzymes secreted into the gut where the physicochemical conditions are not so well controlled as they are within cells, the structure of ribonuclease is reinforced by disulphide bonds. Ribonuclease contains four such bonds. Anfinsen treated the enzyme with a reducing agent, mercaptoethanol, to break these bonds and also with a high concentration of urea, a reagent that disrupts hydrogen bonds. This combined treatment completely inactivated the enzyme. He observed that activity could be restored by gradual removal of the reducing agent and urea, if the conditions were mildly oxidising. Restoration of activity was complete. Since no other agent was present that could have brought the partners in the disulphide bonds together, Anfinsen concluded that the polypeptide chain must have refolded as directed by its primary sequence and that, once refolded, the original disulphide bonds must have formed again.

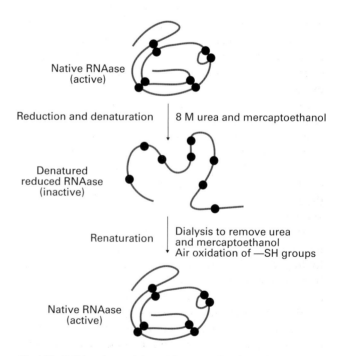

Fig. 13 Anfinsen's experiment (see text for details). The filled circles represent cystine or half-cystine residues.

While the primary structure of a polypeptide defines the way in which it will fold to form an active protein in the cell, the problem of predicting the actual secondary and tertiary structures of proteins from their amino acid sequences has not been solved. The number of ways in which a chain could fold is so enormous that it is currently beyond the power of even the most powerful computer to predict the stable folding that the majority of proteins appear to achieve within a minute after formation of their primary structure. Limited predictions can be made. Some amino acid residues are found more frequently in alpha helixes than in beta sheets and vice versa, so the probable secondary structure of a given section of sequence can often be recognised. Proline cannot be accommodated within an alpha helix and is often found at the junction between one helix and another in globular proteins. The structure of related proteins can also be used as a basis for prediction.

Quaternary structure and subunits

Many proteins contain more than one polypeptide chain. Usually the individual chains fold into subunits that specifically bind to other subunits to make up the complete protein. For example, each molecule of haemoglobin contains four polypeptide chains, each of which is folded to form a subunit that contains a bound haem group. The subunits have complementary binding sites for each other and assemble to form the functional tetramer. The subunits making up a protein are sometimes identical and sometimes not. In the case of the four haemoglobin subunits, there are two alpha chains and two beta chains. Alpha and beta chains have related amino acid sequences and have similar tertiary structures. The related protein myoglobin, which stores oxygen in muscle, exists as a single polypeptide chain with a sequence related to those of the haemoglobin chains. This chain adopts a tertiary structure similar to that of the haemoglobin subunits and binds a haem group but does not assemble into any larger structure.

Multiple subunit proteins are important because they create the possibility of interaction between subunits; the state of one subunit can influence the functioning of another.

The subunits making up a protein are usually held together by specific but non-covalent forces such as hydrogen bonds, hydrophobic forces (see p. 5) and electrostatic attractions. These numerous but weak forces are sometimes reinforced by strong covalent disulphide bonds between the subunits. Immunoglobulin G, a plasma protein that protects the body by recognising antigens ('non-self' macromolecules in the blood), contains four polypeptide chains: two heavy H chains and two light L chains joined by disulphide bonds (see Fig. 170, p. 275).

Domains

Long polypeptides may contain several folding domains. In some very long polypeptide chains, different parts of the sequence adopt tertiary structures that are separate from the tertiary structures adopted by other parts of the sequence, forming structures similar to those seen with multiple subunits. These partial structures or domains are tethered to each other by short flexible polypeptide sequences. The heavy H chains of immunoglobulin G each contain four domains while the light L chains each contain two domains.

2.5 Ligand binding sites

Learning objectives

You should be able to:

- explain how folding of polypeptide chains creates specific binding sites for ligands

- give examples of the importance of ligand binding in biochemistry.

X-ray crystallography and other physical methods can provide information about the ways in which proteins bind their ligands and the effects ligand binding can have on three-dimensional structure. Proteins achieve specific binding of their ligands by means of forces similar to those they use to achieve specific folding. Achievement of a specific tertiary structure does not involve all the side chains in the amino acid sequence. Other amino acid side chains, usually not near to each other in the primary sequence, can be brought together in space in a specific three-dimensional conformation to form a binding site. This binding site has a structure complementary to the structure of the bound ligand. If the ligand has the potential to form hydrogen bonds, the binding site will have hydrogen bond donor and acceptor groups situated to form bonds with the ligand. If the ligand has a hydrophobic region, hydrophobic side chains in the binding site make close contacts with it. A group of opposite charge in the binding site matches a charged group on the ligand. Specificity and affinity of binding are achieved by numerous weak interactions.

Protein function, and hence all of life, depends on the ability of proteins to recognise and bind tightly to their specific ligands even though the ligand molecules may only be present in very small amounts in complex mixtures of similar molecules. For example, the receptor for the protein hormone insulin is present on the surface of many cells. It will recognise, bind and respond to insulin circulating in the blood when blood contains only 10^{-10} moles (6×10^{-7} g) of insulin per litre. Insulin is recognised even though blood plasma contains about 60 g per litre or more of total protein, at least a 100 million-fold excess over the amount of insulin present. Other proteins concerned with controlling the expression of our genes can recognise and bind to a section of DNA sequence which represents about one part in 100 million of the complete DNA sequence in each cell.

Since ligand binding by proteins depends on numerous weak interactions, it is reversible and rapid. Ligands do not have to form the ligand–protein complex in one step; they can collide with and occupy part of the binding site and then trigger changes in protein conformation that create other parts of the binding site and hence increase the affinity of binding. Most protein–ligand interactions do not involve covalent bond formation. Ligand binding is important in enzyme function, the subject of the next chapter.

Self-assessment: questions

Single best answer MCQs

1. Identify the biochemical processes in which proteins play a key role.
   a. Protein synthesis
   b. Digestion of proteins in the digestive tract
   c. Replication of DNA
   d. Two of the above are true
   e. a, b and c are all true

2. Your text has drawn attention to the common principle that proteins recognise and bind other molecules. Which one of the following statements accurately describes ligand binding by proteins?
   a. Specificity of ligand binding means that each protein only binds a single ligand
   b. Enzymes can only recognise ligands that are involved in the reaction that they catalyse
   c. Ligands are non-protein molecules that are bound by proteins
   d. Ligand binding involves the formation of a covalent bond between the ligand and the binding site on the protein
   e. Proteins bind specific base sequences in DNA to control synthesis of other proteins

3. Which of the following statements accurately describes properties of amino acids in proteins?
   a. Proteins are made from a set of 20 amino acids and amino acids not in the set are never found in proteins
   b. Except for glycine, the amino acids found in proteins are chiral because their side chains contain a carbon atom with four different groups attached
   c. All amino acids have one amino group and one carboxyl group
   d. An amino group, a carboxyl group and the side chain are all attached to the same carbon atom, the α-carbon
   e. The α-amino group and the α-carbon are involved in peptide bond formation

4. Which one of the following descriptions of amino acids and their side chains in proteins is accurate?
   a. Arginine and glutamic acid both carry carboxyl groups on their side chains
   b. Cysteine is the only amino acid that has a sulphur-containing side chain
   c. Phenylalanine and alanine have aromatic hydrocarbon rings in their side chains
   d. Lysine, leucine and histidine are the only amino acids with side chains that can carry a positive charge
   e. Glycine is the amino acid with the smallest side chain and proline has a side chain that forms a five-membered ring, which includes the amino nitrogen

5. There are several key statements that recall critical aspects of amino acid groups in proteins. Which one from the following list is correct?
   a. Serine and tryptophan both have hydroxyl groups in their side chains
   b. Glutamine and asparagine have amide groups on their side chains
   c. The most abundant amino acid in collagen is proline
   d. All the amino acids found in proteins, except proline, have a hydrogen atom attached to their α-carbon
   e. In globular proteins, the side chains of the hydrophobic amino acids valine, leucine and isoleucine are likely to be on the surface of the protein

6. Proteins are composed of amino acids joined by peptide bonds. Select from the following the one correct statement concerning the peptide bond.
   a. Joins the α-carboxyl of one amino acid with the amino group of the amino acid next in the polypeptide chain
   b. Shows partial double bond character and is usually found in the *cis* configuration
   c. Allows free rotation
   d. Has an –NH group that can act as a hydrogen bond acceptor
   e. Has a –CO group that can act as a hydrogen bond donor

7. Polypeptide chains in proteins have which one of the following characteristics? They:
   a. Are often branched
   b. Often show regularity in the sequence of amino acids they contain
   c. Have an amino acid sequence that is known as their secondary structure
   d. Have an amino acid sequence that make each protein unique
   e. Have two ends that are identical

8. Identify the single correct statement concerning the varying levels of structure found in proteins.
   a. The secondary and tertiary structures of a protein depend on its amino acid sequence
   b. The secondary structure of a protein is the three-dimensional configuration of all the amino acids in the sequence
   c. The tertiary structure of a protein is the three-dimensional configuration of amino acids close together in the sequence
   d. The primary, secondary and tertiary structures of a protein are destroyed when the protein is denatured
   e. Protein secondary structures are stabilised by disulphide bonds

9. Studies on ribonuclease by Anfinsen were critical to our understanding of protein structure. Which of the following is an accurate description of his study?
   a. The primary structure of a protein is responsible for its tertiary structure
   b. The tertiary structure of a protein can be predicted from its sequence
   c. Anfinsen's experiment showed that peptide chains can only take up their active conformation in the presence of urea
   d. Anfinsen's experiment showed that peptide chains can only take up their active conformation in the presence of reducing agents
   e. The alpha helix and the beta pleated sheet occur in structural proteins but are rarely found as elements of secondary structure in globular proteins

10. Which one of the following statements is correct concerning denaturation or hydrolysis of proteins?
    a. Peptide bonds are readily hydrolysed by exposure to cold dilute hydrochloric acid
    b. The amino acid sequence of a protein is determined by hydrolysis of all the peptide bonds in the protein and analysis of the amino acids in the hydrolysate
    c. Denaturation alters the primary structure of a protein and destroys its biological activity
    d. Proteins can be denatured by exposure to acids, alkalis or concentrated solutions of urea or by elevated temperatures
    e. Most proteins become more soluble when denatured

11. Identify the single correct statement concerning protein structure.
    a. Proline residues are never found at the end of an alpha helix
    b. Lysine and leucine side chains are usually found in the interior of water-soluble globular proteins
    c. Aspartic acid and valine acid side chains are usually found on the exterior of water-soluble globular proteins
    d. Pairs of thiol groups from cysteine side chains are often oxidised to form a disulphide bond, which stabilises the tertiary structure of the protein
    e. Polypeptide chains forming a beta pleated sheet are always antiparallel

12. Select the option that correctly describes protein subunits and domains.
    a. The molecules of many proteins contain two or more separate polypeptide chains
    b. Some long polypeptide chains form two or more folding subunits separated by flexible sections
    c. Separate polypeptide chains within a protein are known as domains
    d. Subunits in a protein are always identical
    e. Multiple polypeptide chains in a protein are never linked by covalent bonds

Short essay question

'Protein function can be largely explained in terms of specific ligand binding.' Discuss.

Self-assessment: answers

Single best answer MCQ answers

1. a. Protein synthesis needs nucleic acid to supply sequence information, but many proteins are also involved: ribosome components, enzymes, etc.
   b. The enzymes that digest dietary protein are proteins.
   c. Enzymes and DNA binding proteins are required for DNA replication.
   d. **False**.
   e. This is the best answer.

2. a. **False**. Many proteins bind multiple ligands.
   b. **False**. Many enzymes bind other ligands, e.g. allosteric effectors.
   c. **False**. Proteins often bind other proteins, e.g. insulin is bound by its receptor.
   d. **False**. Most protein–ligand interactions do not lead to covalent bond formation.
   e. **True**. All organisms use specific recognition of DNA base sequences by proteins to control gene expression.

3. a. **False**. Amino acids not in the set of 20 are sometimes found. Amino acids from the set are incorporated in proteins and modified after incorporation.
   b. **False**. It is the alpha carbon that has four groups attached.
   c. **False**. Some have second amino or carboxyl groups on their side chains.
   d. **True**.
   e. **False**. The alpha amino group, not the alpha carbon, is involved in peptide bond formation.

4. a. **False**. Aspartic acid, not arginine, is the other amino acid with a second carboxyl group.
   b. **False**. Methionine has a sulphur atom in its side chain.
   c. **False**. Tyrosine, not alanine, is very similar to phenylalanine; tyrosine has a phenolic hydroxyl.
   d. **False**. Arginine, not leucine, is the third amino acid that can carry a positive charge on its side chain.
   e. **True**. Glycine has the smallest possible side chain, a hydrogen atom. The side chain of proline loops back to form a ring with the alpha nitrogen.

5. a. **False**. Threonine, not tryptophan, has a hydroxyl group on its side chain.
   b. **True**.
   c. **False**. The most abundant amino acid residue in collagen is glycine.
   d. **False**. Proline has an alpha hydrogen. It does not have a hydrogen on its nitrogen when it forms a peptide bond.
   e. **False**. Valine, leucine and isoleucine side chains are excluded from solvent water, and cluster in the cores of globular proteins.

6. a. **True**.
   b. **False**. It is predominantly found in the *trans* configuration.
   c. **False**. Its partial double bond character precludes rotation.
   d. **False**. The –NH group is a hydrogen bond donor.
   e. **False**. The carbonyl oxygen atom carries a fractional negative charge and is a hydrogen bond acceptor.

7. a. **False**. Peptide chains are always linear.
   b. **False**. Only a few structural proteins, such as collagen with glycine as every third residue, show any repeating pattern.
   c. **False**. The amino acid sequence is also known as the primary structure.
   d. **True**. Sequence controls how the chain folds and is essential for biological activity.
   e. **False**. They can be distinguished from each other; one has an amino group not involved in a peptide bond, the other a carboxyl.

8. a. **True**. The folding of the polypeptide gives the structure minimum energy for its sequence.
   b. **False**. Secondary structure refers only to the folding of residues, which are close together.
   c. **False**. The tertiary structure of a protein is the three-dimensional configuration of all the amino acids in the sequence.
   d. **False**. Denaturation does not affect primary structure.
   e. **False**. Disulphide bonds stabilise the tertiary structure of some proteins.

9. a. **True**. Anfinsen's experiment showed this.
   b. **False**. Prediction needs too many calculations even for modern computers.

c. **False**. Anfinsen used urea to unfold the protein. It only refolded when he removed the urea.

d. **False**. Unstretched keratin fibres contain alpha helix.

e. **False**. About 75% of the residues in haemoglobin are in alpha helical segments. Beta pleated sheets are found in many enzyme molecules.

10. a. **False**. Peptide bonds vary in the ease with which they are hydrolysed but most require heating for hours in strong acid.

b. **False**. This is how the amino acid composition is determined. Sequence information is destroyed by complete hydrolysis.

c. **False**. Denaturation, by definition, destroys biological activity, but it does not alter primary structure.

d. **True**. These are all common methods of denaturing proteins.

e. **False**. Proteins usually become insoluble on denaturation. Coagulation of egg white proteins on heating is the usual example. The major exception is insoluble collagen which is converted to soluble gelatin by heating.

11. a. **False**. Proline nitrogen cannot form hydrogen bonds, so proline can occur at the end of a helix although not within it.

b. **False**. Leucine is hydrophobic and is usually in the core of the protein, but lysine has a hydrophilic ionised amino group on its side chain that will usually be at the protein surface.

c. **False**. Not valine. Aspartic acid and glutamic acid have ionised side chain carboxyl groups that are hydrophilic.

d. **True**. This is how disulphide bonds are formed.

e. **False**. Beta pleated sheets having parallel polypeptide chains are found.

12. a. **True**. Haemoglobin with four chains and insulin with two are examples.

b. **False**. Separately folding lengths within a polypeptide chain are known as domains, not subunits.

c. **False**. Separate polypeptide chains are known as subunits.

d. **False**. For example, the enzyme lactate dehydrogenase is a tetramer of four M type or H type subunits and can exist as M_4, M_3H, M_2H_2, MH_3 or H_4.

e. **False**. For example, the four chains in immunoglobulin G are joined by disulphide bonds and the two chains in insulin have inter- and intrachain disulphide bonds.

Short essay answer

Whether protein molecules are functioning as building blocks for structures, as catalysts, as allosteric or controllable catalysts, as transport proteins in blood, as antibodies, as hormone receptors, as packaging for DNA, as pumps or transport mechanisms across membranes, their function always involves recognition and specific binding of other molecules or of parts of other molecules.

Try to think of a protein that has a function that does not involve specific ligand binding!

3 Enzymes

Overview

Most of the chemical reactions occurring in cells require catalysis by enzymes. These protein catalysts act by binding their substrates at sites containing chemical groups that promote reaction. The rates of enzyme reactions are influenced by many factors, notably by the concentration of substrate. Enzymes are subject to inhibition by specific molecules, particularly by molecules resembling their substrates. Some enzymes are not merely catalysts but are responsible for regulating cellular processes to meet the needs of the cell or to respond to signals from outside the cell.

Learning objectives

You should be able to:

- describe with examples the efficiency, potency and specificity of enzymes

- describe the chemical nature of enzymes and the occurrence of non-protein constituents in some enzymes

- define the following terms: prosthetic group, coenzyme, stereospecificity.

3.1 Proteins as catalysts

The living cell is the site of many chemical reactions, most of which require catalysts if they are to proceed at a sufficient rate under physiological conditions for the requirements of the cell. One of the most important functions of proteins is as protein catalysts or enzymes. Enzymes show remarkable properties compared with the catalysts used by chemists:

- efficiency
- potency
- specificity.

Enzymes are very efficient catalysts

Enzymes do not require elevated temperatures to promote reaction nor do they require that the reactions they catalyse take place in acid, alkali or non-aqueous solution. Enzyme reactions take place at body temperature and, with a few exceptions, take place in aqueous solution near pH 7. No material is wasted in side reactions. The yield from enzyme-catalysed reactions is usually only limited by the equilibrium point of the reaction being catalysed. Enzymes promote reactions that bring chemical systems towards equilibrium but have the ability to couple reactions together so that a 'downhill' (energy-yielding) reaction may appear to drive one that is 'uphill'.

Enzymes are very potent catalysts

Each enzyme molecule is able to promote the conversion of hundreds, thousands or even more substrate molecules to product each second. One molecule of carbonic anhydrase, the enzyme that catalyses the reversible conversion of carbon dioxide and water into bicarbonate and hydrogen ions, can convert about one million molecules of substrate per second.

Enzymes are very specific catalysts

A different enzyme is required for almost every reaction that needs to be catalysed because each enzyme is generally very limited in the range of reactions it can promote. Hexokinase, the enzyme that phosphorylates

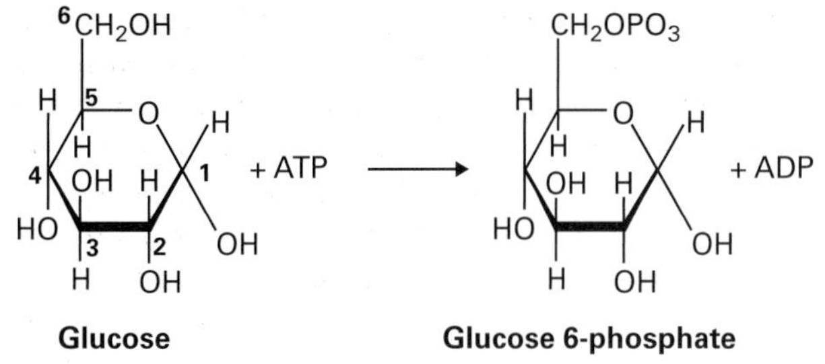

Glucose   **Glucose 6-phosphate**

Fig. 14 Specificity of the reaction catalysed by hexokinase: phosphorylation is confined to the hydroxyl group carried by carbon-6.

glucose in preparation for its further metabolism, can also phosphorylate mannose, but experiments on the enzyme purified from brain show that it has little or no action on any other monosaccharide. It requires ATP (adenosine triphosphate) as a source of the phosphate group, which it transfers only to the hydroxyl group on carbon-6 of the substrate. Although glucose and mannose have other sites where they could be phosphorylated, the specificity of hexokinase is such that glucose (and mannose) is only phosphorylated at this position (Fig. 14).

Enzymes differ in the degree of specificity that they show. Some enzymes concerned with synthetic reactions are very specific and catalyse only one reaction. Other enzymes, especially those concerned with digestion, can catalyse the hydrolysis of a wide range of similar compounds. For example, trypsin, a protein-digesting enzyme that is active in the duodenum, is able to cleave peptide bonds in a large number of proteins and peptides. The structure of most of the substrate molecule does not matter so long as it contains peptide bonds that involve the carboxyl groups of the amino acids arginine and lysine. Trypsin can be considered to be specific for a small part of its substrate. Chymotrypsin, a similar enzyme, can only cleave peptide bonds involving the carboxyl group of amino acids with bulky aromatic side chains, such as phenylalanine, tyrosine and tryptophan. Both of these enzymes can also hydrolyse ester bonds involving these same carboxyl groups, although ester bonds are not found in their natural substrates.

Chemical nature of enzymes

Many enzymes are composed entirely of protein. Others have in addition some non-protein component such as a metal ion or an organic group essential for their catalytic action.

Metalloenzymes

Metalloenzymes have a structure that includes a tightly bound metal ion that is essential for activity. For example, *zinc* is found in carboxypeptidase, carbonic anhydrase and alcohol dehydrogenase, and *copper* is found in many enzymes that use molecular oxygen as a substrate. *Iron, manganese, molybdenum* and *cobalt* have also been found in the structures of some enzymes and are essential for their activity. The metal ion is generally very tightly bound to the enzyme at binding sites that may include cysteine sulphydryl groups, imidazole groups on histidine side chains or other groups on the protein.

Many enzymes have prosthetic groups

Many enzymes contain complex non-protein organic molecules called prosthetic groups which are necessary for their function. These organic molecules provide the enzyme with chemical functional groups that are not available as side chains on amino acids. Some prosthetic groups, such as the haem group found in haemoglobin but also present in many important enzymes, can be completely synthesised in the body. Other prosthetic groups of enzymes cannot be synthesised and are based on *vitamins*: essential organic components of the diet that are required in small amounts (pp. 262–267). For example, flavin adenine dinucleotide, FAD, a prosthetic group found in some enzymes that catalyse oxidation reactions, contains the vitamin *riboflavin*. Enzymes that cleave carbon–carbon bonds to produce carbon dioxide often have a thiamine pyrophosphate prosthetic group. *Thiamine* is a vitamin. Its deficiency in the diet leads to the disease, beri-beri, which affects many organ systems. A prosthetic group remains bound to its enzyme during the complete catalytic cycle.

Coenzymes are often involved in transfer reactions

Coenzymes are small molecules that are changed in an enzyme-catalysed reaction but will eventually be regenerated; by comparison, a substrate usually undergoes further reactions. Many enzyme reactions involve the transfer of a relatively small chemical grouping from one substrate to another: hexokinase transfers a phosphate group from ATP to glucose. ATP is the phosphate donor in many other reactions in which phosphate is transferred. It acts as a common substrate shared by many phosphate-transferring enzymes and is called a coenzyme. Similarly, enzymes catalysing oxidation–reduction reactions usually transfer two hydrogen atoms from a substrate to an acceptor such as NAD^+ (nicotinamide adenine dinucleotide), one of the common substrates or coenzymes of hydrogen transfer. Coenzymes also exist for the transfer of acetyl, acyl, glycosyl and other groups. Coenzymes often have a nucleotide unit within their structure, so most of them contain ribose, phosphate and a nitrogenous base such as adenine. Vitamins are required for the synthesis of some but not all coenzymes. *Nicotinamide*, a B vitamin, is required for the synthesis of NAD^+ and the related coenzyme $NADP^+$.

Coenzymes differ from prosthetic groups in that they need to move from enzyme to enzyme to carry out their function. For example, ATP is converted to ADP during hexokinase action but another phosphate transfer, catalysed by another enzyme, is required to convert the ADP back to ATP so that it can function again as a phosphate donor.

About fifty years after enzymes were purified sufficiently to demonstrate that they were proteins, RNA molecules with catalytic activity were discovered. Such *ribozymes* appear to have very limited catalytic abilities and to be less efficient than enzymes, which are protein. Ribozymes are involved in the processing of other RNA molecules.

Enzymes are stereospecific

Molecules that can exist in distinct left-handed and right-handed forms (i.e. their mirror image cannot be exactly superimposed on the 'real' image in any orientation) are said to be optically active or *chiral*. They will rotate a beam of plane-polarised light to the right (+, dextro rotatory) or to the left (–, laevo rotatory). Lactate and all the amino acids except glycine are examples.

Enzymes that act on such molecules or which produce chiral products from non-chiral substrates always show stereospecificity. If the substrate is optically active, only one of the two optical isomers will react. If the product can show optical activity, only one of its isomers will be formed. Lactate dehydrogenase, which is found in many tissues, can only oxidise the L form of lactate to non-chiral pyruvate. It can also catalyse the reduction of pyruvate and produces only L-lactate when it does so.

3.2 Enzyme nomenclature

Learning objective

You should be able to:

- understand the basis of enzyme nomenclature.

Enzymes are named after the reactions they catalyse. Their names are generally based on the names of their substrates and indicate the nature of the reaction that is catalysed. They almost always end with the suffix '-ase'.

For example, lactate dehydrogenase is the enzyme that oxidises lactate by removing two atoms of hydrogen from it; other *dehydrogenases* will remove hydrogen from other substrates. *Kinases* transfer phosphate groups, often from ATP; thus, hexokinase moves a phosphate group from ATP to the hexoses glucose or mannose. Enzymes that catalyse hydrolytic reactions are often named after their substrates, their class name, *hydrolase*, being assumed. For example, urease hydrolyses urea, sucrase hydrolyses sucrose and maltase hydrolyses maltose. Some digestive enzymes that were discovered before the naming system outlined above came into use have names that do not comply: pepsin, rennin, trypsin, chymotrypsin and thrombin are all *proteases*, which hydrolyse peptide bonds. The names described above are the trivial names, the names used for enzymes in most biochemical writing. An official nomenclature system has been agreed that avoids any ambiguity, but it generates very cumbersome names which are useful only for reference. Each enzyme has a full name and an Enzyme Commission (EC) number derived from its position in the classification scheme. For instance, hexokinase has the full name ATP:D-hexose 6-phosphotransferase and the classification number EC 2.7.1.1. It is a *transferase*, so it is in group 2; it transfers a phosphate group, so it is in subgroup 7; it has an alcohol group as an acceptor, so it is in subsubgroup 1; and it is the first such enzyme to be classified. Further description of the classification is beyond the scope of this book.

3.3 Measurement of enzyme activity

Learning objectives

You should be able to:

- describe in principle how the activities of enzymes are measured

- describe the progress curve for an enzyme-catalysed reaction and the significance of the initial rate, *v*.

The measurement of enzyme activity, or enzyme assay, is a very common operation in biochemical research and medical practice. Assay of enzymes in plasma and other clinical specimens is important for the diagnosis of many diseases. The activity of most enzymes is easy to measure. Even in a sample containing hundreds of enzymes it is possible to measure the activity of an individual enzyme. Enzymes do not have to be purified or separated before they are assayed; indeed, enzyme assay is a powerful and essential tool for following the progress of enzyme purification.

Clinical note:
Enzyme assay in clinical diagnosis

Enzyme assays are performed in hospital laboratories to further the diagnosis of a wide range of clinical conditions. Many of the assays are performed on blood plasma. Cellular enzymes are usually confined to the cells in which they are synthesised and in which they function. However, if tissue damage occurs during disease, cell membranes may be damaged and enzymes may leak from the cell into the blood where they circulate for several days. Because each cell type has its characteristic complement of enzymes, identification of abnormally high levels of activity of some enzymes in plasma can point to damage of particular tissues. Measurement of the amount of enzyme that has leaked gives a measure of the amount of tissue damage that has occurred. For example, several hours after a coronary blood vessel is blocked, oxygen deprivation damages heart muscle, and *lactate dehydrogenase* and *creatine phosphokinase* activities in the blood rise markedly (Fig. 15). These enzymes leak from the damaged tissue. Their assay can confirm the diagnosis and provides an estimate of how much muscle is involved. The occurrence of isoenzymes, described later in this chapter, can be used to make these clinical tests even more discriminating.

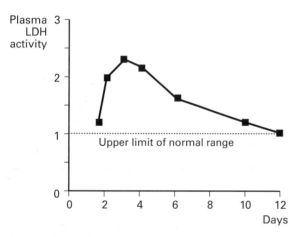

Fig. 15 Use of enzyme assay in clinical diagnosis: lactate dehydrogenase (LDH) appears in plasma a few hours after heart muscle is damaged (given as a multiple of upper limit of normal range).

Enzymes are assayed by incubating them with their substrates under appropriate conditions and measuring the rate of product formation. Because of enzyme specificity, it is almost always possible to devise conditions in which only the enzyme of interest is active. Many other enzymes may be present but they do not interfere because they have no substrates on which to act. Other enzymes that can use the provided substrate need not interfere if the substrate is present in excess amount and if they convert this substrate to a different product not measured by the assay.

The aim of an enzyme assay is to measure the initial rate of the enzyme-catalysed reaction. This can be done by producing a graph of the amount of product formed against time. Such a graph is called the *progress curve* of the reaction. The formation of product can be detected by any suitable analytical method. Spectrophotometry, changes in the absorption of visible or ultraviolet light by the sample, is often used. This technique, available in all biochemistry laboratories, combines sensitivity and convenience and will provide a continuous curve (Fig. 16). For even greater sensitivity, radiochemical methods using substrates labelled with radioactive isotopes may be used. In these methods, the product of the reaction, which also carries the label, must be separated from excess substrate before its radioactivity is measured. Radiochemical methods are even more sensitive than spectrophotometry but are more expensive and less convenient. Radiochemical methods are particularly valuable for assaying enzymes that catalyse the synthesis of polymers such as DNA, RNA and glycogen. They make it possible to distinguish newly synthesised polymer from polymer that may be present at the start of the assay as template, primer or contaminant.

Progress curves, however determined, have the same general form; the graph is approximately linear, having maximum slope shortly after the start of the reaction (Fig. 16). Later the slope decreases. This decrease in slope can be for a variety of reasons:

- the enzyme may begin to run out of substrate
- conversion of product back into substrate may become significant as the reaction system approaches equilibrium
- the catalysed reaction may, as it progresses, change a condition such as pH in the assay, leading to lower efficiency for the enzyme
- the enzyme may lose activity as the assay progresses.

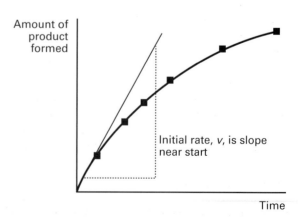

Fig. 16 Progress curve for an enzyme-catalysed reaction.

The only point on the progress curve where all these factors can be controlled is at the very start of the reaction. Hence, during enzyme assay, the rate of the enzyme-catalysed reaction is always calculated from the slope of the progress curve as near to the start of the reaction as is feasible. This is known as the initial rate, v.

3.4 Factors influencing enzyme-catalysed reactions

Learning objectives

You should be able to:

- list the factors that influence the rate of enzyme-catalysed reactions

- describe the effect of varying the substrate concentration and explain what is meant by saturation

- explain what is meant by an enzyme–substrate complex

- define the terms V_{max} and K_m.

Varying enzyme concentration

Since enzyme molecules act independently, the reaction rate measured in an enzyme assay should be proportional to the amount of enzyme present. This proportionality is generally observed and provides a simple test of the validity of the assay method. Any departure from proportionality is almost always an indication of some problem with the assay method.

Enzymes are easily inactivated

The catalytic action of an enzyme is influenced by physicochemical conditions, particularly temperature and pH. Changes in these conditions can have irreversible or reversible effects on the enzyme. Enzymes, being proteins, are usually denatured by high temperatures or by pH values more than a few units away from neutrality. This denaturation is in most cases irreversible. When exploring the effect of changes in temperature and pH on the activity of enzymes, it is best first to define the temperature and pH ranges in which the enzyme is stable. Changes of temperature and pH that do not denature have reversible effects on the enzyme's activity.

Effects of temperature

Enzymes are inactivated by brief exposure to high temperatures. The onset of inactivation occurs over a temperature range of just a few degrees. The actual temperature required for inactivation varies from one enzyme to another but is typically in the range 50–60°C. A few enzymes, notably those from thermophilic microorganisms, can withstand exposure to 100°C. At temperatures below those at which they are inactivated, enzymes show increasing activity with increasing temperature. There is no optimum temperature, and enzyme activity measurements should be made at temperatures that are at least a few degrees below the temperature at which the enzyme is inactivated.

Effect of pH

Within the pH range in which they are stable, the activities of enzymes can be strongly influenced by pH. For many enzymes the graph of activity against pH is bell-shaped with a definite optimum (Fig. 17). Enzyme assays should be carried out at the optimum pH. This is generally achieved by adding a buffer of the appropriate pH to the assay. The optimum pH for an enzyme-catalysed reaction does not necessarily coincide with the pH in the compartment of the cell where it is found.

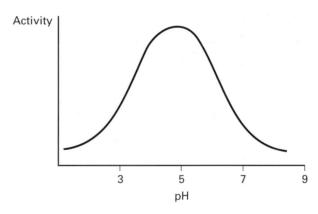

Fig. 17 The effect of pH on the activity of an enzyme, lysozyme. Activity of this enzyme depends on the ionisation state of two carboxyl groups at its active centre; it has a pH optimum of around 5.

Clinical note:
Therapeutic use of enzymes

Preparations of digestive enzymes from the pancreas are used therapeutically in conditions such as cystic fibrosis where natural secretion is inadequate. Such preparations must be formulated or administered in such a way that they reach the duodenum in an active state and do not become inactivated by exposure to the low pH in the stomach.

This variation of activity with pH results from the ionisation of a limited number of groups on the enzyme or substrate. This is well illustrated by studies on the mechanism of action of lysozyme, described later in this chapter.

Effect of varying substrate concentration

Enzyme kinetics is the investigation of enzyme mechanisms by measuring how the initial rate of reaction is affected by varying experimental conditions, particularly by varying substrate concentrations.

At low substrate concentrations, [S], the rate of the enzyme-catalysed reaction is approximately proportional to [S], but as [S] increases the rate approaches a maximum (Fig. 18). This is a consequence of the mechanism of enzymic catalysis.

Most enzyme reactions can be considered to occur in at least three phases. In the first phase, the substrate or substrates bind to a specialised binding site on the enzyme, the active centre, to form an enzyme–substrate complex. In the second phase, chemical change occurs within this complex to generate the products of the reaction, still bound at the active centre. During this second phase, a transient covalent bond may form between an atom in the substrate and an atom in the enzyme. In the final phase, the products dissociate from the enzyme leaving it free to undergo another catalytic cycle. A model devised by Michaelis and Menten represents this mechanism:

$$E + S = E\text{--}S \rightarrow E\text{--}P = E + P$$

where E represents enzyme, S substrate and P product. At high concentrations of substrate, the active centre is fully occupied with substrate, and further increases in substrate concentration cannot increase the occupation further. Under these conditions, the rate-limiting

step in the catalytic process occurs after substrate has bound. The Michaelis equation, which relates the observed initial rate, v, to the substrate concentration, [S], can be derived from this model for enzymic catalysis:

$$v = V_{max}[S]/(K_m + [S])$$

The equation contains two parameters that are characteristic of the rate measurements under the experimental conditions that were used: V_{max}, the maximum reaction rate, and K_m, the *Michaelis constant*. The equation fits the form of the rate versus substrate concentration graph for many enzymes and gives experimental support to the model. V_{max} has the same dimensions as the reaction rate and is the upper limit approached by the reaction rate at high substrate concentrations. The Michaelis constant is the concentration of substrate at which the enzyme gives an observed reaction rate that is one-half of V_{max}. V_{max} should be proportional to the amount of enzyme used in the experiments in which it was determined so it is not a characteristic of the enzyme. If the molecular concentration of enzyme, [E], corresponding to V_{max} is known, it can be used to calculate the value of k_{cat}, since $V_{max} = kcat[E]$. k_{cat} is a measure of the rate at which each enzyme molecule turns over substrate into product.

The value of K_m depends on the relative rates of the reactions involved in the formation of enzyme–substrate complex, its conversion to enzyme–product complex and the dissociation of the enzyme–product complex. It is a characteristic of the enzyme and is a measure of the affinity of the enzyme for its substrate. A low value of K_m indicates that the enzyme has a high affinity for its substrate, and a high value indicates that it has a low affinity.

Although V_{max} and K_m can be estimated from the graph of v against [S] (Fig. 19a), it is usually more accurate to derive them from a linear transformation of the Michaelis equation, such as the *Lineweaver–Burk plot* (Fig. 19b). By plotting the reciprocals of rate and [S], a straight line should be obtained. Estimates of V_{max} and K_m can be calculated from the intercepts of this line on the y and x axes. Other statistically more satisfactory methods of estimating V_{max} and K_m from experimental data can also be used. Estimation of its K_m is usually one of the first investigations carried out with any newly discovered enzyme.

The first justification for determining the value of K_m for an enzyme is a very practical one. What concentration of substrate is appropriate for its assay? It is best to assay enzymes using substrate concentrations that are high enough to approach saturation (Fig. 18), certainly three or four times the K_m value. In these circumstances, slight departures from the intended substrate concentration will give only small errors in the observed rate.

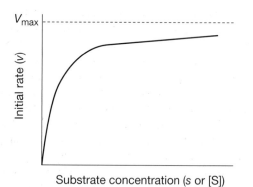

Fig. 18 Effect of varying substrate concentration on a typical enzyme-catalysed reaction.

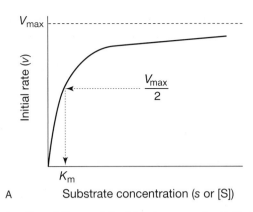 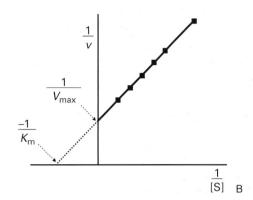

Fig. 19 Estimation of V_{max} and K_m: (a) using a graph of initial rate versus [S], and (b) using a linear plot, the Lineweaver–Burk plot, which provides a more accurate estimate.

At substrate concentrations below K_m, errors in the substrate concentration will have a more serious effect.

A second reason to determine K_m is to characterise the enzyme and possibly to distinguish it from other enzymes catalysing the same reaction. A single biochemical reaction is often catalysed by a different molecular form of enzyme in different tissues, or even in different compartments of the same cell. These multiple molecular forms of an enzyme are known as *isozymes* or *isoenzymes*. They can be distinguished in several ways, notably by study of their kinetics and by gel electrophoresis. While they catalyse a single reaction, they often differ from one another in their kinetics and in the ways in which their activity may be controlled. Isoenzymes have K_m values that fit them for their biochemical role. Hexokinase is found in most tissues that rely on blood glucose and has a low K_m for glucose. This means that the rate of glucose phosphorylation is insensitive to the glucose concentration and does not respond to increased glucose concentrations (Fig. 20). Glucose arriving at the cell is efficiently metabolised. Hexokinase is inhibited by its product and has a low V_{max}, so its rate of phosphorylation of glucose does not increase significantly when the blood glucose concentration rises. In effect, it is insensitive to blood glucose concentration. Glucokinase, an isoenzyme of hexokinase, occurs in liver and in a few other tissues. It has a high K_m and V_{max} and it can respond by increasing the rate of glucose utilisation when large amounts of glucose reach the liver among the products of digestion after a carbohydrate meal. Glucokinase is also the isoenzyme present in the insulin-secreting cells in the pancreas and accounts for the ability of these cells to respond to changing glucose levels in the blood (p. 79).

The final justification for determining K_m is that it is influenced by certain enzyme inhibitors and reveals their mode of action.

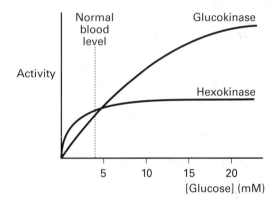

Fig. 20 Hexokinase and glucokinase are isozymes that phosphorylate glucose, the first step in its utilisation. Different K_m values allow hexokinase to supply energy substrates efficiently to cells that rely on blood glucose, while glucokinase (in the liver and the pancreas) responds to high glucose levels.

Enzyme inhibitors

Enzymes show diminished catalytic powers or are inhibited in the presence of a wide range of other molecules. Some inhibitors are quite non-specific; they will inhibit many enzymes. Heavy metal ions such as mercury, lead and copper usually inhibit enzymes, so even traces of these ions must be removed both from water and from chemicals to be used in experiments with enzymes. Other inhibitors show more specificity. Specific inhibitors may block enzyme action by mimicking the substrate in some way or other; others may bind to the enzyme altering its shape and thus the shape of the active site. The inhibitor may bind to and occupy the substrate-binding site, forming a specific enzyme–inhibitor complex in which further chemical change

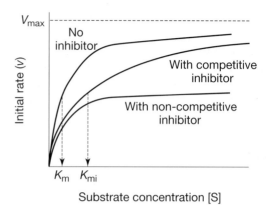

Fig. 21 Competitive and non-competitive inhibitors. A fixed concentration of inhibitor has different effects depending on its mechanism of action.

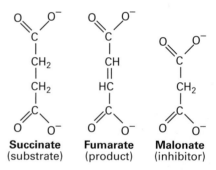

Fig. 22 Competitive inhibition of succinate dehydrogenase by malonate, which has an obvious structural similarity to succinate.

does not occur. Other inhibitors get as far as the phase of enzyme action when chemical change occurs. However, instead of forming a transient covalent bond with the enzyme as the substrate does, the inhibitor forms a stable covalent bond, so blocking further reaction. Inhibitors can be reversible, bound to the enzyme by non-covalent bonds, and so, in principle at least, are able to dissociate from the enzyme, restoring it to activity. Other inhibitors that form a covalent bond with the enzyme are irreversible in their action. Enzyme inhibition can be described as:

- competitive
- non-competitive
- irreversible.

Competitive inhibitors

One particularly common mode of inhibition is reversible competitive inhibition, where the inhibitor molecule resembles the substrate molecule. The active centre can

bind either inhibitor or substrate but not both at once. The amount of enzyme tied up as unproductive enzyme–inhibitor complex depends not only on the concentration of inhibitor but also on the concentration of the substrate with which the inhibitor is competing. At high concentrations of substrate, the effects of competitive inhibitors are greatly diminished (Fig. 21). The effect of the competitive inhibitor is to increase the K_m of the enzyme for its substrate (to K_{mi}); V_{max} remains the same. If the concentration of substrate is increased enough, the active site will be saturated with substrate and the inhibitor excluded. The inhibition of succinate dehydrogenase by malonate is the classic example of competitive inhibition (Fig. 22). The similarity of the succinate and malonate molecules can be easily seen.

Non-competitive inhibitors

Other enzyme inhibitors bind to the enzyme in such a way that the substrate, even though it can still bind to the enzyme, cannot undergo reaction or may react more slowly. In this case, the extent of inhibition will not be diminished by high substrate concentrations (Fig. 21) and the inhibition is said to be non-competitive. With a non-competitive inhibitor, V_{max} is lowered but K_m is unaltered. An example is the inhibition of the membrane-bound Na^+/K^+-ATPase by *ouabain*, a toxic glycoside.

Irreversible inhibition

Any compound that binds to an enzyme and prevents its catalytic action may irreversibly inhibit the enzyme. One molecule of inhibitor is sufficient to knock out one molecule of enzyme. Nerve gas inhibitors such as DIFP (diisopropylfluorophosphate) inhibit serine enzymes (Fig 2.7, p. 38). These compounds form stable phosphate esters with the reactive serine side chain and thus block the action of the enzyme. These inhibitors were discovered as very potent and toxic inhibitors of *acetyl-cholinesterase*, an enzyme involved in nerve action and which also depends on an activated serine side chain.

3.5 Mechanisms of enzyme action

Learning objectives

You should be able to:

- describe the general nature of an enzyme–substrate complex
- explain what is meant by the transition state of a chemical reaction
- list the factors that may be important in the activation of an enzyme's substrate
- describe how the presence of acidic or basic groups in the enzyme–substrate complex can promote catalysis
- give an example of how the interaction between amino acid chains can enhance their reactivity.

As we have seen, the catalytic action of enzymes involves the formation of specific complexes between enzymes and their substrates. This accounts for the efficiency, potency and specificity of enzymic catalysis. Many enzymes have had their structures determined in both the absence and the presence of competitive inhibitors. These models show how the polypeptide chain is folded and the position of all the amino acid side chains. It is usually impossible to determine enzyme structures in the presence of substrates, but plausible models can be built to represent the structures of enzyme–substrate complexes. The position of the active centre can be deduced from the binding site for competitive inhibitors. Models of substrate molecules can be fitted to the enzyme models, giving an insight into the structure of the enzyme–substrate complex. For each enzyme studied, features of the complex can be identified that promote activation of the substrate and direct its reaction to form a specific product. Table 2 lists four of the most studied enzymes and particularly important features that have been identified in the reaction mechanism of each.

Table 2 Four much-studied enzymes, the reactions they catalyse and notable features of their reaction mechanisms

Enzyme	Reaction catalysed	Features of reaction mechanism
Carboxypeptidase A	Hydrolyses polar amino acid from C-terminal of peptide	Induced fit: enzyme changes conformation when substrate binds Water molecule on zinc in enzyme made more reactive
Lysozyme	Hydrolyses polysaccharide in cell walls of some bacteria	Monosaccharide unit next to bond that is cleaved is forced into more reactive transition state for reaction Aspartate side chain stabilises carbcation intermediate Glutamate side chain is proton donor for acid catalysis
Chymotrypsin	Hydrolyses peptide bond involving carboxyl group of amino acids with bulky non-polar side chains, e.g. phenylalanine, tyrosine and tryptophan Also hydrolyses ester bonds	Aspartate, histidine and serine side chains interact to enhance serine hydroxyl as a nucleophile Transient covalent intermediate formed and then hydrolysed
Hexokinase	Transfers phosphate group to glucose from ATP	Two substrates, glucose and ATP, are orientated for reaction Water excluded from reaction to prevent hydrolysis, a side reaction

The nature of the enzyme–substrate complex

The molecular models show features common to all enzymes. The fit between the substrate and its binding site at the active centre of the enzyme is precise. Charged groups on the substrate are attracted by groups of opposite charge on the enzyme. Hydrogen bond donors and acceptors on the substrate can form bonds with appropriately positioned acceptors and donors on the enzyme. Hydrophobic groups on substrates fit into hydrophobic pockets in the enzyme. At one time it was thought that this fit between the enzyme and its substrate was rigid and could be likened to the fit between a lock and key. It is now thought that formation of the enzyme–substrate complex is more dynamic than this. Enzymes can be flexible and many change shape on binding their substrates. Substrates, too, may have to distort and adopt less stable conformations before they fit the binding site on the enzyme. Substrates are forced into a state close to that of the transition state in the reaction they are about to undergo. This concept of enzymes and substrates adapting their structures during complex formation was first described by Koshland and is called *induced fit*.

Proteins can enfold their substrates

Examination of detailed three-dimensional structures determined by X-ray crystallography of enzymes and their complexes with inhibitors or substrates has shown changes in the shape of enzymes when they bind their substrates. These changes in conformation can be used to promote the required reactions and to prevent side reactions. Protein flexibility allows enzymes to enfold their substrates during complex formation, excluding water molecules and thus preventing hydrolysis. Hexokinase shields ATP, its coenzyme substrate, from water while catalysing the transfer of a phosphate group to its other substrate, glucose. ATP hydrolysis is prevented since the only acceptor group accessible to the activated phosphate is on the glucose molecule bound to the enzyme.

Enfolding the substrate can also enhance its reactivity. If a substrate is bound in a region of the enzyme from which bulk solvent water is excluded, electrostatic attractions and repulsions between charged groups on the enzyme and on the substrate are greatly strengthened, increasing the reactivity of the substrate molecule. *Carboxypeptidase*, a zinc-containing protease that hydrolyses an amino acid from the C-terminal end of its peptide substrate, was one of the first enzymes for which clear evidence of a change in conformation on binding of substrate was obtained. A tyrosine side chain in the enzyme swings over the bound substrate, shielding it from solvent water. A single water molecule within the complex has its reactivity enhanced by the zinc atom and cleaves the peptide bond between the C-terminal amino acid and the rest of the substrate.

Bond cleavage

Before we can consider how complex formation can bring about reaction, we need to describe the nature of the chemical reactions important in biochemistry. A covalent bond is the sharing of two electrons by the two atoms involved in the bond. During chemical reaction, a covalent bond is cleaved and a new bond or bonds are formed. In almost all biochemical reactions, both shared electrons remain with one atom after bond cleavage and the other atom takes none. The products of the cleavage are usually unstable and quickly rearrange or form covalent bonds with new partners. Cleavage of a covalent bond is an energetically unfavourable process: an energy barrier exists between the initial and final states and this barrier must be surmounted. If it were otherwise, covalent bonds would not exist. To cleave the bond it is necessary to stretch it until it reaches the transition state, the peak on the bond length versus energy graph (Fig. 23). This can be represented in an energy diagram for the reaction. Without a catalyst, the energy for bond stretching must come from thermal collisions with solvent molecules and other molecules in solution. Even if the bond length reaches the critical transition state and cleavage occurs, the molecular fragments produced may recombine, producing no net reaction. The presence of an enzyme lowers the energy barrier between reactants and products but has no effect on the overall energy change of the reaction: the rate of reaction is increased but the equilibrium constant remains the same. How can the presence of an enzyme promote the reaction? Two important factors are activation of the substrate and stabilisation of the products.

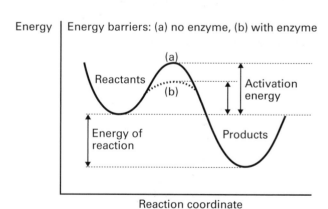

Fig. 23 Energy diagram for a reaction in the absence and the presence of any enzyme. The reaction coordinate is a measure of the progress of the reaction. It might, for instance, represent the length of a bond that is being broken.

Activation of the substrate

Several factors seem to be involved in the activation of substrates. The distortion of the substrate towards the transition state, the proximity of chemical groups on the enzyme that can promote reaction, the orientation of the substrate for reaction with another molecule and alteration of the molecular environment of the substrate have all been suggested as activation mechanisms.

Binding to an enzyme can weaken the critical bond in the substrate. As we have seen, substrates and enzymes have to adjust their structures when forming a complex. Substrates are often distorted towards the transition state structure. This is seen in the enzyme *lysozyme*, a widely distributed enzyme that kills some bacteria by hydrolysis of their polysaccharide cell wall material. The substrate-binding site on lysozyme lies in a cleft on the surface of the enzyme. This site binds six monosac-

---

Clinical note:
Discovery of lysozyme

Lysozyme was discovered by Alexander Fleming who later discovered penicillin. The antibacterial action of lysozyme has not been used therapeutically. Its presence in tears and other secretions is part of the natural defences of the body.

---

charide units in the long polysaccharide chain of the substrate. Five of these six units are not distorted during binding to the enzyme but the other unit is distorted before it can bind (Fig. 24). The monosaccharide units all contain a six-membered ring containing five carbons and an oxygen atom. This ring is most stable in a puckered configuration, the chair configuration (Fig. 25), with one atom above and one below the plane defined by the other four atoms. This configuration is retained by five of the six bound units. When the other unit binds to lysozyme its ring is forced into the half-chair configuration. Carbon-1 of this ring, the atom that is a partner in the carbon–oxygen bond that is cleaved during reaction, is forced up into the plane of the ring. This weakens the carbon–oxygen bond.

Stabilisation of the products

Once the substrate has bound to the active site with possible activation, the second effect, the promotion of the reaction by nearby chemical groups on the enzyme, comes into play. If the carbon–oxygen bond were to cleave in the lysozyme example, the products would be a carbon atom carrying a positive charge (i.e. an unstable carbcation) and an oxygen carrying a negative charge, also unstable (Fig. 26). There are two carboxyl groups on lysozyme near to where the substrate is bound. One of these, the side chain of an aspartate

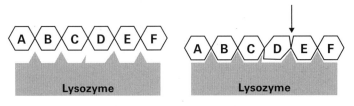

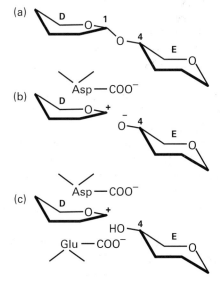

Fig. 24 Binding of substrate to the active centre of lysozyme. Notice how the D ring of the substrate must distort before substrate binding can occur. This ring must assume the half-chair configuration to fit the active centre. The bond cleaved during the reaction is between the D and E rings.

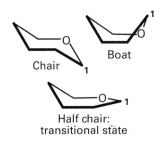

Fig. 25 Transition state in lysozyme catalysis. Ring D in lysozyme substrate adopts the less stable half-chair conformation prior to the cleavage of the glycosidic bond to carbon-1 of the ring.

Fig. 26 Stabilisation of the products of bond cleavage during lysozyme catalysis. (a) The D and E rings before bond cleavage. (b) The D and E rings after cleavage. There is a carbcation at carbon-1 of the D ring, which is stabilised by the negatively charged carboxyl group on an aspartate side chain at the active centre. (c) The negatively charged oxygen on carbon-4 of the E ring is stabilised by transfer to it of a proton from a protonated glutamate side chain, also at the active centre.

residue, is ionised and has a negative charge. It is close to the carbon atom of the substrate that gains the positive charge on bond cleavage and this favours the production of this unstable intermediate. The second carboxyl group involved in the catalytic process is on a glutamate side chain. This group must be in the undissociated or protonated state to promote reaction. It gives its proton to the negatively charged oxygen produced by bond cleavage, converting it to the stable hydroxyl group found in the product of the reaction. This is an example of *acid catalysis*. An appropriately positioned amino acid side chain on the enzyme acts as a proton donor to provide the hydrogen ion (proton) needed for facile reaction. The position of such a proton donor may be critical in deciding which of two possible chiral products is formed by the enzyme reaction; this determines the stereospecificity of the enzyme.

Proximity and orientation of substrates

Enzymes that have more than one substrate bind these substrates in an orientation suitable for reaction. When the critical bond breaks, new partners are nearby so that the molecular fragments can form new bonds. One of the factors making uncatalysed reactions between two molecules in solution so slow is that collisions between the molecules, although frequent, are almost always in unsuitable orientations for reaction. An enzyme by binding first one substrate and then another can ensure that they are in the optimal orientation for reaction.

Formation of the enzyme–substrate complex explains the stereochemical specificity of enzymes. Substrate-binding sites, being three-dimensional, will distinguish between the two optical isomers of a chiral substrate, one of which will fit the binding site and react, the other will not fit and therefore remains unchanged. Enzymes are chiral, so, even when a non-chiral substrate is bound, new chemical groupings to be attached to this substrate will always approach from the same direction in space and so produce only one of the two possible stereoisomers of the product.

Interaction between side chains can enhance their reactivity

Many proteases with different specificities are involved in the digestion of proteins in the gut. One class of digestive protease, the *'serine' proteases*, have been studied in great detail and shown to have a common mechanism of action. This class of proteases includes trypsin, chymotrypsin and elastase. Thrombin, a protease involved in blood clotting, has a similar mechanism. All these enzymes contain a serine side chain that is uniquely reactive. The hydroxyl group on the side

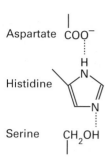

Fig. 27 Activation of the serine side chain of the active site in serine proteases by a charge relay system, allowing the negatively charged carboxylate of the aspartate to share its charge with the serine oxygen.

chain displaces the amino group involved in the peptide bond, which is cleaved, and forms a transient ester intermediate with the carboxyl group. The ester intermediate is then hydrolysed, leaving the protease free for another round of catalytic action. The enzyme forms an unstable covalent intermediate with part of the substrate. When this intermediate is hydrolysed, the catalytic process is complete.

The serine hydroxyl on its own would not be sufficiently reactive to displace part of the substrate and form a covalent bond with the remainder. In the serine proteases, it has its reactivity enhanced by interaction with an imidazole group on a histidine side chain, which in turn interacts with a negatively charged carboxyl group on an aspartate side chain (Fig. 27). The carboxylate 'shares' its negative charge with the serine oxygen, making this atom a stronger nucleophile, more able to attack the carbonyl carbon of peptide and ester substrates. This group of side chains has been called a *charge relay system*. The amino acids contributing to the system are widely separated in the polypeptide sequence but are brought together by the tertiary structure. Nerve gases such as diisopropylfluorophosphate inhibit acetylcholine esterase by forming a stable covalent bond between the phosphorus atom of the inhibitor and the oxygen atom on the reactive serine side chain. They do not react with unactivated serines.

3.6 Control of enzyme activity

Learning objectives

You should be able to:

* explain what is meant by allosteric control of enzyme activity

- explain how enzyme activity can be controlled by reversible covalent modification

- explain how active enzymes can be formed by irreversible covalent modification of precursor zymogens.

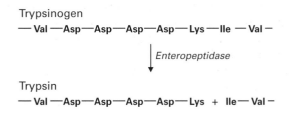

Fig. 28 Activation of trypsin. Enteropeptidase is specific for trypsinogen, which is cleaved at the sequence shown above and thereby activated.

In every metabolic pathway, the activity of at least one enzyme is subject to regulation so that the flux of material through the pathway can be controlled.

Allosteric control

Some enzymes are reversibly inhibited or activated by the presence of metabolites that are not their substrates or products. These metabolites, if inhibitory, are usually distant products of the pathway, so providing negative feedback for the activity of the pathway. Enzymes controlled in this way have binding sites additional to those at which they bind their substrates. Binding of inhibitors or activators at these sites changes the shape of the enzyme molecule, decreasing or increasing its catalytic ability. This form of control is known as allosteric. Allosteric enzymes are always composed of subunits and have multiple interacting active centres. While they can be saturated with their substrates, they often show *sigmoid* graphs of initial rate versus substrate concentration and, therefore, do not obey strict Michaelis kinetics.

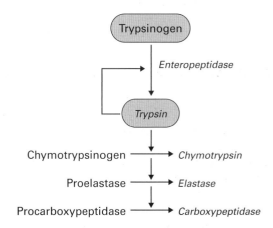

Fig. 29 Activation of digestive proteases.

Control by reversible covalent modification

This regulation is often in response to a signal coming from outside the cell, such as response to a hormone. In this case, the enzyme is itself the substrate of other enzymes. One of these modifies the enzyme, making it active, while another reverses the modification, making it inactive again. *Glycogen phosphorylase*, the enzyme that mobilises carbohydrate fuel reserves in animal cells, is activated by addition of a phosphate group to a serine side chain and is inactivated when this phosphate group is removed. The hormones *adrenaline (epinephrine)* and *glucagon* trigger the activation of phosphorylase in their respective target cells (pp. 246–248).

Control by irreversible covalent modification

Some digestive enzymes are potentially so damaging to the cells that synthesise them that they are secreted as inactive precursors or *zymogens*. Once secreted, these zymogens are converted into their active forms. This activation process is irreversible. Trypsin, a major protease involved in protein digestion in the duodenum, is secreted as the inactive precursor trypsinogen in the pancreatic juice. Once in the duodenum, it is acted on by a specialised peptidase, *enteropeptidase*, secreted by cells in the duodenal wall. Enteropeptidase cleaves a peptide bond in trypsinogen, converting it to trypsin (Fig. 28). Trypsin, once formed, can act on further molecules of trypsinogen, so the activation process is autocatalytic. Trypsin also activates other protease precursors from the pancreas, particularly chymotrypsinogen, proelastase and procarboxypeptidase (Fig. 29). Pepsin, the major protease active in the stomach, is secreted as its inactive precursor, pepsinogen. This is activated by an autocatalytic process in the acid conditions of the stomach. Blood clotting also depends on the appropriate activation of protease precursors in the plasma by limited specific proteolysis (Ch. 19).

3.7 Membrane transport

Learning objective

You should be able to:

- describe how proteins involved in membrane transport processes share many properties with enzymes.

As well as catalysing chemical reactions, proteins can also promote transport processes. Ions and hydrophilic molecules cannot, on their own, penetrate the lipid bilayer that is the basis of all biological membranes. Proteins in membranes can form channels that will selectively allow ions to cross the membrane. Transporter proteins can form lipid-soluble complexes with hydrophilic molecules such as glucose. These complexes can pick up their ligands on one side of the membrane and release them on the other side, thus promoting transport. Proteins can also couple transport processes to chemical reactions, so allowing differences in ionic concentration on opposite sides of the membrane to be built up. Proteins involved in transport processes share many of their properties with enzymes. They show specificity, including stereospecificity, they show saturation when the ligand concentration is high and they are susceptible to inhibition, particularly by compounds similar to the ligands they transport.

The involvement of enzymes and other proteins in membrane transport processes will be mentioned again in Chapter 4.

Self-assessment: questions

Single best answer MCQs

1. Your text has emphasised the vital role of enzymes in the body since they allow reactions to proceed at rates sufficient to support physiologic processes. Which one of the following statements about enzyme catalysis is correct?
   a. Enzymes convert all available substrate into product because they do not waste material on side reactions
   b. An enzyme molecule is a true catalyst and remains unchanged during catalysis
   c. In an equilibrium reaction system, an enzyme that catalyses the forward reaction will also catalyse the back reaction
   d. An enzyme cannot convert a substrate that is not optically active into a product that is optically active
   e. An enzyme cannot convert a substrate that is optically active into a product that is not optically active

2. As you will read later in this text when we discuss protein digestion in the gut, several proteases have key roles and their specificities are key. Identify the correct statement about the digestive proteases.
   a. Trypsin can cleave peptide bonds involving the carboxyl function of leucine residues
   b. Trypsin can cleave peptide bonds involving the carboxyl function of alanine residues
   c. Chymotrypsin can cleave peptide bonds involving the amino groups of phenylalanine and tyrosine
   d. Trypsin and chymotrypsin can cleave ester bonds as well as peptide bonds
   e. Chymotrypsin is active in the duodenum while trypsin is active in the stomach

3. Coenzymes and prosthetic groups are found in all the key metabolic pathways. Which one of the following statements is accurate about these key molecules?
   a. Carbonic anhydrase contains a tightly bound zinc ion that is essential for its structure but not its activity
   b. Some enzymes contain organic molecules called prosthetic groups that are essential for activity; prosthetic groups are vitamins and cannot be synthesised in the body
   c. Coenzymes are small polypeptides that are involved in transfer reactions catalysed by enzymes

   d. Coenzymes carry acyl or phosphate groups in many enzyme-catalysed reactions that involve the transfer of these groups
   e. Coenzymes transfer oxygen in most cellular oxidation–reduction reactions

Enzyme assays are carried out every day in clinical chemistry laboratories. Questions 4–6 deal with enzymes and their assay. In each case identify the single correct statement.

4. a. Enzymes must be purified before their activity can be measured
   b. Enzymes are assayed by measuring the maximum amount of substrate they convert into product under standardised conditions
   c. The observed rate in an enzyme reaction should be proportional to the amount of substrate present
   d. The catalysed reaction can be followed by measuring the rate of appearance of product or the rate of substrate consumption
   e. A graph of the rate of reaction against substrate concentration is known as a progress curve

5. a. The use of radioactive substrates provides a convenient and sensitive technique for the assay of many enzymes. Such techniques are used wherever feasible
   b. Enzymes that catalyse the formation of polymers such as nucleic acids or glycogen are often assayed using spectrophotometry
   c. The catalysed reaction must be stopped before the amount of product formed is measured
   d. Since the rate of the catalysed reaction tends to decrease with time during the course of an assay, the rate of reaction is always measured as close to the start of the reaction as possible
   e. Enzymes are usually assayed at pH 7 with saturating concentrations of substrate present

6. a. Enzyme assay is much used in biochemical research but has no practical importance
   b. Enzymes often have an optimum temperature so they should be assayed close to the temperature of the tissue or cell in which they occur
   c. Enzymes often have an optimum pH for activity so they should be assayed at a pH value close to this optimum

d. Enzymes are denatured if they are not kept close to their optimum pH
e. Enzymes are inactive outside the pH range 4–9

7. Identify the single correct statement about the effect of varying substrate concentration, [S], on the rate, v, of an enzyme-catalysed reaction.
   a. K_m, the Michaelis constant, is equal to one-half of V_{max}
   b. At [S] values below K_m, v is approximately independent of [S]
   c. At [S] values well above K_m, v is approximately proportional to [S]
   d. At high [S] values, v approaches V_{max} as [S] increases
   e. The parameters v, V_{max}, [S] and K_m are related by the Michaelis equation as follows:

$$v = (V_{max} + [S])/(K_m + [S])$$

8. Which one of the following statements is correct concerning the Michaelis constant, K_m?
   a. Is measured in the same units as the rate of the enzyme-catalysed reaction
   b. Varies with the amount of enzyme used in measuring the reaction rate
   c. Can be considered to be a measure of the affinity an enzyme has for its substrate
   d. Has a low value to indicate a low affinity for substrate
   e. Has the same value for differing isozymes

9. Which one of the following statements is correct concerning the inhibition of enzymes?
   a. Many enzymes are activated by heavy metal ions such as mercury and lead
   b. Competitive inhibitors of enzymes bind irreversibly to the active centre and form an unproductive enzyme–inhibitor complex
   c. Some specific inhibitors of enzymes bind covalently to the enzyme that they inhibit
   d. Decreasing the concentration of substrate relieves inhibition by inhibitors that bind reversibly at the active centre
   e. Many drugs act as non-specific enzyme inhibitors

10. Identify the single accurate statement concerning the mechanism of action of enzymes.
    a. Enzymes have rigid structures that fit their specific substrates
    b. Substrates are often distorted during formation of the enzyme–substrate complex
    c. Enzymes bind the substrates but not the products of the reactions that they catalyse

d. Only amino acid side chains at the active centre have a role in the catalytic process
e. Amino acid side chains involved in the formation of the active centre are usually close together in the amino acid sequence of the enzyme protein

11. Which one of the following statements accurately describes enzyme-catalysed reactions?
    a. One of the two electrons that formed the bond cleaved in an enzyme-catalysed reaction remains with each of the atoms previously joined by the bond
    b. Acidic and basic amino acid side chains often play an important role in catalysis but not in substrate binding
    c. The state of ionisation of acidic and basic groups near the active centre does not affect the catalytic activity of the enzyme
    d. Nerve gases react with serine residues on many enzymes but only inhibit those that have a serine side chain essential for the catalytic process
    e. Some enzymes form temporary covalent bonds with part of the substrate

12. Allosteric enzymes feature in many key metabolic pathways and the special features of such enzymes are important for your understanding of metabolism. Which one of the following statements concerning allosteric enzymes is correct?
    a. Allosteric enzymes bind allosteric effectors at their active centre; these ligands, metabolites or other signal molecules switch the enzyme on or off when they bind
    b. Enzymes that have subunits and multiple active centres are allosteric
    c. Allosteric enzymes do not show saturation with substrate because they do not obey Michaelis kinetics
    d. Allosteric control is irreversible
    e. Allosteric enzymes are often involved in negative feedback control mechanisms

13. Which of the following statements is accurate about zymogens?
    a. Zymogens are inactive precursors of enzymes and are activated by specific cleavage of critical disulphide bonds
    b. Zymogen activation is important in the digestion of proteins and in blood coagulation
    c. Chymotrypsin is produced from chymotrypsinogen by the action of enteropeptidase

d. The zymogens of pepsin, trypsin, chymotrypsin and elastase are synthesised in the pancreas and reach the duodenum before they are activated

e. Pepsin is secreted as pepsinogen, and activated by trypsin action

14. Identify the single correct statement about the control of enzyme activity by reversible covalent modification.

a. Enzymes subject to control by reversible phosphorylation are activated by being phosphorylated on a serine or threonine side chain

b. Enzymes subject to control by reversible phosphorylation are inactivated by dephosphorylation

c. Phosphorylation of serine side chains to control enzyme activity is catalysed by enzymes known as protein phosphatases, which require ATP

d. Dephosphorylation of serine side chains to control enzyme activity is catalysed by enzymes known as protein kinases

e. Control of enzyme activity by reversible phosphorylation is an important cellular response to some hormonal signals

True/false questions

Are the following statements true or false?

1. Coenzymes are small, heat-stable molecules containing a nucleotide grouping that are often involved in enzyme-catalysed transfer reactions.

2. Enzymes that contain prosthetic groups can often be separated into a protein part, the holoenzyme, which is inactive, and a non-protein part.

3. Enzymes may have one or more active centres where their substrates bind and undergo chemical change.

4. Phosphatases are enzymes that synthesise phosphate esters.

5. Liver and heart lactate dehydrogenase are identical.

6. Isoenzymes are distinct molecular forms of enzymes catalysing the same reaction and controlled in the same way.

7. The addition of a competitive inhibitor to an enzyme reaction will increase the apparent K_m for substrate.

8. The value of V_{max} determined for an enzyme is proportional to the amount of enzyme used when measuring values of the initial rate, v.

9. The value of K_m determined for an enzyme is independent of the amount of enzyme used when measuring values of the initial rate, v, but will vary from one isoenzyme form to another.

10. Trypsin, chymotrypsin, elastase and thrombin all act outside cells and are all secreted as inactive proenzymes or zymogens.

Short essay question

What is the evidence that an enzyme forms a complex with its substrate during the course of an enzyme-catalysed reaction? How does this complex formation account for the specificity of enzymes and their potency as catalysts?

Self-assessment: answers

Single best answer MCQ answers

1. a. **False**. Material is not wasted on side reactions, but some substrate may not be converted to product because an equilibrium mixture of substrate and product is produced.
   b. **False**. Enzyme molecules are often chemically modified during the catalytic process but are returned to their original state when the round of catalysis is complete.
   c. **True**. Otherwise the enzyme would not bring the system to equilibrium.
   d. **False**. For example, pyruvate to L-lactate by lactate dehydrogenase in muscle.
   e. **False**. For example, L-lactate to pyruvate by lactate dehydrogenase in muscle.

2. a. **False**. Trypsin needs a positively charged side chain such as that of lysine in its substrate. Leucine has an uncharged side chain.
   b. **False**. Alanine has an uncharged side chain. Arginine is the second amino acid recognised by trypsin.
   c. **False**. These amino acids have the bulky hydrophobic side chains needed for substrate binding, but it is peptide bonds involving their carboxyl group that are cleaved.
   d. **True**. Esters are cleaved by the same mechanism and are used as substrates in some assays for these enzymes.
   e. **False**. Trypsin is active in the duodenum. It is pepsin that is active in the stomach.

3. a. **False**. The zinc ion is essential for activity.
   b. **False**. Many prosthetic groups are synthesised from vitamins but some prosthetic groups, notably haem, can be made in the body.
   c. **False**. Coenzymes are involved in transfer reactions but usually have a nucleotide moiety in their structures. They are not polypeptides.
   d. **True**. Transfer reactions of acyl groups often involve coenzyme A. Phosphate transfers often involve ATP.
   e. **False**. Oxidation reactions in cells are predominantly by hydrogen transfer and involve NAD or NADP.

4. a. **False**. Enzymes do not need to be purified before being assayed. Assay conditions should be such that only the target enzyme is active.

   b. **False**. It is the rate of product formation that is measured, not the total amount of product formed.
   c. **False**. The rate should be proportional to the amount of enzyme present.
   d. **True**. It is usually better to follow product formation, but for some enzymes substrate consumption is easier to measure.
   e. **False**. A progress curve is a graph of the amount of product formed against time.

5. a. **False**. Isotopic assays are expensive and rarely convenient. Spectrophotometry is generally used if it is applicable.
   b. **False**. Isotopic methods are generally used since they can measure the amount of new polymer formed in the presence of polymer present at the start of the assay.
   c. **False**. By using optical methods it is often possible to follow an enzyme-catalysed reaction without stopping it.
   d. **True**. The reaction rate almost always decreases as the reaction proceeds.
   e. **False**. No standard pH is used for enzyme assay since enzymes differ in their optimal pH.

6. a. **False**. For instance, enzyme assay is much used in clinical diagnosis.
   b. **False**. Enzymes have no true optimum temperature for their action; the best temperature for an assay depends on several factors.
   c. **True**. At this pH, the rate is least sensitive to small changes in pH.
   d. **False**. Enzymes vary greatly in their stability to changes in pH.
   e. **False**. Many enzymes are stable outside this range; for example, pepsin is stable below pH 4 and alcohol dehydrogenase is active at pH 10.

7. a. **False**. It is the substrate concentration that gives v equal to half V_{max}.
   b. **False**. At values of [S] well below K_m, v is proportional to [S].
   c. **False**. If [S]>K_m, the enzyme is saturated with substrate and v is independent of [S].
   d. **True**. At high values of [S], the value of v is a useful working estimate of V_{max}.
   e. **False**. The Michaelis equation should be $v = (V_{max} \times [S])/(K_m + [S])$. The numerator is the product of V_{max} and [S], not their sum.

8. a. **False**. K_m has the same units as [S]. Remember K_m and [S] are added together in the denominator of the Michaelis equation.
   b. **False**. V_{max} is proportional to the amount of enzyme present but K_m is independent.
   c. **True**. Enzymes with low K_m values are active at low [S] values.
   d. **False**. A low value of K_m indicates a high affinity for substrate.
   e. **False**. Measuring K_m values is one way of distinguishing isoenzymes.

9. a. **False**. They are non-specifically inhibited. This is one reason why such metals are environmental poisons.
   b. **False**. Inhibitor binding is generally reversible.
   c. **True**. For example, nerve gases form covalent derivatives of acetylcholinesterase.
   d. **False**. Inhibition is relieved by increasing [S].
   e. **False**. To be useful as a drug, an enzyme inhibitor must be specific. This is a basis for rational drug development.

10. a. **False**. Enzymes are often flexible and many can engulf their substrates. This is the concept of 'induced fit'.
    b. **True**. The enzyme often forces the substrate towards the transition state for reaction.
    c. **False**. Think about the many enzymes that catalyse reversible reactions. Enzymes are frequently inhibited in the presence of their products.
    d. **False**. Side chains remote from the substrate binding site are sometimes involved, e.g. an aspartate side chain in 'serine' proteases.
    e. **False**. Folding the polypeptide chain to bring together side chains from widely separate positions in the amino acid sequence creates the active centre.

11. a. **False**. Both electrons generally remain with one of the atoms in the bond.
    b. **False**. Often they are essential for binding charged substrates.
    c. **False**. Acidic or basic groups cannot play their role in catalysis unless they are in the appropriate state of ionisation.
    d. **False**. Nerve gases only react with the single serine side chain at the active centre of 'serine' enzymes that has an enhanced reactivity.
    e. **True**. For example, covalent bonds with the serine side chains in serine proteases.

12. a. **False**. The binding sites for allosteric effectors are distinct from the substrate binding sites.
    b. **False**. All allosteric enzymes have subunits, but many other enzymes have subunits.
    c. **False**. They do show saturation; the graph of initial rate v against [S] is usually sigmoid.
    d. **False**. Allosteric control is reversible; the activity of an allosteric enzyme depends on the concentrations of allosteric activators and inhibitors present at any time.
    e. **True**. Allosteric control with negative feedback is found in many metabolic pathways.

13. a. **False**. Zymogens are activated by cleavage of specific peptide bonds.
    b. **True**. These are the major processes in which zymogens are found.
    c. **False**. Enteropeptidase acts on trypsinogen only.
    d. **False**. Pepsinogen is activated in the stomach. It is not synthesised in the pancreas.
    e. **False**. Pepsinogen is activated by the acidic conditions in the stomach. Trypsin is not active in the stomach.

14. a. **False**. Some such as glycogen phosphorylase are activated by phosphorylation, others such as glycogen synthetase are inactivated.
    b. **False**. See answer to (a).
    c. **False**. Protein kinases transfer phosphate groups from ATP to hydroxyl groups on the side chains of serine, threonine or tyrosine residues.
    d. **False**. Protein phosphatases remove phosphate groups from proteins.
    e. **True**. Control of glycogen synthesis and breakdown by glucagon in liver and by adrenaline (epinephrine) in muscle are notable examples.

True/false answers

1. **True**.
2. **False**. The protein part without the prosthetic group is called the apoenzyme. The holoenzyme is the protein part plus the prosthetic group.
3. **True**.
4. **False**. They hydrolyse phosphate esters.
5. **False**. Different isoenzymes of lactate dehydrogenase are present in these two tissues.
6. **False**. They catalyse the same reaction but they are usually controlled in different ways.
7. **True**.
8. **True**. Enzyme assay depends on this proportionality.
9. **True**.
10. **True**. This prevents unwanted and possibly damaging reactions occurring in cells.

Short essay answer

Several lines of evidence point to complex formation. The phenomenon of saturation with substrate is most easily explained in this way, as is the phenomenon of competitive inhibition. Also, the formation of some enzyme–substrate complexes can be detected by optical and other physical methods. Models of enzyme molecules often show plausible binding sites for their substrates.

Complex formation explains enzyme specificity if the substrate binding site on the enzyme makes a large number of specific non-covalent interactions with many parts of the substrate molecule. Complex formation can also explain the potency of enzymes as catalysts. By binding two reactants in a complex, optimal orientation can be achieved for their reaction. Reactants can also be made more reactive within the complex by distortion towards the transition state for the reaction.

4 Cell membranes

Overview

Membranes form the boundary of the cell and have other important functions. They regulate conditions inside the cell by the specific import and export of materials. They mediate the response to many hormonal signals. They carry molecules identifying the cell to the immune system and allowing the cell to take part in cell–cell interactions.

4.1 Membrane structure

Learning objectives

You should be able to:

- define a lipid and list the lipids commonly found in membranes
- describe how lipid molecules can be organised to form monolayers and bilayers
- describe the properties of a phospholipid bilayer
- list the functions of membrane proteins
- indicate the location of carbohydrate groups on membranes.

Cells need a structure at their boundary to confine what must be kept in the cell and to exclude potentially toxic substances from outside. The boundary structure of the cell is the cell membrane, referred to in animals as the *plasma membrane*. Anything inside this membrane is intracellular and anything outside is extracellular. Functions of the membrane include:

- control of intracellular conditions by import and export of materials
- secretion of materials for use outside the cell
- reception of signals from other cells
- identification of the cell to other cells so that cells can interact, e.g. adhere to form structures.

Eukaryotic cells have internal membranes

As well as having plasma membranes, most eukaryotic cells have other membranes within them so that most cells are divided into functional compartments (Fig. 30). For instance, the cell nucleus is surrounded by the nuclear membrane. Every mitochondrion is delimited by two membranes, an outer and an inner membrane, separated by an intermembrane space. Other cellular organelles such as lysosomes and the Golgi apparatus are membranous structures. Table 3 lists some of the more important biochemical processes associated with different cellular compartments, organelles and other structures.

Cellular membranes are associated with other structural components in a cell: the *cytoskeleton*, a system of protein filaments and microtubules. No attempt has been made to represent the cytoskeleton in Figure 30.

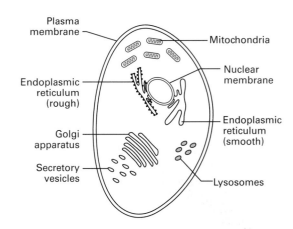

Fig. 30 Membranes of the cell.

Table 3 The main cellular compartments and their functions

Compartment or organelle	Main biochemical functions
Nucleus	Contains DNA DNA replication and packaging RNA synthesis RNA processing
Mitochondrial matrix	Most enzymes of the citric acid cycle and fatty acid oxidation
Mitochondrial inner membrane	Oxidative phosphorylation Succinate dehydrogenase Fatty acyl CoA dehydrogenase
Ribosomes	Protein synthesis
Endoplasmic reticulum	Transport of newly synthesised proteins to the Golgi apparatus
Golgi apparatus	Sorting and modifying newly synthesised proteins for transport within the cell and for export
Lysosomes	Hydrolytic enzymes, e.g. proteases, carbohydrases, lipases, nucleases Processing of imported macromolecules
Secretory vesicles	Proteins and other materials for export, en route from Golgi to plasma membrane
Cytosol	Glycolysis Fatty acid synthesis Pentose phosphate pathway

Cell membrane structure

Lipid components

Cell membranes are based on a phospholipid bilayer. Lipids are defined as materials that are extracted from living material by non-polar solvents such as chloroform. They are not water-soluble although, as we shall see, they can interact with water in important ways. Lipids have diverse chemical structures. Lipids found in membranes include *phospholipids* and *cholesterol* (Fig. 31). Phospholipids such as phosphatidylcholine are the main constituents of most membranes. The fluidity of the membrane depends on the length and degree of unsaturation of the fatty acid hydrocarbon chains. Short chains and unsaturation increase the fluidity. Fluidity of the membrane is also influenced by temperature: membranes are less fluid at low temperatures. The fatty acid content of membrane lipids varies from one organism

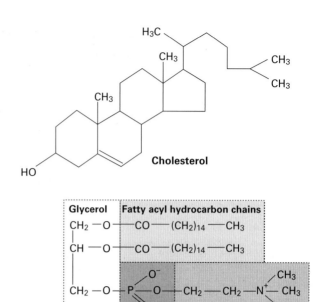

Fig. 31 Membrane lipids. Phosphatidylserine and phosphatidylethanolamine are also commonly found.

to another depending on the temperature at which the organisms live. Cholesterol is found in the plasma membrane of animal cells, where it reduces fluidity. It is not present in the membranes of bacteria.

Membrane lipid molecules are *amphipathic*: each has a hydrophobic part and a hydrophilic part (see p. 5). Such molecules are surface active: they will line up at an air/water or water/oil interface to form a monolayer with the hydrophilic part of the molecule in contact with the water phase and the hydrophobic part projecting into the non-aqueous phase. If no surface is available, the molecules may form *micelles*, spherical aggregates with hydrophobic cores and hydrophilic exteriors. Another stable configuration that these molecules can adopt is a *bimolecular leaflet*: two monolayers back to back with the hydrophobic surfaces in contact (Fig. 32). This structure allows the hydrophilic groups

Clinical note:
Lung surfactant

Dipalmitoylphosphatidylcholine is a major constituent of lung surfactant which covers the alveolar surfaces in the lung. It exerts a surface pressure which prevents complete collapse of the alveoli when air is expelled from the lung. It is normally first secreted about the time of birth and its absence is responsible for respiratory distress syndrome seen in newborn, especially premature, infants.

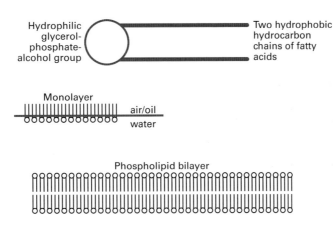

Fig. 32 Phospholipid molecules in water. A phospholipid molecule (top) is represented as a hydrophilic head (circle) and two hydrophobic hydrocarbon chains (lines). Such molecules will form a monolayer (middle) at any unoccupied air/water or oil/water interface. They can also form bilayers (bottom). In all these states the hydrophilic head groups are in contact with water, whereas the contact between water and the hydrophobic hydrocarbon chains is minimal.

on the molecules to stay in contact with water while minimising contact between the hydrophobic groups and water. Such a planar structure is stable except at its edges. It can become completely stable by forming a closed surface such as a sphere. Cell membranes are based on *lipid bilayers* in the form of closed surfaces. The lipid bilayer is flexible and self-sealing. It is a dynamic structure, rather like a two-dimensional liquid. Individual molecules in the bilayer are able to diffuse laterally within the plane of the bilayer; they can also rotate about an axis perpendicular to the bilayer. However, they cannot move their hydrophilic head groups from one side of the membrane to the other; such a 'flip-flop' motion is energetically impossible. Membrane lipids remain in the orientation in which they are inserted in the membrane and cannot move from one layer of the bilayer to the other. As a result, the lipid compositions of the two layers can be, and indeed are, distinct.

The lipid bilayer forms a barrier to the passage of many molecules, particularly hydrophilic and charged molecules such as glucose and amino acids. Any materials that can cross the bilayer itself by diffusion are usually small uncharged molecules such as oxygen, carbon dioxide, short-chain fatty acids in their undissociated forms and water itself.

Phospholipid bilayers are impermeable to polar molecules

A lipid bilayer has at its core a hydrophobic layer that is about 4 nm deep. This core is a barrier that prevents small hydrophilic molecules and ions from entering or leaving the cell. A glucose molecule or an amino acid would have to break its hydrogen bonds with water while it was crossing the bilayer, so the bilayer is impermeable to glucose and amino acids. Similarly, potas-sium, sodium and chloride ions are insoluble in the lipid layer and cannot pass through it. Macromolecules are also unable to cross the membrane on their own. However, transport of all these materials across the membrane does occur. It depends on the presence of specific protein *transporters* in the membrane. In addition, the plasma membrane has oligosaccharide groups attached covalently to protein residues on its exterior.

Protein components

Proteins are found associated with the membrane. The amount of protein and the nature of membrane proteins vary from one membrane to another. The inner mitochondrial membrane is about 75% protein by weight; most membranes have much less. Membrane proteins have many functions, which include:

- transport of materials across the membrane
- reception and transmission of signals from other cells
- structural, giving shape to the cell or binding the cell to others to form tissues.

Different membrane proteins are associated with the membrane in different ways (Fig. 33). Some proteins are inserted into the lipid bilayer and have regions that are accessible to both the extracellular and intracellular phases; they are said to 'span' the membrane. Others are anchored in the lipid bilayer so that they remain associated with the membrane but have contact with only one side of the membrane. Still further proteins are on the outside or inside of the bilayer but attached to more embedded proteins. Membrane proteins are sometimes classified as integral or peripheral: the former cannot be removed from the membrane without destroying it, while the latter can be removed still leaving the membrane intact.

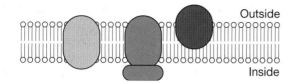

Fig. 33 Proteins in the membrane. Membrane proteins may span the membrane or only be accessible from one side.

The orientation of membrane proteins with respect to the membrane is important; regions of a protein must remain in contact with the same phase all the time. While proteins may be mobile within the plane of the membrane and may also be able to rotate around an axis perpendicular to the plane of the membrane, they cannot by themselves flip-flop or rotate about an axis parallel to the plane of the membrane.

Complex carbohydrate groups

Complex carbohydrate groups are covalently linked to membrane proteins on the outer surface of cells. They are involved in cell–cell interactions and allow the *immune system* to distinguish between cells that are 'self' and cells that are 'non-self' and which are therefore targets. *Blood group substances*, carbohydrates on the surface of the red cell, differ among individuals according to blood group and must be matched between the donor and the recipient of a blood transfusion.

4.2 Transport across membranes

Learning objectives

You should be able to:

- explain the essential features of transport by diffusion, by facilitated diffusion and by active transport

- describe how ATPases are involved in active transport

- explain the concept of cotransport

- explain how transport of ions across a membrane can produce or dissipate electrical potentials

- define receptor-mediated endocytosis and give examples of macromolecules imported by this process

- describe how macromolecules and neurotransmitters are exported from cells.

Transport of molecules across membranes may occur in three ways:

- diffusion: free passage from a high to a low concentration
- facilitated diffusion: transport along a concentration gradient by a carrier system without the expenditure of energy
- active transport: involves carrier proteins and requires energy; often occurs against concentration gradients.

Small molecules

Transport proteins facilitate the transport of molecules that would otherwise be unable to cross the membrane. Every cell that uses glucose as a fuel has *glucose transporter* proteins embedded in its membrane. These proteins bind glucose molecules from the extracellular fluid on the outside of the membrane and release them on the inside of the cell. Amino acids and ions such as chloride, bicarbonate, sodium, potassium and calcium are also transferred across the membrane by specific transport proteins.

Transport proteins resemble enzymes:

- they bring about a process which would otherwise be much too slow because it involves a large energy barrier
- they show specificity, including stereospecificity
- they show saturation kinetics
- they are inhibited by specific inhibitors
- their absence owing to a genetic mutation can give rise to an inherited disease
- they occur in distinct forms: just as distinct molecular forms of enzymes, or isozymes, occur within an organism to catalyse the same reaction but have different kinetic properties or control mechanisms, so also do transport proteins occur in distinct molecular forms. The glucose transporters in animals mentioned on pages 78–79 are an example of this.

Active membrane transport

Transport processes can occur to decrease or increase a concentration difference between one side of the membrane and the other. Transport is energetically favourable when it is downhill: that is, from a region where the transported molecule is present in high concentration to a region where its concentration is low. But transport in the opposite direction can occur if the transport protein is able to use metabolic energy to move the transported molecule uphill. Transport of a molecule against a concentration difference or electrical gradient is often referred to as *active transport*. Some transport

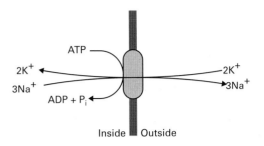

Fig. 34 Active transport: ATPase in the cell membrane acting as an ion pump.

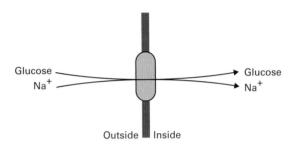

Fig. 35 Cotransport of sodium and glucose is important during the absorption of glucose in the gut. Glucose, at low concentration in the lumen of the gut, is taken into cells, which may contain a higher concentration.

proteins are also ATPases and use the energy from the hydrolysis of ATP; they are often referred to as *pumps* (Fig. 34). ATP hydrolysis and the transport of ions are tightly coupled in ion pumps; one cannot occur without the other. Another way of achieving uphill transport is by cotransport, moving one molecule uphill but at the same time moving another molecule downhill (Fig. 35). This process is referred to as *secondary active transport*. An example is the cotransport of sodium and glucose, which is important during the absorption of glucose in the gut. Glucose, at low concentration in the lumen of the gut, is taken into cells, which may contain a higher concentration. Uphill transport of glucose is achieved by its cotransport with sodium ions, which are moving from a high sodium concentration region to a low sodium concentration region within the cell. This explains why starvation victims are better treated with glucose solutions that contain salt than with glucose solutions in water alone.

Transport of charged molecules

Materials that are transported are sometimes electrically neutral like glucose but may be charged like sodium or potassium ions; transport of the charged molecules is influenced by membrane potentials. Membranes are barriers to the movement of ions and can act as electrical insulators if ion transport is not allowed. If the distribution of ions is not the same on each side of a membrane,

then an electrical potential difference can be established across the membrane. When a charged particle moves across a membrane it will be influenced by the electrical potential that exists across the membrane as well as by any concentration difference. Ions can be transported from regions of low concentration to regions where the concentration is higher if there is a sufficiently large electrical potential gradient that favours the movement. Ionic movement from a region of high concentration to a region where the concentration is low may be energetically unfavourable if the transport is opposed by an adverse electrical potential. Potential differences will be dissipated if ion transporters allow ion transport down the gradient.

Transport and energy conversion

A pump transporting a charged ion can use the chemical energy of ATP hydrolysis to build up a membrane potential. For example, energy from the oxidation of foodstuffs is used to pump hydrogen ions across the mitochondrial inner membrane. This builds up a proton concentration gradient and electrical potential across this membrane. Energy stored in this way is used to drive the synthesis of ATP from ADP and inorganic phosphate (see p. 89).

Linked transport

Transport of different molecules is sometimes linked, as, for example, the cotransport of sodium and glucose in the gut.

Classification of transporters

Membrane transport proteins can be classified according to the nature of the transport process that they promote (Fig. 36). The simplest type of transporter moves a single molecule at a time. The glucose transporters found on the plasma membranes of most cells are of this nature.

Symporter

This is required by its mechanism to transport two different molecular species at the same time; neither species can be transported on its own. The glucose transporter involved in the uptake of glucose from the gut is a symporter; it can only transport glucose while it simultaneously transports a sodium ion. Energy from the concentration difference for sodium ions (high sodium concentration outside cells and low inside) is used to move glucose from a region where its concentration may be low, in the lumen of the gut, to a region where its concentration is higher, inside the mucosal cell (p. 79).

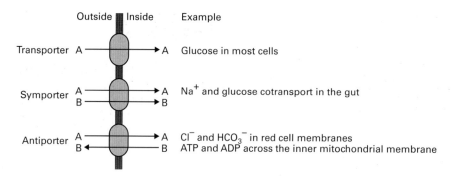

Fig. 36 Transporters classified by the nature of the transport process.

Antiporter

This, like the symporter, involves the transport of two molecular species at the same time, but in this case the species move in opposite directions. There is an antiporter in the red cell membrane that brings about the exchange of chloride and bicarbonate ions. Another antiporter, this time in the mitochondrial inner membrane, allows ATP made inside the mitochondrion to leave by exchanging it for ADP, which enters the inner mitochondrial compartment and can then be phosphorylated to form more ATP.

Macromolecules

Import of macromolecules

Other receptor proteins are involved in the import of macromolecules into the cell by the process known as *receptor-mediated endocytosis*. Lipoproteins, which distribute cholesterol to cells (see Ch. 9, p. 134), and transferrin, which carries iron, are examples of macromolecules that enter cells in this way. These molecules bind to specific receptor molecules that have binding domains on the outside of the plasma membrane. Once loaded, these receptor molecules move in the plane of the membrane to form a cluster. Internal domains of the receptors interact with intracellular proteins, notably *clathrin*, which builds up a structure that makes the membrane invaginate, forming what is known as a *coated pit*. Eventually, part of the membrane pinches off inside the cell to form an *endosome*, which contains both the receptors and the receptor-bound molecules. The endosome is then taken apart, making the imported molecules available to the cell and releasing the receptors for recycling or for breakdown (Fig. 37) (see also Ch. 9, p. 134).

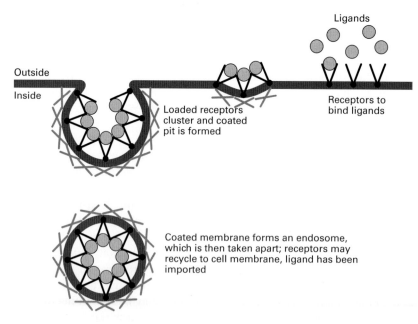

Fig. 37 Receptor-mediated endocytosis, used to import macromolecules into the cell.

Export of macromolecules

Secretion of macromolecules through the plasma membrane also occurs. Pancreatic cells synthesise the precursors of digestive proteases and secrete them into the pancreatic juice. Other pancreatic cells in the islets synthesise the peptide hormones insulin and glucagon and secrete them as required into the blood. Proteins for secretion are packaged into intracellular membrane-bounded vesicles by the Golgi apparatus. The membranes of these vesicles fuse with the plasma membrane of the cell and the contents of the vesicles are released outside the cell.

Membrane functions such as those described above are vital to the functioning of the nervous system. Secretion of neurotransmitters by nerve endings involves the fusion of vesicles that contain the transmitter with the plasma membrane. Detection of these neurotransmitters by another neuron involves receptor proteins. These in turn may activate transport of ions down a potential gradient, resulting in a nerve impulse.

4.3 Hormone receptors

Learning objective

You should be able to:

* describe how membranes are involved in the cellular responses to water-soluble hormones.

Membrane proteins are involved in the cellular response to some water-soluble hormones, such as

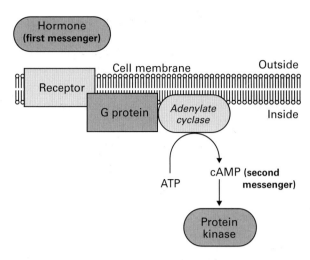

Fig. 38 Role of membrane proteins in the cyclic AMP-mediated cellular response to hormones.

adrenaline (epinephrine), and the peptide hormones glucagon and insulin. Target cells that can respond to a particular hormone have receptor proteins for that hormone on the outside of their plasma membranes. These proteins have an extracellular domain that carries binding sites for the hormone. When hormone molecules circulating in the plasma are recognised and bind, a conformational change that occurs in this external domain is transmitted through another domain that spans the lipid bilayer to the inside of the membrane (Fig. 38). This triggers enzymic events inside the cell that amplify and transmit the hormonal message to influence metabolic events. Related mechanisms and receptors are used for growth and differentiation factors (Ch. 17).

Self-assessment: questions

Single best answer MCQs

1. Identify the single correct statement concerning the function of cell membranes.
   a. Cell membranes carry molecules that are specific for cell type
   b. Cell membrane proteins are not involved in responses to water-soluble hormones
   c. Cells can export macromolecules but cannot import them
   d. Cells can import small molecules such as building blocks and some metabolites but cannot export them
   e. Cell membranes separate regions with identical ionic compositions

2. Identify a correct statement about the composition of membranes.
   a. Phosphatidylcholine is a common constituent of membranes in animals and contains two fatty acyl chains and a glycerol moiety
   b. Cholesterol occurs in animal and plant bacterial membranes
   c. Triacylglycerol is found in animal membranes but not in plants
   d. Oligosaccharides are commonly attached to the inside surface of membranes
   e. Membranes contain up to 50% protein by weight

3. Identify a correct statement about the phospholipid components of membranes.
   a. Have their hydrophilic groups orientated towards the cell exterior
   b. Phospholipids in each layer are able to rotate freely about axes perpendicular to the plane of the membrane
   c. Do not diffuse laterally within each layer of the bilayer
   d. Move freely between the two layers of the bilayer
   e. Contain only saturated fatty acyl groups

4. Identify a correct statement about the protein components of membranes.
   a. Membranes contain more phospholipid than protein
   b. Protein molecules in membranes can rotate and move laterally; they can also change their direction of insertion in the membrane
   c. Some membrane protein molecules are in contact with the aqueous phase on both sides of the membrane

   d. Membrane proteins act as receptors and transporters but not catalysts (enzymes)
   e. Integral membrane proteins can be removed leaving the membrane intact

5. Identify a correct statement about the permeability of cell membranes.
   a. Cell membranes are freely permeable to oxygen but not to carbon dioxide
   b. Glucose can only cross membranes by active transport
   c. Cell membranes are freely permeable to hydrogen ions
   d. Sodium ions can only cross membranes in exchange for potassium ions
   e. Chloride ions can be exchanged for bicarbonate ions across the red cell membrane

6. Which statement accurately describes protein-mediated transport across membranes?
   a. Like enzyme reactions it shows stereospecificity but it does not show saturation
   b. Like enzyme reactions it can be linked to the hydrolysis of ATP
   c. Like an enzyme reaction it can be inhibited by a specific inhibitor but this inhibition is irreversible
   d. Like enzymes, proteins involved in transport processes can be altered by genetic mutation but this does not give rise to inherited disease
   e. It never involves chemical change

7. Select the process in which membrane transport is directly involved.
   a. The absorption of monosaccharides but not amino acids from the gut
   b. The uptake but not the export of nutrients by cells
   c. The movement of ATP but not ADP across the mitochondrial inner membrane
   d. The generation of ATP from the oxidation of foodstuffs
   e. The replication of DNA

8. Identify the single correct statement concerning mechanisms of membrane transport.
   a. Transporters that are responsible for movement of a single molecule or ion can only carry out transport down a gradient of concentration or potential between the two sides of the membrane

b. An antiporter is responsible for the linked movement of molecules or ions in opposite directions; the species transported must carry the same charge

c. A symporter is responsible for the linked movement of two molecules or ions in the same direction; the species transported must carry equal but opposite charges

d. Transport of ions across membranes can set up but not dissipate membrane potentials

e. Transport of ions or molecules across membranes can set up or dissipate concentration differences between the two sides of the membrane

9. Receptor-mediated endocytosis involves the following steps: (1) receptor molecules cluster; (2) formation of a coated pit; (3) transported molecule binds to receptor on membrane; (4) endosome formation; (5) clathrin binds to internal domains of receptors. In which order do these steps occur?

a. 1, 2, 3, 4, 5
b. 3, 1, 5, 2, 4
c. 3, 4, 5, 1, 2
d. 2, 3, 5, 4, 1
e. 4, 5, 3, 2, 1

Short essay question

Write about the similarities between enzymes and the proteins that are responsible for transport processes in membranes.

Self-assessment: answers

Single best answer MCQ answers

1. a. **True**. Membranes contain transporter proteins and carry hormone receptors and recognition molecules that are specific to each cell type.
   b. **False**. Water-soluble hormones cannot enter through cell membranes. They influence their target cells by binding to specific receptors on membranes.
   c. **False**. Cells can both export and import macromolecules. Macromolecules that are imported by cells include transferrin and low-density lipoprotein.
   d. **False**. Some cells, such as those in liver, export small molecules including glucose.
   e. **False**. Cell membranes contain ion pumps, which maintain higher potassium and lower sodium ion concentrations inside cells than in the surrounding fluid.

2. a. **True**. This phospholipid is the main constituent of the bilayer. It also contains a phosphorylcholine moiety.
   b. **False**. Cholesterol is ubiquitous in animals but absent from most prokaryotes.
   c. **False**. Triacylglycerol is not found in membranes. It is the energy-storage material of adipose tissue cells and is non-polar, not amphipathic.
   d. **False**. Membrane glycoproteins are found on the outer surface.
   e. **False**. Some membranes, e.g. the inner mitochondrial membrane, have up to 75% protein.

3. a. **False**. The hydrophilic groups of membrane lipids are orientated towards the aqueous phases on the two sides of the membrane.
   b. **True**. Phospholipid molecules are free to rotate about their long axis.
   c. **False**. Phospholipid molecules can diffuse in the plane of the membrane.
   d. **False**. Phospholipid molecules remain in whichever layer, inner or outer, they were first inserted.
   e. **False**. The degree of unsaturation of fatty acyl side chains in the phospholipids controls membrane fluidity.

4. a. **False**. Membranes vary; the mitochondrial inner membrane is 75% protein.
   b. **False**. They cannot change their direction of insertion.
   c. **True**. They are said to span the membrane.
   d. **False**. Some very important enzymes are membrane-bound. Many membrane-bound enzymes are involved in transport processes.
   e. **False**. Removal of integral proteins disrupts the membrane; proteins that may be removed leaving it intact are described as peripheral.

5. a. **False**. Carbon dioxide is sufficiently lipid soluble to cross without the aid of a carrier.
   b. **False**. Most glucose transporters facilitate downhill transport only.
   c. **False**. The impermeability of the inner mitochondrial membrane to hydrogen ions is important in energy conversion in cells.
   d. **False**. Exchange for potassium ions is only one of the ways in which sodium ions are moved across membranes by specific transporters.
   e. **True**. This exchange is important for the transport of carbon dioxide by the blood.

6. a. **False**. Saturation is observed in transport processes.
   b. **True**. Membrane-bound ATPases are involved in many transport processes.
   c. **False**. Such inhibition is often reversible.
   d. **False**. Many inherited diseases, cystic fibrosis is an example, are due to inherited defects in transport proteins.
   e. **False**. Chemical change is sometimes involved, e.g. ATP hydrolysis.

7. a. **False**. Membrane transporters are needed for almost all nutrients.
   b. **False**. Membrane transport is needed for both processes.
   c. **False**. ADP and inorganic phosphate must be imported and ATP transported out.
   d. **True**. Most ATP production is powered by the transport of hydrogen ions down a potential and concentration gradient into mitochondria.
   e. **False**. The replication of DNA does not involve membrane transport.

8. a. **False**. The sodium pump responsible for movement of sodium ions out of many cells, links ATP hydrolysis to transport and can set up concentration and potential differences.

b. **False**. The species may differ in charge; for instance, the ATPase in membranes that exchanges sodium and potassium exports 3Na$^+$ and imports 2K$^+$.

c. **False**. For example, the symporter that cotransports glucose and sodium ions in the gut.

d. **False**. For example, the establishment of a resting membrane potential in nerves and its dissipation during an action potential.

e. **True**. This is how cells control the composition of their contents and the internal environment of the body.

9. a. **False**.

b. **True**. This is the correct order: (3) transported molecule binds to receptor on membrane; (1) receptor molecules cluster; (5) clathrin binds to internal domains of receptors; (2) formation of a coated pit; (4) endosome formation.

c. **False**.
d. **False**.
e. **False**.

Short essay answer

Points which should be mentioned include: (1) both promote processes made slow by a large energy barrier; (2) both can promote uphill as well as downhill processes by coupling their action to ATP hydrolysis; (3) both show great specificity, including stereospecificity, in the molecules that they can convert or transport; (4) both show saturation kinetics; (5) both can be inhibited by competitive inhibitors; (6) both show distinct molecular forms in different cells and tissues. The absence of an enzyme or a transport process caused by a genetic mutation can give rise to an inherited disease.

5 Gas transport by the blood

Overview

Red cells carry oxygen to the tissues at a rate necessary to supply the energy needs of the body. They also transport carbon dioxide to the lungs for excretion. The transport processes for oxygen and carbon dioxide are highly integrated and very efficient.

5.1 Red cells

Learning objective

You should be able to:

- list the macromolecules in the red cell that carry out gas transport.

In this chapter, we shall see how red cells circulating in the blood, supply oxygen to the tissues and eliminate carbon dioxide. These relatively simple cells contain a few components directly involved in gas transport and not much else. The mature red cell has minimal metabolism, no mitochondria, no nucleus and no ribosomes or protein synthesis. The macromolecules involved in gas transport are:

- haemoglobin: a protein with a haem prosthetic group
- carbonic anhydrase: an enzyme
- chloride/bicarbonate transporter: a membrane protein.

Because the oxygen supply to the tissues limits the rate at which most organisms can use energy, the components of the gas transport system have evolved to become as efficient as possible. The transport processes for oxygen and carbon dioxide are highly integrated.

5.2 Oxygen transport

Learning objectives

You should be able to:

- describe how haemoglobin is adapted for the efficient transport of oxygen by the blood
- sketch the oxygen dissociation curve for human blood
- list the factors influencing the affinity of haemoglobin for oxygen
- describe how carbon monoxide inhibits the transport of oxygen.

The supply of oxygen to the tissues is our most immediate physical need. A human adult at rest needs a continuous supply of energy equivalent to about 150 watts, enough to power a large light bulb. Oxidising foodstuffs with molecular oxygen generates this energy. We take in about 250 ml of oxygen gas per minute. If our oxygen supply is interrupted for more than a few minutes, irreversible damage is done to some tissues, notably the brain. Ensuring that the subject is breathing is a top priority in first aid. Oxygen is abundantly available in the air around us but cannot diffuse into our tissues at a sufficient rate to meet our needs. It must be transported by the blood, from the lung, the specialised organ for gas exchange, to all other tissues.

The problem of transporting oxygen

Oxygen is only slightly soluble in water. A litre of water in equilibrium with air at atmospheric pressure dissolves about 5 ml of oxygen. To transport 250 ml of oxygen each minute in solution in water would involved pumping 50 litres of water per minute, a major undertaking that would increase our energy need and hence our oxygen need even further. It is much more efficient to increase the oxygen-carrying capacity of the blood (the pumped liquid) and to pump at a lower rate.

Haemoglobin

Haemoglobin greatly increases the oxygen-carrying capacity of the blood. Blood can carry about 200 ml of oxygen per litre because it contains a large amount of haemoglobin, about 150 g per litre. This amount of protein dissolved directly would make a very viscous solution, which would need much energy to pump it around the body. This is avoided by carrying the haemoglobin in red cells, which are suspended in plasma. The biconcave disc shape of most mammalian red cells is possibly an adaptation to make them more flexible for passing through capillaries. Even though the red cells account for about 45% of the blood volume, the blood is not much more viscous than plasma.

Haemoglobin is a remarkably soluble protein. Red cells contain about 350 g of haemoglobin per litre. *Sickle cell anaemia* is a disease caused by a mutant form of haemoglobin that has a lowered solubility when deoxygenated. It precipitates if the partial pressure of oxygen becomes too low. This deforms the red cells and makes them less flexible so that they block capillaries. The red cells are also more fragile than normal and have a decreased lifetime in the circulation.

Haemoglobin has been much studied. This is not only because of its important physiological role, but also because it is so readily available. Red cells are easily isolated from blood by centrifugation and washing with isotonic saline. Haemoglobin accounts for more than 95% of the soluble proteins released from red cells when they are lysed with distilled water. The supernatant from such a lysate has been used for many studies in physical biochemistry. Many studies on haemoglobin are facilitated by its red colour; haemoglobin absorbs blue light very strongly and the binding of some ligands influences its absorption of light. The study of haemoglobin has revealed many features later discovered in other proteins.

Haemoglobin structure and function

The 20 amino acid side chains available in proteins include no group with any capacity for binding oxygen. Haemoglobin has haem groups as binding sites for oxygen: haemoglobin is said to have a *haem* prosthetic group. Haem can be removed from haemoglobin leaving the colourless protein known as *globin*; haemoglobin can be reconstituted by adding haem to globin.

Haemoglobin has a molecular weight of about 65 000 and contains about 600 amino acid residues. These form four polypeptide chains: two identical alpha chains and two identical beta chains. Alpha chains and beta chains are similar in size and have distinct but related sequences. Each chain is folded to form a subunit with a binding site for a haem group. The folded chains or subunits also bind to each other to form the complete molecule (Fig. 39). No covalent bonds are involved in the binding of haem to the globin chains or the assembly of the globin subunits to form the tetrameric haemoglobin molecule. There are two alpha and two beta subunits. Alpha and beta subunits are similar but not identical; they have similar tertiary structures with eight sections of alpha helix. The haemoglobin molecule can be considered as two equivalent pairs of alpha–beta subunits that lock together. The relative positions of the two pairs of subunits change on oxygenation of the haemoglobin.

The structure of haem is shown in Figure 80 (p. 121). It is an iron-containing organic group that can combine with oxygen. On its own, it would not be a satisfactory oxygen carrier. It is virtually insoluble in water and it can react with oxygen in more than one way. The oxidation state of the iron atom in haem corresponds to ferrous (Fe^{II}) and in this state it can bind molecular oxygen. The complex that is formed is quickly and irreversibly converted to a compound containing ferric iron (Fe^{III}). Haem on its own can combine with oxygen but it does not give it up again. To be a successful carrier,

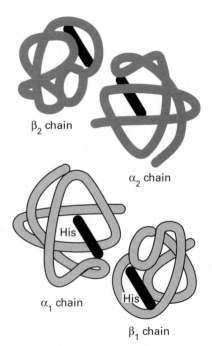

Fig. 39 The subunit structure of haemoglobin. The two pairs of subunits are shown separated for clarity. Normally, the $\alpha_2\beta_2$ pair (shaded) interlock with the $\alpha_1\beta_1$ pair (outlined). The relative positions of the two alpha–beta pairs changes on oxygenation of the haemoglobin.

haem must release its oxygen when oxygen levels are low; that is, it must be oxygenated not oxidised.

Oxygenation, not oxidation

Haem forms a water-soluble complex when it is bound to globin. It is bound by the protein in such a way that one of the coordination positions on the iron is still available to bind oxygen. It is also held in a chemical environment where the oxidation of its iron atom by molecular oxygen is almost completely inhibited. The iron of each haem group is linked to the side chain of a so-called proximal histidine residue. These histidine residues are shown in two of the subunits depicted in Figure 39. The ligands oxygen and carbon monoxide can bind to the iron of each haem on the other side of the haem from the proximal histidine. There is another histidine side chain, that of the distal histidine, positioned near the ligands. As a result, haem bound to globin can pick up oxygen in the lungs and release it in the tissue capillaries. The iron atom in haem remains in the ferrous state during oxygen transport. Haemoglobin is said to be capable of *reversible oxygenation*.

Allosteric effects in haemoglobin

The globin parts of the molecule can bind other molecules as well. The binding of oxygen by haemoglobin is influenced by changes of pH and carbon dioxide concentration. Sites that bind hydrogen ions and carbon dioxide mediate this influence. A further binding site, formed in the crevice between the two beta subunits, binds 2,3-bisphosphoglycerate (2,3-BPG), which, when bound, decreases the affinity of haemoglobin for oxygen.

Haemoglobin is said to show *allosteric* interactions between its ligand-binding sites. Allosteric means 'at another place'. If the other binding site(s) interacts with an identical ligand the effect is said to be *homotropic*; if the other ligand is a different molecule, the effect is *heterotropic*.

Homotropic allosteric effects

The binding of an oxygen molecule at one haem group influences the affinity with which oxygen is bound at another haem group. Since the ligands are identical, this is a homotropic effect. Its occurrence can be seen when the oxygen dissociation curve of haemoglobin is examined. This curve is a graph of how the amount of oxygen bound by haemoglobin varies with the concentration or partial pressure of molecular oxygen with which it is in equilibrium. Such a graph (Fig. 40) is useful to demonstrate some of the adaptations that have evolved in haemoglobin to make oxygen transport more efficient. Notice that the dissociation curve is *sigmoid* or

S-shaped. Its slope increases as we move away from the origin and reaches a maximum value near the point where the haemoglobin is 50% saturated. Beyond that point, the slope decreases again until at high partial pressures of oxygen, such as the pressure in the atmosphere at sea level or in a ventilated lung, haemoglobin is nearly saturated, with almost every haem group having an oxygen bound to it. Increasing the oxygen pressure beyond this point does not significantly increase the amount carried by the blood.

The sigmoid dissociation curve of haemoglobin shows that the four haem groups on a haemoglobin do not bind oxygen independently. They interact and show a *positive cooperativity*. The affinity with which oxygen is bound at any haem group is influenced by the binding of other oxygen molecules at the other three haem groups. With all four haem groups unoccupied by oxygen, it is difficult for the first oxygen molecule to bind. However, once it does bind, it changes the shape of the whole haemoglobin molecule making it much easier for the other three haem groups to react. So for each haemoglobin tetramer, the fully deoxygenated and fully oxygenated states are favoured over the partially oxygenated intermediate states. The change in shape of the tetramer is brought about by an amplification of a slight movement of the iron atom when oxygenation occurs. In the deoxygenated state, the iron atom is too large to fit in the space between the four nitrogens of the haem group so it is displaced from the plane of the haem. On oxygenation it shrinks and is held in the haem plane.

The allosteric effect that produces the sigmoid dissociation curve is an important adaptation of haemoglobin to increase the efficiency of oxygen transport. Oxygen is delivered to the tissues without the oxygen concentration in the tissues having to fall too low. Enzymes that use oxygen, particularly cytochrome oxidase, have oxygen delivered to them at concentrations

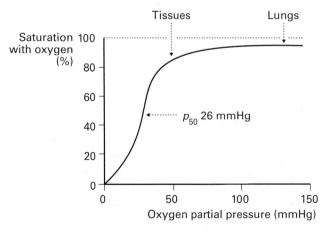

Fig. 40 The oxygen dissociation curve of human blood.

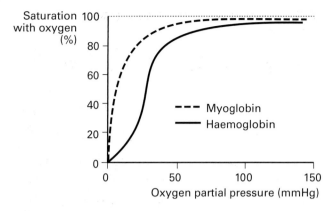

Fig. 41 The oxygen dissociation curves of haemoglobin and myoglobin. Notice how very low partial pressures of oxygen are necessary for appreciable dissociation of oxymyoglobin.

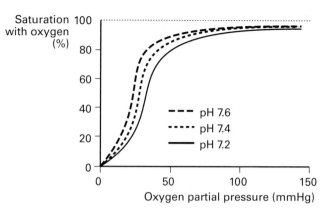

Fig. 42 Effect of pH on the oxygen dissociation curve of haemoglobin (Bohr effect). Notice that acidification, lowering the pH, decreases the affinity of haemoglobin for oxygen, moving the dissociation curve to the right.

sufficient for them to work efficiently. An oxygen transport protein such as myoglobin with a single haem group would need a high oxygen affinity if it is to be fully oxygenated in the lungs. Not much oxygen dissociates from such a protein unless it is exposed to a very low oxygen concentration (Fig. 41). Were myoglobin to be used instead of haemoglobin, it would deliver oxygen to the tissues at a much lower concentration.

Heterotropic allosteric effects

Haemoglobin also shows heterotropic allosteric interactions, i.e. between the binding sites for different ligands. If oxygen dissociation curves are determined at different pH values or in the presence of different concentrations of carbon dioxide, both of these variables are seen to affect the equilibrium between oxygen and haemoglobin.

Figure 42 shows that at low pH values haemoglobin has a lower affinity for oxygen than it has at high pH values. This is known as the *Bohr effect*. This is a physiological adaptation; it results in an increase in the unloading of oxygen by the blood in tissues where increased energy use has resulted in an increase in the production of carbon dioxide or lactic acid, the respective end-products of aerobic and anaerobic metabolism for the production of ATP.

Regulation by 2,3-BPG

The affinity of haemoglobin for oxygen is affected by the concentration of 2,3-BPG in the red cell (Fig. 43). This substance is produced metabolically from glucose in the red cell (Fig. 174, p. 280). It binds to a site between the beta subunits in deoxyhaemoglobin but not to oxyhaemoglobin. Its presence moves the oxygen dissociation curve to the right. The affinity of haemoglobin for oxygen can thus be altered to optimise oxygen transport at high altitude.

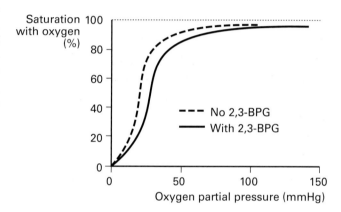

Fig. 43 Effect of addition of 2,3-BPG to the oxygen dissociation curve of haemoglobin. 2,3-BPG binds only to the deoxy form of haemoglobin, stabilising it. In the absence of 2,3-BPG, the dissociation curve is moved to the left.

2,3-BPG is also important in promoting oxygen transport across the placenta. Fetal haemoglobin has the two beta subunits of normal adult haemoglobin replaced by two gamma subunits, which do not form any binding site for 2,3-BPG. It therefore has a higher oxygen affinity than maternal haemoglobin and oxygen transfers readily from mother to fetus (Fig. 44).

Haemoglobin was the first protein studied that showed allosteric effects. These effects are also important in many other proteins as we will discover when we consider how the catalytic activity of enzymes is controlled in metabolism.

Carbon monoxide binding to haemoglobin

A few other small molecules, notably carbon monoxide, can bind to the haem groups in competition with oxygen. Haemoglobin has a 250-fold higher affinity for

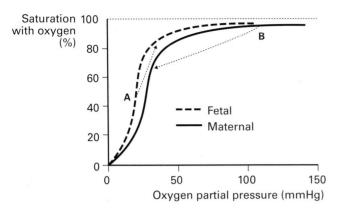

Fig. 44 Oxygen exchange in the placenta. Fetal haemoglobin, HbF, has no binding site for 2,3-BPG, so it has a higher affinity for oxygen than the HbA of the mother. This is essential for efficient transfer of oxygen from mother to fetus. Maternal arterial blood (point B) loses oxygen while fetal blood (point A) gains oxygen until they both have the same partial pressure of oxygen.

Clinical note:
Carbon monoxide poisoning

A patient with 30% of their haemoglobin gas binding capacity occupied by carbon monoxide is much more seriously incapacitated than a patient who has lost 50% of their haemoglobin through anaemia. Bound carbon monoxide triggers the allosteric effect, and the remaining haem groups have such a high affinity for oxygen that its transport to the tissues is seriously compromised.

---

carbon monoxide than it has for oxygen, so exposure to low concentrations of carbon monoxide, from car exhaust fumes or from badly ventilated gas heaters, can have fatal results. Therapy for carbon monoxide poisoning includes treatment with pure oxygen to increase the partial pressure of oxygen in the lungs, allowing it to compete with and displace the carbon monoxide.

About 1% of the oxygen binding sites in the blood are normally occupied by carbon monoxide, even in non-smokers not exposed to exhaust fumes. This carbon monoxide is produced in the body from the breakdown of haem itself (see Fig. 148, p. 228). In haemoglobin and myoglobin, the binding of carbon monoxide is hindered relative to oxygen by the distal histidine side chain that is close to these ligands when they bind. Model haem compounds bind carbon monoxide so that it is perpendicular to the plane of the haem, while oxygen binds at an angle. By preventing carbon monoxide binding in its preferred orientation, the distal histidine in haemoglobin reduced affinity by about 100-fold. Without this effect, endogenous carbon monoxide would occupy many more oxygen binding sites.

5.3 Carbon dioxide transport

Learning objectives

You should be able to:

- list the forms in which carbon dioxide is carried in the blood

- describe the reaction of carbon dioxide with water and explain the role of carbonic anhydrase

- explain how the bicarbonate/chloride transporter in red cell membranes increases the efficiency of carbon dioxide transport

- explain how haemoglobin can transport carbon dioxide as carbamino compounds.

While oxygen has to be transported from lungs to tissues, carbon dioxide must be transported from the tissues for exhalation by the lungs. Carbon dioxide has physicochemical properties that make its transport less difficult than the transport of oxygen. Nevertheless, haemoglobin has adaptations that facilitate this process. Carbon dioxide can be transported in the blood in three ways:

- in simple solution ($\approx$10%)
- by reversible conversion to bicarbonate and hydrogen ions (> 50%)
- by reversible combination with amino groups on haemoglobin to form carbaminohaemoglobin ($\approx$30%).

Simple solution

Carbon dioxide is much more soluble than oxygen and about 10% of its transport can be accounted for as transport of the dissolved gas.

Bicarbonate and hydrogen ions

Carbon dioxide can also react with water to form bicarbonate and hydrogen ions:

$$CO_2 + H_2O \rightleftharpoons HCO_3^- + H^+$$

The reaction is reversible and slow, taking minutes to approach equilibrium even at body temperature. In pure water, the equilibrium is very much in favour of carbon dioxide, only about one part in a thousand being converted to carbonic acid. As carbonic acid is a stronger acid than acetic acid, it ionises to form *bicarbonate* ions and hydrogen ions. At pH 7.4, the pH of blood, if a buffer species is present that can take up the hydrogen ions then more than 90% of carbon dioxide can be converted to bicarbonate before equilibrium is achieved. One of the adaptations of haemoglobin is that it is a powerful buffer at pH 7.4, so carbon dioxide can be converted to bicarbonate in the red cell. More than one-half of the carbon dioxide transported from the tissues to the lungs is transported as bicarbonate ions.

Carbonic anhydrase

The uncatalysed reaction between carbon dioxide and water to form bicarbonate and hydrogen ions is reversible but slow. It would be unable to produce enough carbon dioxide from bicarbonate during the second or less that the red cell spends in the lung capillary. Red cells contain an enzyme, *carbonic anhydrase*, which catalyses the reversible hydration of carbon dioxide to form bicarbonate ions and hydrogen ions. Carbonic anhydrase is a zinc protein with a molecular weight of about 30 000. The single zinc atom is essential for activity. The enzyme is very active in red cells but absent from the plasma. Production of bicarbonate and hydrogen ions is, therefore, confined to the red cells so that negligible change in pH of the plasma occurs as a consequence of carbon dioxide transport. Haemoglobin, as well as its other adaptations for gas transport, has a high content of the amino acid histidine. This amino acid has an imidazole group on its side chain that acts as a powerful buffering group, so that the pH change within the red cell owing to carbonic anhydrase action is minimised. Some imidazole groups on haemoglobin are oxygen-linked, their buffering action being influenced by the state of oxygenation of the haem groups. When protonated they facilitate the release of oxygen. This accounts for the Bohr effect, the effect of pH on the oxygen dissociation curves of haemoglobin (Fig. 42). Increased carbon dioxide concentrations lower the pH and promote the dissociation of oxygen from combination with haemoglobin. Tissues that are metabolically most active, and which produce the most carbon dioxide, therefore receive the greatest supply of oxygen.

Clinical note:
In vivo inhibition of carbonic anhydrase

Patients with glaucoma, a condition in which the intraocular pressure is increased, can be treated with acetazolamide, a potent carbonic anhydrase inhibitor which lowers bicarbonate concentration in the aqueous humor. Such patients can adequately transport carbon dioxide from their tissues to their lungs, presumably by carrying more of it in solution and as carbaminohaemoglobin.

Chloride/bicarbonate transporter

The amount of carbon dioxide that can be converted into bicarbonate in the red cell is also increased by the ability of the red cell to 'share' its bicarbonate ions with the plasma. The red cell membrane contains an ion transporter that promotes the exchange of chloride and bicarbonate ions between the red cell and plasma. In tissue capillaries, when carbon dioxide is converted to bicarbonate in the red cell, some of the bicarbonate ions can leave the red cell and enter the plasma (Fig. 45). Chloride ions must move in the opposite direction to avoid any net transport of charge. In the lung capillaries, some of the bicarbonate in the red cell is converted to carbon dioxide, which is exhaled, and more bicarbonate enters the red cell from the plasma. There is a corresponding movement of chloride ions from red cell to plasma. The carbon dioxide–bicarbonate system, as well as accounting for removal of about 60% of carbon dioxide produced by the body, is also important in regulation of acid–base balance.

Combination with haemoglobin

Carbon dioxide can react with some N-terminal amino groups on haemoglobin directly (no enzyme is required) to form labile carbamino compounds or *carbamates*, which release carbon dioxide in the lungs:

$$Hb\text{-}NH_2 + CO_2 \{ReversReact\} Hb\text{-}NH\text{-}COO^- + H^+$$

The reaction only involves N-terminal groups, which must be unprotonated. Lysine side chain amino groups, which are much more basic, are fully protonated at physiological pH values.

This process is allosterically linked to oxygenation, so that combination of haemoglobin with carbon dioxide favours deoxygenation and combination with oxygen favours release of carbon dioxide. Carbamate formation accounts for about 30% of carbon dioxide transport.

5.4 Abnormal haemoglobins and haemoglobinopathies

Learning objectives

You should be able to:

- describe what is meant by a haemoglobinopathy and give an example.

The prevalent inherited disease sickle cell anaemia is caused by a change in the structure of the haemoglobin molecule. This change makes sickle cell haemoglobin,

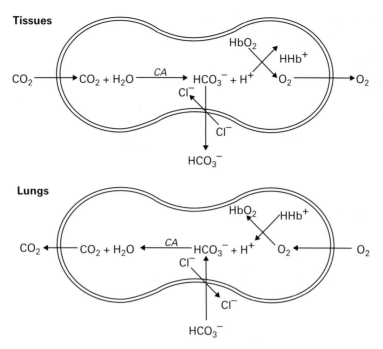

Tissues

Lungs

Fig. 45 Movement of bicarbonate and chloride ions during gas transport. Chloride ions enter the red cell to keep electrical balance. When hydrogen ions are produced in the tissues by hydration of carbon dioxide, they promote the dissociation of oxyhaemoglobin (HbO_2). CA, carbonic anhydrase.

Clinical note:
HbS confers resistance to malaria

The presence of HbS in red cells, even with HbA also present as in heterozygotes, makes them less likely to be invaded by the malaria parasite. This gives the individual a significant resistance to malaria and accounts for the high incidence of the gene for this form of haemoglobin in areas of the world where malaria is rife.

HbS, electrophoretically distinguishable from the normal adult form of haemoglobin, HbA. Haemoglobin is readily obtained from human subjects so many samples have been screened by electrophoresis and hundreds of mutant haemoglobins discovered. Some of these haemoglobins are associated with disease states, particularly anaemia; others show normal function. In many cases, the amino acid sequence of the mutant haemoglobin differs from the normal at only two positions in the 600 or so of total sequence. For example, HbS has the same amino acid sequence as HbA except at position 6 in each of its two beta chains, where it has valine residues instead of the glutamates found in HbA. This seemingly slight change creates a 'sticky' patch on the molecule which promotes aggregation of the deoxy form and decreases its solubility. The resulting aggregates distort the red cell, shortening its lifetime, and make the cell less flexible and thus unable to negotiate tissue capillaries. Replacing a glutamate residue, which has a negatively charged side chain, with a valine residue, which has no charge on its side chain, incidentally alters the charge and the electrophoretic mobility of the protein.

Much has been learnt about the relationship between haemoglobin structure and function by identifying the differences between HbA and a large number of mutants. The role of two histidine residues in each sub-unit is particularly important. The side chains of these residues are close to the haem iron and their replacement by tyrosine side chains gives forms of haemoglobin (HbM) in which the haem group is instantly oxidised to the ferric state when it reacts with oxygen. Oxidised haemoglobin is known as methaemoglobin and is not able to act as an oxygen carrier.

Self-assessment: questions

Single best answer MCQs

1. Identify the single correct statement about general aspects of gas transport by the blood.
   a. An adult at rest uses about 250 ml of oxygen per hour
   b. Red cells account for about 45% of the blood volume
   c. A litre of water in equilibrium with air at atmospheric pressure dissolves about 50 ml of oxygen
   d. The oxygen-carrying capacity of normal blood is about 20 ml of oxygen per litre
   e. Normal blood contains about 375 g of haemoglobin per litre

2. Knowledge of the structure of the haemoglobin molecule is critical to your understanding of its role in oxygen and carbon dioxide transport in the circulation. Which one of the following statements accurately describes haemoglobin structure?
   a. It contains four atoms of iron which must be in the Fe^{III} oxidation state for it to bind oxygen
   b. Each iron atom is combined in a haem group and coordinated to a nitrogen atom in a histidine side chain
   c. It contains four identical polypeptide chains per molecule
   d. Each polypeptide chain has a haem group linked to it covalently
   e. The four polypeptide chains are linked by disulphide bonds

3. Identify the correct description of the physicochemical properties of haemoglobin.
   a. It is the only protein contained in red blood cells
   b. This protein is contained in red cells because it is not very soluble in water
   c. Appears red because the haem groups strongly absorb red light
   d. Changes in its colour occur when it reacts with oxygen or carbon monoxide
   e. When the iron atoms in haemoglobin are oxidised from the Fe^{II} to the Fe^{III} state, the resulting compound is a denatured protein that cannot be reconverted to the Fe^{II} state

4. Identify the single correct statement about the haem component of haemoglobin.

   a. Contains one atom of iron in the Fe^{II} state and is surrounded by four nitrogen atoms
   b. Does not react with oxygen unless combined with globin
   c. Is very soluble in water
   d. Is not a prosthetic group since haemoglobin is not an enzyme
   e. Haem groups in haemoglobin are not influenced by the binding of oxygen to the other haem groups

5. The subunit structure of haemoglobin is critically important to its function in gas transport. Identify from the following the single correct statement about haemoglobin subunits.
   a. Adult human haemoglobin molecules contain two alpha and two beta subunits
   b. Fetal human haemoglobin molecules contain two beta and two gamma subunits
   c. The subunits are connected by covalent bonds
   d. Each subunit has about 600 amino acid residues in its polypeptide chain
   e. The tertiary structure of each subunit contains eight sections of beta sheet

6. Identify the single correct statement concerning ligand binding by haemoglobin.
   a. Oxygen and carbon dioxide compete for the same binding sites
   b. Carbon monoxide binds irreversibly to haemoglobin and prevents it from carrying oxygen
   c. Carbon dioxide binds directly to amino groups on lysine side chains but not to N-terminal amino groups
   d. 2,3-bisphosphoglycerate binds to adult haemoglobin but not to fetal haemoglobin
   e. When 2,3-bisphosphoglycerate binds to haemoglobin its affinity for oxygen is increased

7. Knowledge of the sigmoid oxygen dissociation curve of haemoglobin allows one to have an understanding of physiological aspects of gas transport. Identify the single correct statement about that curve.
   a. It is due to a heterotrophic allosteric interaction between the haem groups
   b. It is due to negative cooperativity between the haem groups
   c. Changes of pH have no effect on the curve

d. It moves to the left in the presence of 2,3-bisphosphoglycerate

e. It involves a change in the shape of the whole haemoglobin molecule

8. Which one of the following statements accurately describes oxygen haemoglobin association?

a. The first oxygen molecule binding to a haemoglobin molecule decreases the oxygen affinity of the other haem groups

b. Oxygen dissociation from one haem group in fully saturated haemoglobin makes it more difficult for oxygen to dissociate from the other haem groups

c. Increases in carbon dioxide concentrations in the red cell decrease the affinity of the haemoglobin for oxygen

d. Binding of 2,3-bisphosphoglycerate to haemoglobin makes it bind oxygen with higher affinity

e. Increase in pH in the red cell makes haemoglobin bind oxygen with lower affinity

9. Which one of the following statements describes accurately carbon dioxide transport in the blood?

a. Carbon dioxide is more soluble in water than oxygen; dissolved carbon dioxide accounts for about 30% of its transport in the blood

b. Most of the carbon dioxide carried in the blood is in the form of bicarbonate

c. The interconversion of carbon dioxide and bicarbonate cannot occur unless catalysed by carbonic anhydrase

d. Carbonic anhydrase is present in the plasma and not in the red cell

e. Carbon dioxide binds to the haem groups on haemoglobin

10. Identify the single correct statement about sickle cell haemoglobin.

a. It differs from normal adult haemoglobin in every subunit

b. It is less soluble than normal adult haemoglobin when oxygenated

c. It is only found in subjects suffering from sickle cell anaemia

d. Individuals possessing sickle cell haemoglobin are less likely to contract malaria

e. It does not have a sigmoid oxygen dissociation curve

Short essay question

Haemoglobin has been called an 'honorary' enzyme. Write about the properties that haemoglobin shares with enzymes.

Self-assessment: answers

Single best answer MCQ answers

1. a. **False.** 250 ml per minute is required.
    b. **True.** Lower values indicate anaemia.
    c. **False.** It only dissolves about 5 ml of oxygen.
    d. **False.** Blood carries about 200 ml of oxygen per litre.
    e. **False.** Blood contains about 150 g of haemoglobin per litre.

2. a. **False.** Haemoglobin cannot function as an oxygen carrier unless its iron atoms are in the Fe^{II} oxidation state.
    b. **True.** The sixth coordination position on the iron can bind an oxygen molecule.
    c. **False.** Each molecule contains two alpha and two beta chains.
    d. **False.** No covalent bonds are involved in binding the haem group.
    e. **False.** Haemoglobin contains no disulphide bonds.

3. a. **False.** It is by far the most abundant but not the only protein in the red cell.
    b. **False.** Haemoglobin is very soluble in water; haem is almost insoluble.
    c. **False.** Haemoglobin has a very strong absorption band in the blue.
    d. **True.** The colour changes are useful to show the state of the haemoglobin.
    e. **False.** It is not denatured. Methaemoglobin, the oxidised form of haemoglobin, occurs in some clinical conditions. It can be detected by spectrophotometry. An enzyme in the red cell returns the haemoglobin to its functional state.

4. a. **True.**
    b. **False.** Haem is oxidised irreversibly by oxygen.
    c. **False.** It is almost completely insoluble.
    d. **False.** The term prosthetic group is used for an organic group attached to any protein.
    e. **False.** They are greatly influenced; they are said to interact.

5. a. **True.**
    b. **False.** Fetal haemoglobin contains two alpha and two gamma subunits.
    c. **False.** Only non-covalent forces are involved in the aggregation of the four subunits.
    d. **False.** Each subunit contains about 150 amino acid residues.

e. **False.** About 75% of the amino acid residues are contained in the eight alpha helical segments, the A, B, C, D, E, F, G and H helices.

6. a. **False.** It is carbon monoxide that competes with oxygen for the binding sites on haem.
    b. **False.** Carbon monoxide binds with higher affinity than oxygen, but it can be displaced by high oxygen concentrations. Oxygen therapy is used to treat carbon monoxide poisoning.
    c. **False.** Carbon dioxide binds to the N-terminal amino groups.
    d. **True.** 2,3-bisphosphoglycerate binds to adult deoxyhaemoglobin, lowering its affinity for oxygen.
    e. **False.** Its affinity for oxygen is decreased.

7. a. **False.** It is described as a homotropic effect since one ligand, oxygen, is influencing the binding of other oxygen molecules.
    b. **False.** The cooperativity is positive. Binding one oxygen facilitates the binding of others.
    c. **False.** pH greatly influences the affinity with which oxygen is bound.
    d. **False.** The curve is moved to the right denoting reduced affinity for oxygen.
    e. **True.** Oxygenation produces a small movement of the iron atom in the haem group; this is amplified to alter the shape of the whole haemoglobin molecule.

8. a. **False.** It makes it easier for further oxygen molecules to bind.
    b. **False.** Dissociation of oxygen from one haem group makes it easier for the other oxygen molecules to dissociate.
    c. **True.** This makes the transport of oxygen by haemoglobin more efficient.
    d. **False.** 2,3-bisphosphoglycerate stabilises deoxyhaemoglobin and reduces the affinity.
    e. **False.** Removal of hydrogen ions by reaction with bicarbonate to produce carbon dioxide in the lung increases affinity of haemoglobin for oxygen.

9. a. **False.** About 10% of the total carbon dioxide is carried in solution under normal conditions.
    b. **True.** About 60% of the total.
    c. **False.** Unless it is catalysed, this reaction is too slow to allow carbon dioxide to be unloaded by the blood in the lungs.

d. **False**. Carbonic anhydrase in the blood is confined to the red cells.

e. **False**. It reacts reversibly with the N-terminal alpha amino groups.

10. a. **False**. Only the beta subunits are affected.
   b. **False**. The deoxygenated form of sickle cell haemoglobin has the low solubility.
   c. **False**. Subjects with one sickle gene have approximately 50% mutant and 50% normal haemoglobin in each red cell. They have no clinical symptoms.
   d. **True**. Possession of one sickle gene is an advantage in malarial areas. This accounts for the high incidence of the gene.
   e. **False**. Its oxygen affinity is very similar to that of normal haemoglobin.

Short essay answer

The following points should be mentioned. Haemoglobin and enzymes have binding sites where small molecules are bound reversibly. Both show specificity of binding and exhibit saturation. Both can occur as different molecular forms in different tissues and at different stages of development. These forms often show different affinities for their ligand. Both can have their binding sites blocked by competitive inhibitors. Some enzymes have binding sites like those on haemoglobin that interact or show cooperativity. Some enzymes have allosteric sites like those on haemoglobin. When these sites are occupied they can alter the affinity with which the protein binds its main ligand. Both occur as mutant forms in which function is altered or lost.

6 Carbohydrate and fat catabolism

- illustrate compartmentalisation in cells in connection with the organisation of metabolic pathways
- list the coenzymes used by various types of enzymatic reactions.

Overview

Glucose and fatty acids are the major fuels (suppliers of ATP) for the body. Glucose is utilised by all cells and is especially important for tissues such as the brain. Fatty acids are the major fuel for the heart and are used by skeletal muscle to support long-term exercise. The metabolism of glucose and fatty acids converge at the level of the tricarboxylic acid cycle and oxidative phosphorylation.

6.1 Basic concepts of intermediary metabolism

Learning objectives

You should be able to:

- define the terms metabolism, catabolism and anabolism
- give several examples of how ATP is utilised in the body
- describe how the metabolic pathways for carbohydrates, amino acids and fatty acids are integrated
- explain the importance of free energy change in metabolic pathways

Intermediary metabolism is an enormous topic within biochemistry and Chapters 6–9 of this 'core' text present essential material that will explain the design of the major metabolic pathways so that their control in the fed and fasted states (Ch. 10) can be understood. The first question to answer is: 'What is metabolism?'

Metabolism is the sum of two contrasting processes: *catabolism* and *anabolism*.

Catabolism

Catabolism consists of the pathways where complex nutrient molecules (lipids, carbohydrates and amino acids) are broken down to simpler end-products such as carbon dioxide, water and ammonia, accompanied by the synthesis of ATP (Fig. 46). ATP is frequently described as the 'energy currency' of cells as it can be transported to those sites in the cell where it is utilised for various cellular functions, such as:

- synthesis of proteins, RNA, DNA for growth, adaptation and repair
- synthesis of lipids and glycogen
- performance of mechanical work
- transport of ions against a gradient
- absorption of nutrients against a gradient.

The reaction ATP $\rightleftharpoons$ ADP + P$_i$ (inorganic phosphate) is displaced far from equilibrium in cells in favour of ATP; this enables otherwise unfavourable reactions in metabolic pathways to proceed. It does not depend on special properties of the pyrophosphate bonds (so-called 'high-energy' bonds) in ATP! The very high ratios of ATP to ADP are possible because of the very efficient synthesis of ATP in cells.

The oxidation of fuels such as glucose and fatty acids (Fig. 47) results in the production of the reduced coenzymes NADH and FADH$_2$. Electrons and hydrogens are lost by the substrates being oxidised and are gained by the coenzymes produced. Electrons provide a means for

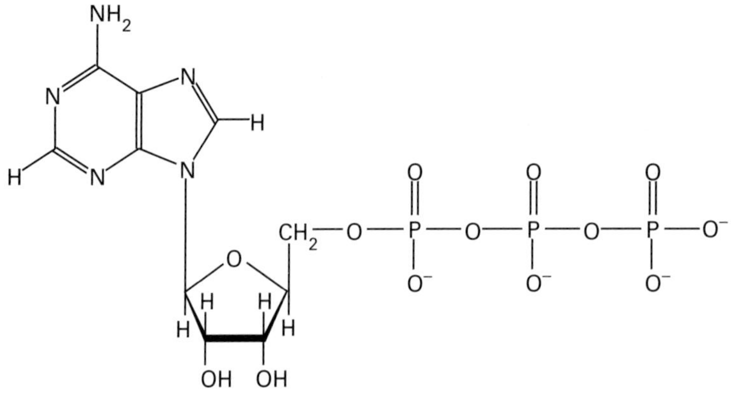

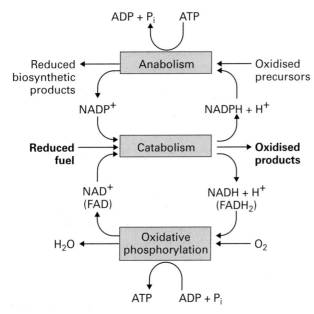

Fig. 46 The structure of ATP.

Fig. 47 Transfer of reducing power in the overall strategy of metabolism.

transfer of chemical energy from the energy-yielding reactions of catabolism to the energy-requiring reactions of ATP synthesis and the biosynthesis of hydrogen-rich molecules such as fatty acids. Within mitochondria, the oxidation of NADH and $FADH_2$ by the electron transport chain (see section 6.6) establishes a proton gradient that drives the reverse reaction $ADP + P_i \rightarrow ATP$.

Anabolism

Anabolism refers to biosynthetic processes in which simple precursor molecules are enzymatically converted into the molecular components of cells, such as nucleic acids, proteins, complex lipids and polysaccharides. Biosynthesis requires the input of chemical energy (usually ATP), which is provided by coupling to catabolism. To synthesise reduced biosynthetic products such

as fatty acids there is requirement for 'reducing power' in the form of NADPH (Fig. 47) produced in the pentose phosphate pathway (Ch. 7).

The source of our dietary fuels

We are *heterotrophs*, which means that we 'feed on others' and can synthesise our organic molecules only from other organic compounds that we obtain from *autotrophs* (plants), which are 'self-feeding'. Autotrophs and heterotrophs live together in a symbiotic relationship where autotrophs use solar energy and atmospheric carbon dioxide to build complex organic molecules. Heterotrophs use these complex molecules as fuel and, in the case of aerobic organisms, return carbon dioxide to the atmosphere. Hence, carbon and oxygen are continuously cycled between the plant and animal worlds.

Stages of metabolism

Although metabolism involves hundreds of different compounds (metabolites) and enzymes, the central pathways are few in number and common to most forms of life. Krebs and Kornberg showed the simplicity of this arrangement when they placed all of the major metabolic pathways within a scheme called 'the three stages of metabolism' (Fig. 48).

- Stage 1: digestion of complex dietary fuels to monomeric units which are absorbed from the gut
- Stage 2: conversion of the monomeric units into simple molecules within cells
- Stage 3: simple molecules oxidised to carbon dioxide and water.

The monomeric units within Stage 2 are *amino acids, glucose* and *fatty acids*; they have a common key metabolic product, acetyl-coenzyme A (acetyl-CoA). Figure 48 outlines these stages and shows how biosynthetic pathways can be superimposed upon the catabolic pathways. Stage

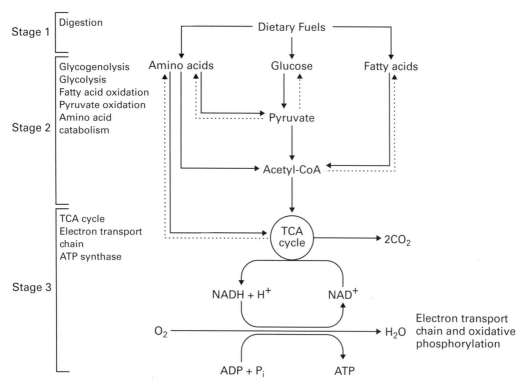

Fig. 48 Integration of carbohydrate, amino acid and fatty acid metabolism. Pyruvate, acetyl-CoA and the tricarboxylic acid (TCA) cycle have central roles for all three fuels. The dashed lines indicate biosynthetic pathways.

3 constitutes an *amphibolic* pathway in that it can be used catabolically to degrade small molecules from Stage 2 or can be used anabolically to provide precursor molecules for biosynthesis. Stage 3 is where most ATP is generated.

Enzymatic and thermodynamic aspects of metabolism

You should review Chapter 3 as a basis for understanding the operation and control of the key metabolic pathways in the body. Although every reaction in a metabolic pathway *need not* have a free energy change (ΔG) that is negative, the ΔG for the entire pathway *must be* negative! Thus, on purely thermodynamic grounds, it should be clear that a catabolic pathway such as glycolysis and an anabolic pathway such as gluconeogenesis couldn't simply be the reverse of each other. Glycolysis and gluconeogenesis are *parallel pathways*, and three of the steps are unique to each pathway (Ch. 7). The advantage of parallel pathways to the control of metabolism (Ch. 10) is that, if the catabolic pathway is 'turned on', the anabolic pathway is 'turned off' and vice versa.

Compartmentalisation is critical for regulation

Metabolic regulation is enhanced by compartmentalisation, in which opposing reactions/pathways are physi-

cally separated. For example, fatty acid synthesis occurs within the cytosol of the cell whereas fatty acid oxidation occurs in the mitochondria.

Energy charge

ATP-yielding pathways can be independently controlled by the *energy charge* of the cell. When ATP levels are adequate, ATP-yielding pathways should be, and are, 'switched off'. Logically, when ATP is consumed, such pathways should be 'turned on'. The compounds involved in calculating energy charge, ATP, ADP and AMP, are allosteric effectors for many enzymes. *Adenylate kinase* is a key enzyme since it catalyses the regeneration of one ATP plus AMP from two ADP. The ATP is used to perform work, but the (relatively) large increase in [AMP] that occurs activates both glycogen breakdown (p. 99) and the first controlled step in glycolysis (see p. 81), leading to production of more ATP.

Coenzymes and prosthetic groups contain water-soluble vitamins

Coenzymes and prosthetic groups are special molecules (Table 4) in that they act along with enzymes in many metabolic reactions. They increase the types of reaction that can occur in the body and provide links by which

Table 4 Coenzymes in intermediary metabolism

Enzymatic reaction	Coenzymes/cofactors
Oxidation–reduction	Nicotinamide adenine dinucleotide (NAD*) Nicotinamide adenine dinucleotide phosphate (NADP$^+$) Flavin adenine dinucleotide (FAD) Flavin mononucleotide (FMN) Lipoic acid
Amino acid catabolism	Pyridoxal phosphate
Oxidative decarboxylation	Thiamine pyrophosphate
Carboxylation	Biotin
Reductive biosynthesis	NADPH Tetrahydrobiopterin NADH
Acyl transfer	Coenzyme A Acyl carrier protein
One-carbon metabolism	Tetrahydrofolate (FH$_4$)
Methylation reactions	S-Adenosylmethionine Tetrahydrofolate (FH$_4$) Methylcobalamin (B$_{12}$)

energy and reducing power can be transferred from reaction to reaction. An important point to recognise is that most of the coenzymes and prosthetic groups are derivatives of water-soluble (B) vitamins. Patients with deficient intake of certain B vitamins will have defects in metabolic pathways, leading to altered metabolism that can have serious consequences (Ch. 18).

6.2 Digestion and absorption of dietary carbohydrates and fats

Learning objectives

You should be able to:

- describe the chemical nature of the dietary carbohydrates

- describe the action of salivary and pancreatic amylases and brush border carbohydrases on dietary carbohydrates

- explain the glucose–sodium symport system involved in glucose and galactose absorption in the gut and the role of the sodium pump

- describe the chemical nature of the dietary fats

- outline the products of action of pancreatic lipase, cholesteryl hydrolase and phospholipase A2 on dietary lipids

- explain the role of bile salts and phospholipids in micelle formation and the absorption of lipids in the gut.

Digestion of dietary carbohydrates, fats and proteins in the gut give rise to products that can be absorbed across intestinal mucosal cells and then absorbed into the body.

Dietary carbohydrate

About 50–60% of the calories consumed by the average Western adult is in the form of carbohydrate. Only a small fraction of the total carbohydrate of the plant world can be utilised for nutrition by humans since we lack the digestive enzymes for the degradation of cellulose and some other plant polysaccharides that are present in our diets.

Polysaccharides

The major digestible dietary polysaccharides are *starch* and *glycogen*, which are polymers of glucose (Fig. 49). Starch has amylose (approx. 20%) and amylopectin (approx. 80%) components, the former being a long chain of glucoses joined by α-1:4-linkages. Amylopectin has α-1:4- and also α-1:6-linkages, which result in branching. Glycogen (animal starch) is similar in structure to amylopectin but with a greater frequency of branching. Only a single glucose residue in amylopectin and glycogen will have a free reducing group on carbon-1. The glucose moieties at the ends of branches are referred to as *non-reducing ends*.

Disaccharides

Disaccharides include: *sucrose*, consisting of one fructose and one glucose; *lactose*, made up of one galactose and one glucose; and *maltose*, made up of two glucoses.

Monosaccharides

Monosaccharides found in our dietary carbohydrates include *glucose*, *fructose* and *galactose*. All of the monosaccharides are reducing sugars since they possess a reducing group at carbon-1 or carbon-2.

> **Clinical note:**
> Urinary sugar
>
> If a patient has lots of reducing sugar in his/her urine it is important to establish whether or not this is glucose. Significantly urinary glucose is suggestive of diabetes mellitus, but fructosuria or galactosuria are indicative of other metabolic disorders.

Monosaccharides

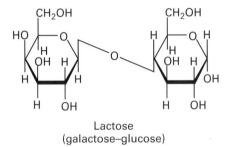

α-D-Glucose   α-D-Galactose   α-D-Fructose

Disaccharides

Lactose
(galactose–glucose)

Sucrose
(glucose–fructose)

Maltose
(glucose–glucose)

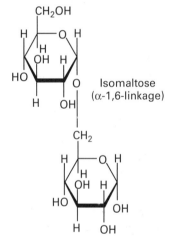

Isomaltose
(α-1,6-linkage)

Amylopectin or glycogen

$$—\; \text{Glucose} \xrightarrow{1\text{-}4\alpha} \text{Glucose}$$

$$\Big|\, 1\text{-}6\alpha$$

$$—\; \text{Glucose} \xrightarrow{1\text{-}4\alpha} \text{Glucose} \xrightarrow{1\text{-}4\alpha} \text{Glucose} \xrightarrow{1\text{-}4\alpha} \text{Glucose} \xrightarrow{1\text{-}4\alpha} \text{etc}$$

Amylose

$$—\; \text{Glucose} \xrightarrow{1\text{-}4\alpha} \text{Glucose} \xrightarrow{1\text{-}4\alpha} \text{Glucose} \xrightarrow{1\text{-}4\alpha} \text{Glucose} \xrightarrow{1\text{-}4\alpha} \text{etc}$$

Fig. 49 The structures of carbohydrates in the diet.

Carbohydrate digestion

Carbohydrates are digested by a process of glycoside hydrolysis, with the resultant monosaccharides being absorbed by the intestinal mucosal cells (Fig. 50). Dietary polysaccharides are hydrolysed to disaccharides and oligosaccharides within the lumen of the gastrointestinal tract by *salivary α-amylase* and by *pancreatic α-amylase*. Since both of these enzymes have a pH optimum around 7.0, the action of salivary amylase is quickly stopped by the acidity in the stomach. However, in the small intestine, buffering action of pancreatic juice and bile

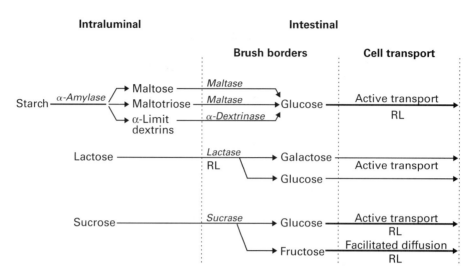

Fig. 50 The overall scheme of carbohydrate digestion and absorption. RL indicates a rate-limiting step in the process.

> **Clinical note:**
> Lactose intolerance
>
> Lactase is quite different from the other carbohydrases in that it catalyses the hydrolysis of a β-1:4-linkage, as found in lactose. Many people have delayed-onset lactose intolerance caused by a significant fall in the levels of intestinal lactase by the early teens. If such individuals consume a large lactose load (e.g. milk) it leads to abdominal fullness, bloating, cramping, pain and profuse watery diarrhoea since the unhydrolysed disaccharide is an osmotic load. Metabolites of lactose produced by colonic bacteria increase the osmotic load further and include acids and gases. Eliminating lactose from the diet prevents these problems.

allows pancreatic amylase to continue the digestion of starch and glycogen in the food. Products include the disaccharide maltose and various oligosaccharides, which include limit dextrins (which are small branched oligosaccharides that contain α-1:6- and α-1:4-linkages) and maltotriose (Fig. 50).

Oligosaccharides and disaccharides are then hydrolysed to monosaccharides by brush border carbohydrases of the intestinal epithelial cells, with a specific digestive enzyme, α-dextrinase, being required to deal with the α-1:6-linkages in amylopectin and glycogen. The brush border carbohydrases are *sucrase-α-dextrinase*, *glucoamylase* and *lactase*. The products of their action upon α-limit dextrins, maltotriose, maltose, sucrose and lactose are the three monosaccharides, glucose, fructose and galactose (Fig. 50).

Carbohydrate absorption

The monosaccharides in the diet and those produced by the digestion of dietary carbohydrates are absorbed into the intestinal epithelial cells by several types of transport mechanisms. Fructose moves into the cell on a membrane carrier (GLUT5) by *facilitated diffusion*. Glucose and galactose are actively transported; this is accomplished by a *sodium-dependent symport system* (SGLT1) (Fig. 51). This transport process ensures that the intracellular glucose concentration is maintained at a higher level than that in the intercellular space on the vascular side of the cell. The carrier-bound sodium ions and glucose enter the cell down a sodium electrochemical gradient which results from the low intracellular sodium concentration and negative membrane potential on the inside of the cell. On the luminal side, one molecule of glucose and two molecules of sodium bind to SGLT1. Presumably the binding of the sodium ions produces a conformational change such that glucose now binds with greater affinity to SGLT1. Inside the cell, the sodium ions are released from SGLT1, and diminished affinity allows the glucose to dissociate. Na^+/K^+-ATPase allows the sodium ions to be transported into the lateral intercellular spaces against an electrochemical gradient using the free energy of ATP hydrolysis. Since glucose transport does not involve ATP directly, it can be considered as *secondary active transport*. Glucose, galactose and fructose are transported from the mucosal cell into the intercellular space by a high-capacity glucose transporter (GLUT2).

> **Clinical note:**
> Cholera and dysentery
>
> A practical use of co-transport is the administration of a mixture of NaCl and glucose by mouth to subjects with cholera or dysentery who are sodium depleted as a result of diarrhoea. The provision of glucose along with the NaCl enables them to re-establish their sodium levels.

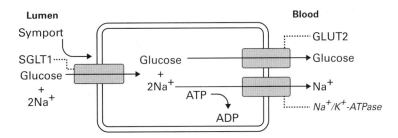

Fig. 51 Glucose–sodium symport system (see text for details).

Saturated fatty acid $\quad CH_3 - (CH_2)_n \overset{3}{-} \underset{\beta}{CH_2} - \overset{2}{\underset{\alpha}{CH_2}} - \overset{1}{COO^-}$

Examples: Butyrate C_4
           Palmitate C_{16}
           Stearate C_{18}

Monounsaturated fatty acid $\quad CH_3 - (CH_2)_n - CH = CH - (CH_2)_n - COO^-$

Examples: Palmitoleate $C_{16:1;9}$ (or Δ^9)
           Oleate $C_{18:1;9}$ (or Δ^9)

Polyunsaturated fatty acid

Examples: Linoleate $C_{18:2;9,12}$
           α-Linolenate $C_{18:3;9,12,15}$
           Arachidonate $C_{20:4;5,8,11,14}$

Triacylglycerols (triglycerides)

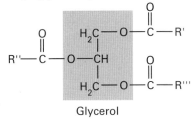

Glycerol

Fig. 52 Structures of fatty acids and triacylglycerols. Two different systems of nomenclature are shown for fatty acids. In one, the carboxyl carbon is carbon-1 and the rest of the carbons follow from that, with the terminal methyl group carbon having the number corresponding to the number of carbons in the fatty acid. The other scheme uses Greek letters, starting from the carbon following the carboxyl carbon. The terminal methyl group is referred to as the omega (ω) carbon. In unsaturated fatty acids, the number that follows the colon (:) refers to the number of double bonds; this is followed by numbers that refer to the locations of the double bonds. In most unsaturated fatty acids found in the body, the double bonds are *cis*.

Dietary fats

Fats are hydrophobic molecules. The major dietary fats are triacylglycerols (triglycerides), which are esters of an alcohol (glycerol) and fatty acids (Fig. 52). Naturally occurring fats usually have different long-chain fatty acids in all three ester positions. The fatty acids can be saturated (e.g. palmitate or stearate) or monounsaturated (e.g. oleate). Other fatty acids are polyunsaturated.

Fat digestion and absorption

Dietary triglycerides are absorbed after undergoing *partial hydrolysis*, with bile salts playing a key role. The key steps are:

1. *Salivary and lingual lipases* preferentially hydrolyse triglycerides composed of short- and medium-chain fatty acids (as found in cow's milk). The 2-monoacylglycerols produced help emulsify other fat in the diet.

2. In the small intestine, bile salts emulsify fats.
3. *Pancreatic lipase* and *co-lipase* are secreted from the pancreas. Co-lipase provides an anchor for *pancreatic lipase* at the triglyceride/bile salt/water interface. In the small intestine, pancreatic lipase catalyses the hydrolysis of triglycerides to 2-monoacylglycerols by removing fatty acids from the 1 and 3 positions.
4. Bile salt micelles are formed which contain triglycerides, monoglycerides, fatty acids and fat-soluble vitamins; they allow for the lipids to be absorbed into the mucosal cells.
5. Fatty acids of fewer than 10–12 carbons go directly to the liver via the portal vein.
6. Triglycerides are re-formed in intestinal mucosal cells from long-chain fatty acids and 2-monoacylglycerols and are then incorporated into chylomicrons, which are lipoproteins involved in the transport of triglycerides in the lymph and blood (p. 131). Apolipoprotein B-48 is required for chylomicron synthesis.
7. Cholesteryl esters in the diet are hydrolysed by the action of *cholesteryl ester hydrolase*. Unesterified cholesterol and cholesteryl esters are included in the bile salt micelles and also end up in chylomicrons.
8. Phospholipids in the diet are hydrolysed by the action of *pancreatic phospholipase A_2*, which removes the fatty acid at the carbon-2 position leaving a lysophospholipid, which is a powerful detergent. The fatty acids released and the lysophospholipids are incorporated into micelles and transported into mucosal cells and appear in chylomicrons.

Gastrointestinal hormones have an important role in digestion

Gastrointestinal hormones ensure that digestive enzymes are present in sufficient quantity in the stomach or small intestine and that the conditions are correct for the action of these enzymes. Key points include:

- *Gastrin*, made in the G cells found in the pyloric glands of the antrum and the proximal duodenum, stimulates acid and pepsinogen secretion in the stomach (see Ch. 8, p. 111). Protein meals, distension of the stomach and vagus nerve stimulation increase gastrin secretion.
- *Secretin*, made in S cells, which are found between crypts and villi of the upper intestine, stimulates water and bicarbonate secretion by pancreatic ductal cells and liver, therefore ensuring that the acidity produced in the stomach is neutralised. Acidification, achieved when the acid chyme enters the small intestine during the digestion of a meal, is the major known stimulus for its secretion.

- *Cholecystokinin*, made by I cells, chiefly in the duodenum and proximal jejunum, stimulates pancreatic acinar cells to secrete digestive enzymes such as amylase and lipase as well as the zymogen forms of proteolytic enzymes. It also brings about dilation of the sphincter of Oddi and contraction of the gallbladder, allowing bile to flow from the gallbladder into the duodenum. Thus, it has a very important role to play in dietary fat digestion and absorption. Cholecystokinin secretion is increased by fats, peptides and amino acids present in the lumen of the small intestine.

6.3 Carbohydrate catabolism

Learning objectives

You should be able to:

- describe the roles of the various transporters involved in glucose transport into cells, focusing on location, K_m and insulin dependence (if any)
- identify the key steps in glycolysis and how they are controlled
- explain the difference between aerobic and anaerobic metabolism of glucose
- give an account of the reactions of the pyruvate dehydrogenase complex and how it is controlled.

Carbohydrates, mainly in the form of the monosaccharide glucose, are important fuels for tissues in the body. An important concept is that glucose can be used as a fuel by all tissues, but there is considerable variation in the ability of different tissues to use other fuels (Ch. 10).

Glucose transport into cells

Following a meal that contains carbohydrate, there is efficient digestion and absorption leading to a significant increase in blood glucose concentration, especially in the portal vein. Glucose is taken up by all tissues in the body, with a high percentage entering liver and muscle where it can be stored as glycogen. The transport of glucose across animal cell membranes involves transport proteins that span the plasma membrane.

Glucose transporters

There are two distinct gene families of glucose transporters. In addition to SGLT1 involved in glucose and galactose absorption in the intestine, there is a family of

Na$^+$-independent facilitated-diffusion glucose transporters (GLUTs) which are ubiquitously expressed in mammalian cells. These proteins have 12 membrane-spanning segments. They are responsible for the movement of glucose from the blood into cells. Glucose uptake into cells is of great physiological significance and GLUTs facilitate the achievement of glucose homeostasis in the fed and fasting states (Ch. 10).

The key points (summarised in Table 5) are:

- GLUT1 is the 'housekeeping' glucose transporter functioning in all tissues, including those that are dependent solely upon glucose for their fuel (such as erythrocytes). It has a K_m of around 1 mM.
- GLUT2 has a high K_m for glucose (10–20 mM). Its presence in the liver means that the liver will take up glucose effectively only when the blood glucose concentration is raised, such as after a meal. It also allows for the export of glucose from the liver in the fasted state. GLUT2 is also significant in the beta cells of the pancreas, where its high K_m contributes to appropriate control of insulin secretion, and in intestinal mucosal cells, where it transports glucose, galactose and fructose.
- GLUT3 is another low K_m glucose transporter also present in the brain. It transports glucose from the cerebrospinal fluid across the plasma membranes of neuronal cells and is very effective.
- GLUT4 occurs in adipose tissue and muscle cells, tissues that are not glucose manufacturers/exporters and have no need for a glucose transporter present in the plasma membranes during the fasting state.

GLUT4 transporters are sequestered in membranes of intracellular vesicles until an increase in blood insulin concentration leads to recruitment of GLUT4 molecules to the plasma membrane; this is complete within 5 minutes and increases glucose uptake 20-fold.

- GLUT5 is a fructose transporter present in the small intestine and the liver.

Glycolysis

The glycolytic pathway is the series of reactions that occurs in the cytosol of cells and allows glucose to be converted to pyruvate (Stage 2 reactions). Glycolysis results in limited ATP synthesis but, in addition, some of the intermediates have critical roles in other pathways and systems.

Relative importance in tissues and organs

This should be obvious since glucose is a fuel for all tissues in the body and under normal conditions is the only fuel for the brain. Glycolysis is an essential precursor to the oxidative phase of glucose metabolism that occurs in the mitochondria of cells. Also the pyruvate formed can provide the oxaloacetate required for operation of the vitally important TCA cycle. Clearly, in cells that lack mitochondria (such as erythrocytes), glycolysis is the only pathway that has the potential to generate ATP for these cells.

The glycolytic pathway

The glycolytic pathway is shown in Figure 53. It is convenient to divide glycolysis into phases.

In the first phase of glycolysis, glucose is converted to fructose 1,6-bisphosphate (F-1,6-BP). The two kinases involved are *hexokinase* or *glucokinase* and then *phosphofructokinase-1* (PFK-1). Hexokinase and glucokinase have differing kinetic properties (Fig. 20). Hexokinase has a low K_m for glucose and catalyses the conversion of glucose to glucose 6-phosphate (Reaction 1) in all tissues of the body. Glucokinase is present in the liver and in the beta cells of the islets of Langerhans in the pancreas. The product of the reaction, glucose 6-phosphate, inhibits hexokinase but not glucokinase. Glucokinase has a K_m much higher than the normal blood glucose concentration. This ensures that during the fasting state the liver is not metabolising blood glucose. Additionally, the high K_m is consistent with the role of the liver in the fed state where the liver takes up glucose and stores it as glycogen. PFK-1 catalyses a second phosphorylation (Reaction 3) which is often described as the first committed step of glycolysis, and is subjected to allosteric control.

Table 5 Glucose transport into cells

Transporter	Location	Characteristics
Na$^+$/glucose transporters	Gut	Glucose-sodium symport
Facilitated-diffusion transporters		
GLUT1	Brain All cells	Low K_m
GLUT2	Liver, beta cells of pancreas, kidney, intestine	High K_m
GLUT3	Most cells	Low K_m
GLUT4	Muscle Adipose tissue	Insulin-dependent translocation to plasma membrane
GLUT5	Intestine, liver	Fructose absorption

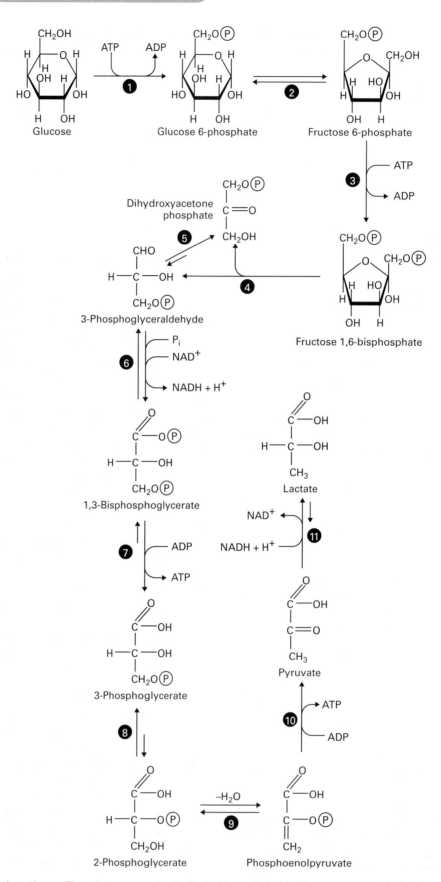

Fig. 53 The glycolytic pathway. Phosphate groups are indicated by a circled P. The enzymes catalysing the numbered reactions are discussed in the text.

In the second phase of glycolysis, F-1,6-BP is converted to two interconvertible triose phosphates (Reaction 4); one of these, 3-phosphoglyceraldehyde, is oxidised in the single oxidative step of glycolysis (Reaction 6). The enzyme involved, *3-phosphoglyceraldehyde dehydrogenase*, is NAD$^+$-dependent. It is important to recognise that there are limited amounts of NAD$^+$ in cells and, therefore, it has to be regenerated if glycolysis is to proceed. Because NADH cannot cross the inner mitochondrial membrane, 'shuttles' serve to carry this out during oxidative metabolism (see section 6.6). During vigorous exercise in muscle, *lactate dehydrogenase* serves to regenerate NAD$^+$ in a reaction in which pyruvate is reduced to lactate (Reaction 11).

In the third phase of glycolysis, reactions occur in which ATP is synthesised by a process known as substrate-level phosphorylation, contrasting with ATP formation in oxidative phosphorylation in mitochondria.

PFK-1 and pyruvate kinase (PK) are important in the control of glycolysis

Flux control through the glycolytic pathway is 'distributed' (it is invalid to consider that one of the steps is the rate-limiting step!) and involves the reactions catalysed by hexokinase, PFK-1 and PK, each of which have large negative $\Delta G^{0\prime}$ values. Understandably, it is these reactions that are subjected to some degree of regulation. In addition, control of glucose transport into the cell will affect the potential maximum flux through the pathway. Most attention has been given to PFK-1 since it catalyses the first committed step in glycolysis.

Regulation of PFK-1 and PK

PFK-1 is inhibited by ATP and citrate and activated by AMP and fructose-2,6-bisphosphate (F-2,6-BP). Under resting conditions, the level of ATP in a cell is sufficient to inhibit PFK-1. An increase in AMP is a signal that ATP is being used at a high rate and that catabolism is necessary to replenish ATP used for whatever reason. The AMP effect is insufficient to activate PFK-1 unless F-2,6-BP levels also increase and the latter occurs when more F-6-P is available. Increased citrate in a cell is a signal that fatty acids are being utilised as fuel and, logically, this should lead to decreased need for glucose catabolism. PFK-1 is also inhibited by an increase in hydrogen ion concentration, [H$^+$], and this safeguards cells against overaccumulation of pyruvate or lactate. The rationale for the effects of F-2,6-BP on glycolysis and the opposing reactions of gluconeogenesis in the liver are discussed in Chapter 7. PK is also inhibited by ATP. The control of PK in the liver is discussed in Chapter 7 in the context of the control of gluconeogenesis.

Net reactions of glycolysis

Summation of all of the reactions gives the following equations for aerobic and anaerobic glycolysis. Note that, under anaerobic conditions, the equation shows that lactate formation leads to oxidation of NADH.

Aerobic glycolysis

$$\text{Glucose} + 2ADP + 2P_i + 2NAD^+ \rightarrow 2\text{Pyruvate} + 2ATP + 2NADH + 2H^+ + H_2O$$

Anaerobic glycolysis

$$\text{Glucose} + 2ADP + 2P \rightarrow 2\text{Lactate} + 2ATP + 2H_2O$$

Aerobic metabolism of pyruvate

Pyruvate enters the mitochondria along with H$^+$ using a symporter. Within mitochondria, it can be completely oxidised to carbon dioxide and water with the associated production of ATP, but first it has to be oxidised to acetyl-CoA. The *pyruvate dehydrogenase complex* (PDC) is huge: it comprises three enzymes involved in the actual reaction (Fig. 54) plus enzymes involved in its control (Fig. 55). There is a core of 60 E$_2$ monomers plus 30 E$_1$ dimers and 6 E$_3$ dimers. PDC is frequently referred to as pyruvate dehydrogenase but it is clear that the first reaction is a decarboxylation catalysed by E$_1$ that has thiamine pyrophosphate (TPP) as cofactor. E$_2$, which has lipoate covalently linked, has two functions: one is the dehydrogenation of the two-carbon unit to give an acetyl group and the second is the transfer of the acetyl group to a third coenzyme, coenzyme A (CoA). If the acetyl group (which serves as a precursor of, amongst others, fatty acids and cholesterol) remained attached to the lipoate that is covalently linked to E$_2$, it would be less available for other metabolic pathways. In the last group of reactions, lipoate is regenerated to its oxidised form by E$_3$, a flavoprotein that utilises FAD as cofactor. Finally, the FADH$_2$ is reoxidised to FAD using NAD$^+$, giving the final products of the reaction: acetyl-CoA, carbon dioxide and NADH.

The PDC reactions have three important features:

1. The PDC-catalysed reaction is irreversible. This has very important consequences for intermediary metabolism in that acetyl-CoA cannot be converted to pyruvate and, therefore, fatty acids are not glucogenic (cannot be used to make glucose).
2. The activity of PDC is the major determinant of glucose oxidation in well-oxygenated tissues in vivo. The conversion of the glycolytic metabolites of glucose to acetyl-CoA enables them to enter Stage 3 of metabolism, leading to the generation of several molecules of ATP.

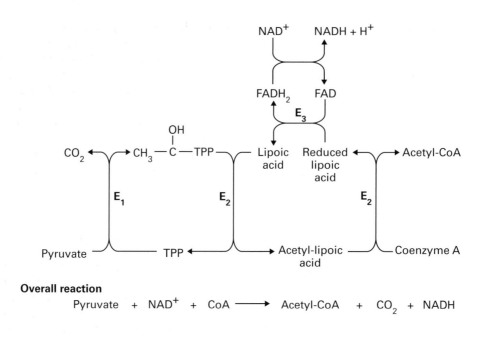

Overall reaction

$$\text{Pyruvate} \; + \; \text{NAD}^+ \; + \; \text{CoA} \longrightarrow \; \text{Acetyl-CoA} \; + \; \text{CO}_2 \; + \; \text{NADH}$$

Participating enzymes	
E_1	Pyruvate dehydrogenase (PDH)
E_2	Dihydrolipoyl transacetylase
E_3	Dihydrolipoyl dehydrogenase

Participating cofactors/coenzymes

TPP, thiamine pyrophosphate (B_1)

Lipoic acid

CoA, pantothenate-containing factor

FAD, flavin adenine dinucleotide (B_2)

NAD, nicotinamide adenine dinucleotide (niacin)

Fig. 54 Reactions of the pyruvate dehydrogenase complex.

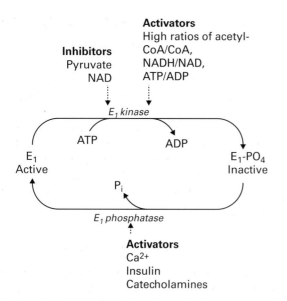

Fig. 55 Control of the pyruvate dehydrogenase complex by both covalent modification and allosteric mechanisms.

3. The control of PDC is multi-faceted in that the reaction is critical to energy metabolism, thus it responds to nutritional state and hormones and also to levels of intrinsic metabolites (Fig. 55). A mixture of covalent and allosteric mechanisms is involved. E_1 of the complex is inhibited by phosphorylation and activated when dephosphorylated. An E_1 kinase (PDK) and an E_1 phosphatase (PDP) are involved and their activities are affected by the ratios of acetyl-CoA/CoA, NADH/NAD$^+$ and ATP/ADP. As one could predict, high ratios activate PDK leading to decreased PDC activity and vice versa. In addition, Ca^{2+} enhances PDP activity both by facilitating the association of PDP with the complex and by decreasing the K_m for the protein substrate, the phosphorylated E_1 component. Insulin (in adipocytes) and catecholamines (in cardiac tissue) increase pyruvate conversion to acetyl-CoA by activation of PDP. There is 'physiological wisdom' in the control of PDC, both short-term and long-term, as will become apparent in Chapter 10.

6.4 Fat catabolism

Learning objectives

You should be able to:

- outline the pathways of fat mobilisation and the roles of hormone-sensitive lipase and albumin

- describe the role of carnitine in the entry of long-chain fatty acids into mitochondria

- explain the beta-oxidation pathway for fatty acids and its control

- outline pathways for ketone body synthesis and catabolism.

Fatty acids have higher energy content per gram than glucose since they are more reduced. The body has limited carbohydrate storage capacity but enormous capacity to store fats (see Ch. 10). This means that fatty acids are usually available as fuel and, if a tissue can utilise them (e.g. the heart), then less glucose is required. Also, when undergoing long-term exercise, a worker or athlete will use fatty acids as a preferred fuel. This occurs particularly in muscles that have a high content of mitochondria (red, slow-twitch muscle).

Fatty acids are mobilised from stored triacylglycerols

Fatty acids are stored as triglycerides mainly in adipose tissue. Their mobilisation as fuels for use by other tissues involves the action of several lipases with the end-products of their action being glycerol plus three fatty acids (Fig. 56). One of the lipases, *triacylglycerol lipase*, is active when phosphorylated; it is called 'hormone-sensitive lipase' because phosphorylation occurs when hormones such as glucagon, growth hormone and adrenaline (epinephrine) are produced in increased amounts in the fasting state or during exercise (Ch. 10). Glycerol, the other product of triacylglycerol hydrolysis, can be phosphorylated in the liver and then metabolised as a glycolytic intermediate or converted to glucose.

Oxidation of fatty acids

The overall design of the beta-oxidation pathway is shown in Figure 56. The key points are:

- Fatty acids are taken up by tissues in which they can be oxidised and the action of *fatty acyl-CoA synthase* generates fatty acyl-CoA derivatives.

- This introduces a problem: the impermeability of the inner mitochondrial membrane to long-chain fatty acyl-CoA derivatives. This is solved by converting them to acyl-carnitines catalysed by *carnitine palmitoyltransferase I* (CPTI) and transferring the acyl-carnitines using a membrane translocase; *carnitine palmitoyltransferase II* (CPTII) then catalyses the regeneration of the fatty acyl-CoA derivatives, now located in the proximity of the enzymes of the beta-oxidation pathway. Fatty acids with less than 12 carbons enter the mitochondria directly and are then activated and beta-oxidised.

- Beta-oxidation reactions are similar to the sequence succinate→fumarate→malate→oxaloacetate of the TCA cycle.

- $FADH_2$ and NADH are formed in the two oxidation steps (Reactions 1 and 3). The final step involves the cleavage of the β-ketoacyl-CoA with a second molecule of CoA (Reaction 4), which yields acetyl-CoA and a fatty acyl-CoA shortened by two carbons. Hence, activation is only required once.

The oxidation of palmitate, a 16-carbon fatty acid, would result in the following:

$$Palmitoyl\text{-}CoA + 7FAD + 7NAD^+ + 7CoASH + 7H_2O \rightarrow 8Acetyl\text{-}CoA + 7FADH_2 + 7NADH + 7H^+$$

Seven (not eight!) oxidation cycles will be required in the degradation of palmitoyl-CoA to eight molecules of acetyl-CoA.

The oxidation of $FADH_2$ and NADH involves the electron transport chain and is coupled to ATP synthesis (see Ch. 6, p. 88).

Beta-oxidation is controlled by malonyl-CoA

All the evidence points to CPTI being an important control point. Malonyl-CoA, an intermediate in fatty acid biosynthesis, inhibits CPTI and this provides an understandable link between these opposing pathways. However, another determinant of the amount of fatty acid that can be utilised by, for example, liver, cardiac or skeletal muscle, must be the supply of fuel to these tissues from fat stores in adipose tissue. Here is another example of control of flux through a pathway being distributed rather than focused on a single rate-limiting step.

Oxidation of odd-numbered fatty acids

Beta-oxidation of a fatty acid with an odd number of carbon atoms yields successive molecules of acetyl-CoA and one equivalent of propionyl-CoA; the propionyl group has three carbons. The major pathway of

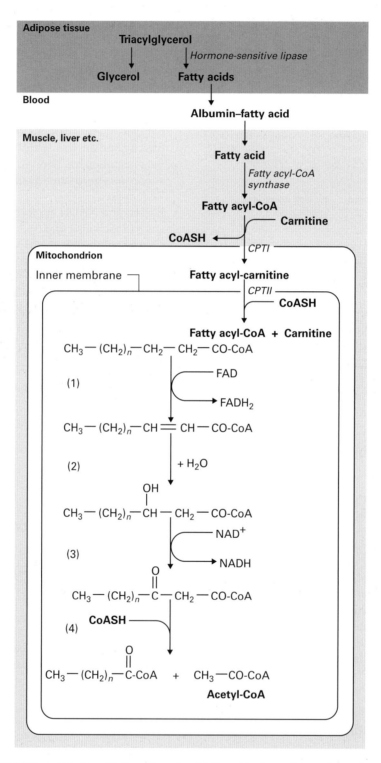

Fig. 56 Fat mobilisation and fatty acid beta-oxidation. The rate of fatty acid release from adipose tissue affects the total amount of fatty acid available as a fuel for tissues such as liver and muscle (see text for further details).

propionyl-CoA metabolism occurs in mammalian mito-chondria and involves its conversion to a TCA cycle intermediate, succinyl-CoA, by three steps, one of which requires a vitamin B_{12} coenzyme. One difference between propionyl-CoA and acetyl-CoA is that the former is glucogenic.

Oxidation of unsaturated fatty acids

Most unsaturated fatty acids in biology have *cis* double bonds. This means that one has to have special reactions (not dealt with in this text) to deal with such compounds. Modified beta-oxidation again yields acetyl-CoA.

Ketone body biosynthesis and metabolism

Ketone bodies were originally thought to be interme-diates of fatty acid oxidation that could only accumulate under abnormal conditions, such as in diabetes mellitus. It is now clear that ketone bodies are important fuels made from fatty acids in the liver under normal condi-tions and then transported via the blood to many tissues to be used as fuels. In effect, this enables the energy of fats to be utilised by many tissues. The ketone bodies are acetoacetic acid, β-hydroxybutyric acid and acetone (Fig. 57). In contrast to the fatty acids from which they are derived, they provide an alternative fuel for the brain.

Key points on ketone body synthesis and metabo-lism are:

- They are formed in the mitochondria of the liver with β-hydroxy-β-methylglutaryl-CoA (HMG-CoA) being a key intermediate (Fig. 57).
- Acetoacetate is the primary ketone body, but in the liver some is reduced to β-hydroxybutyrate by the action of *β-hydroxybutyrate dehydrogenase*; the proportion of these two ketone bodies secreted is dependent upon several factors, including the glycogen status of the liver and the ratio of NADH to NAD^+.
- Acetoacetate can also be decarboxylated (spontaneously) to yield acetone. Acetone is not a fuel; as it is volatile its production will be indicated by the presence of its characteristic odour in expired air.

Clinical note:
Type 1 diabetes mellitus

Impaired utilisation resulting from deficiency of insulin (or reduced effectiveness) is associated with excessive formation of ketone bodies. Patients with type 1 diabetes mellitus have the potential to develop ketoacidosis. Acetone production gives the breath a characteristic odour. If untreated, ketoacidosis can result in coma and death.

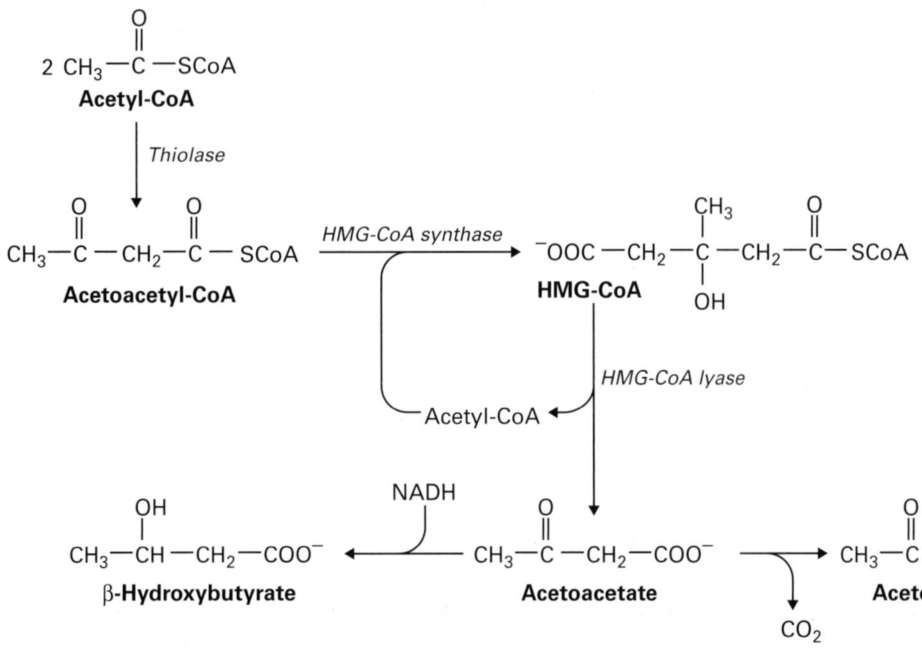

Fig. 57 Ketone body biosynthesis pathway in liver mitochondria.

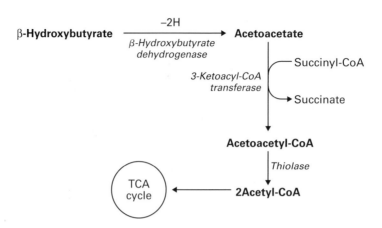

Fig. 58 Ketone body utilisation in extrahepatic tissues.

- The key enzyme of ketone body utilisation is *3-ketoacyl-CoA transferase*, which catalyses the reaction where CoA is transferred from succinyl-CoA to acetoacetate (Fig. 58).
- Ketone body production is directly related to the rate of fatty acid mobilisation from adipose tissue and their oxidation in liver. Also, low levels of oxaloacetate in the liver, associated with low rates of glucose metabolism, increase the potential for acetyl-CoA to be converted to ketone bodies rather than enter the TCA cycle.

6.5 The tricarboxylic acid cycle

Learning objectives

You should be able to:

- explain the design of the TCA cycle and its roles
- explain how the TCA cycle functions in energy metabolism in cells
- describe the role of the TCA cycle in anabolism.

The tricarboxylic acid (TCA) cycle (Krebs cycle, citric acid cycle) is a part of Stage 3 metabolism. It allows for intermediates derived from carbohydrate, fat or amino acids to be completely oxidised to carbon dioxide and water. The pathway occurs in mitochondria where the electron transport chain and ATP synthase are also located.

The reactions of the TCA cycle accounting for the oxidation of the acetyl group of acetyl-CoA to carbon dioxide and water are shown in Figure 59. Citrate formed by the interaction of acetyl-CoA and oxaloacetate is subjected to a series of reactions, four of which are oxidations catalysed by dehydrogenases.

In addition to acetyl-CoA, other metabolites, including those derived from amino acids, can feed into the TCA cycle at various points (see Ch. 8, p. 114). Also, the TCA cycle provides intermediates for the synthesis of biomolecules; it is amphibolic.

Key points about the TCA cycle are:

- Oxaloacetate, which reacts with acetyl-CoA to form citrate to enter the cycle, is regenerated in the last step of the cycle so it functions like a catalyst.
- All the reactions of the TCA cycle are catalysed by enzymes dissolved in the fluid of the mitochondrial matrix with the exception of *succinate dehydrogenase*, which is an integral protein of the mitochondrial inner membrane.
- *Isocitric dehydrogenase* (Enzyme 3) catalyses the oxidative decarboxylation of isocitrate to α-ketoglutarate (2-oxoglutarate).
- α-Ketoglutarate dehydrogenase (Enzyme 4) catalyses an oxidative decarboxylation by a mechanism similar to that of PDC (Fig. 54). α-Ketoglutarate represents a significant point of convergence in metabolism. Several amino acids can be converted to glutamate, which if transaminated or oxidatively deaminated yields α-ketoglutarate. Conversely, these amino acids can be synthesised from α-ketoglutarate (see Ch. 8, p. 114).
- The 3 NADH and 1 $FADH_2$ molecules produced per acetyl-CoA molecule are, in turn, oxidised via the electron transport chain coupled to *ATP synthase*, resulting in the production of 11 ATP; a single GTP is produced by substrate-level phosphorylation in Reaction 5.

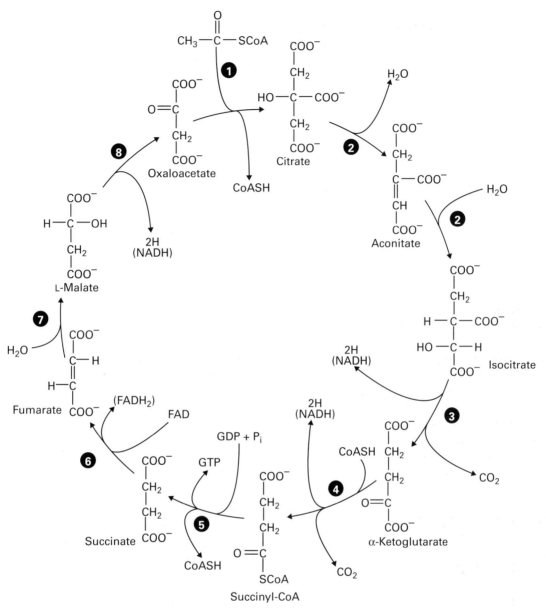

Fig. 59 The reactions of the TCA cycle. Enzymes 1–8 are described in the text.

Net reaction

The net reaction of acetyl-CoA metabolism in the TCA cycle is:

$$Acetyl\text{-}CoA + 3NAD^+ + FAD + GDP + P_i + 2H_2O \rightarrow 2CO_2$$
$$+ 3NADH + 2H^+ + FADH_2 + GTP + CoASH$$

Citrate synthase, isocitrate dehydrogenase and a-ketoglutarate dehydrogenase are control points of the TCA cycle

Flux through the TCA cycle will be determined by several parameters. Within the actual pathway, isocitrate dehydrogenase and α-ketoglutarate dehydrogenase are sensitive to energy charge and to the ratio $NAD^+/NADH$.

However, the flux through the pathway is more complicated and is related to the activity of pathways that supply acetyl-CoA, including PDC and fatty acid beta-oxidation.

6.6 Electron transport and oxidative phosphorylation

Learning objectives

You should be able to:

- explain oxidation of fuels and the production of ATP

- describe how NADH and FADH₂ are handled in the electron transport chain
- outline the role of the proton gradient in ATP synthesis in mitochondria and how it can be dissipated by uncouplers
- calculate ATP yield from glucose and fatty acids.

Transfer of energy-rich molecules

Products of the TCA cycle include NADH + H⁺ and FADH₂, which are 'energy-rich' molecules because they contain a pair of electrons of high transfer potential. Transfer of these electrons to oxygen through a series of carriers has the potential to generate ATP. Oxidative phosphorylation is the process in which ATP is formed as electrons are transferred by this series of carriers from NADH + H⁺ and FADH₂ to oxygen. The formation of a proton gradient is critical to this process.

Shuttles are used for NADH generated in the cytosol

NADH is also generated in the glycolytic pathway. If aerobic metabolism of glucose is to occur, for example to support the performance of muscular work, then cytosolic NADH must be reoxidised to NAD⁺. The obvious pathway using the respiratory assemblies that are located in the inner membrane of the mitochondria is not directly available since neither NAD⁺ nor NADH can pass across the inner mitochondrial membrane. Reoxidation of NADH formed in the cytosol occurs by the operation of two shuttles. The principle of both shuttles is that NADH reduces a metabolite in the cytosol and therefore NAD⁺ is regenerated. Then, the reduced metabolite is oxidised by a mitochondrial enzyme, but in this case the FADH₂ or NADH produced can be oxidised via the electron transport chain. The shuttles in question are the *glycerol 3-phosphate shuttle*, with the net reaction being:

NADH (cytosol) + FAD (mitochondria)→NAD⁺
(cytosol) + FADH₂ (mitochondria)

and the *malate–aspartate shuttle*, with the net reaction being:

NADH (cytosol) + NAD⁺ (mitochondria)→NAD⁺
(cytosol) + NADH (mitochondria)

Mitochondrial electron transport

The mitochondria of the cell consist of two membranes: the outer and inner membranes (Fig. 60). The outer membrane is 6–7 nm thick and is freely permeable to

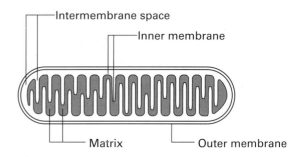

Fig. 60 Compartments and membranes in mitochondria.

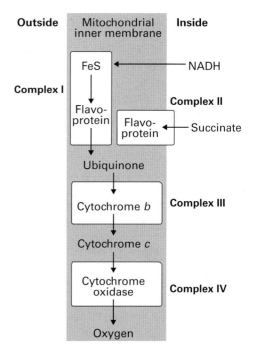

Fig. 61 Respiratory chain complexes of mitochondria.

molecules with molecular weights under 10 000. The intermembrane space contains the enzymes that catalyse the interconversion of adenine nucleotides. The inner membrane is 6–8 nm thick and has many folds directed towards the mitochondrial matrix. These invaginations (called *cristae*) increase the surface area of the inner membrane and are increased in cells with high rates of respiratory activity. Much of the lipid in the inner membrane consists of phospholipid, with phosphatidylcholine predominating on the cytoplasmic side and phosphatidylethanolamine on the matrix side. Most of the cardiolipin is on the matrix side.

The *electron transport system* is composed of four protein–lipid–enzyme complexes, which contain flavins, ubiquinone (coenzyme Q₁₀), iron–sulphur clusters, cytochromes (haem proteins) and protein-bound copper (Fig. 61). Complexes I and II are the 'electron gatherers', transferring electrons to ubiquinone. Then the electrons are transferred through the complexes containing cytochromes and eventually react with molecular oxygen in the reaction catalysed by cytochrome c oxidase.

Characteristics of these complexes include:

- Complex I: accepts reducing equivalents in the form of NADH derived from the action of NAD^+-linked dehydrogenases in the major pathways of intermediary metabolism. The transfer of electrons to *ubiquinone* involves FMN and multiple iron–sulphur (FeS) clusters.
- Complex II: derives reducing equivalents in the form of $FADH_2$ from succinate dehydrogenase and, among others, fatty acyl-CoA dehydrogenase of fatty acid beta-oxidation. Electrons are transferred to ubiquinone.
- Complex III: the cytochrome $b–c_1$ complex which receives electrons from ubiquinone and passes them on to complex IV.
- Complex IV: comprises *cytochrome c oxidase* (COX), which donates the electrons that have traversed the electron transport chain to oxygen, producing water. COX consists of 13 polypeptide subunits. Subunits I, II and III are encoded by the mitochondrial genome and the others by nuclear DNA. Subunits I and II contain the two copper atoms of COX as well as haems a and a_3. COX is inhibited by carbon monoxide, which binds to the Fe(II) form, and also by cyanide, which binds to the Fe(III) form.

ATP synthesis makes use of a proton gradient

The chemiosmotic hypothesis of Mitchell states that oxidation and phosphorylation are coupled by a proton gradient (a proton motive force). In this model, it is proposed that an electrochemical gradient is generated by a proton pump in the inner membrane of the mitochondria. The proton pump is operated by electron flow and causes protons to be expelled through the membrane from the matrix space. Protons flow back into the matrix down their electrochemical gradient and the energy released is used to drive the synthesis of ATP (Fig. 62). Protons are pumped across the inner mitochondrial membrane into the intermembrane space at complexes I, III and IV. This generates a proton gradient, and the potential energy of this gradient is used in complex V (*ATP synthase*) to drive the formation of ATP from $ADP + P_i$.

- Complex V: here, ATP synthesis is carried out by a molecular assembly in the inner membrane shown schematically in Figure 63. The spheres, which project on the matrix side of the inner membrane of

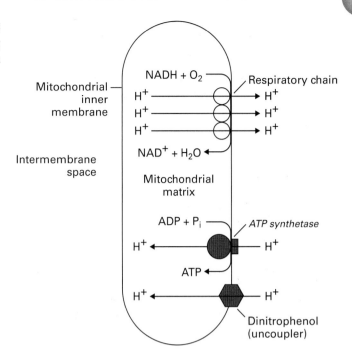

Fig. 62 The proton circuit in oxidative phosphorylation. Note that the electron transport chain and ATP synthase are separate entities in the inner mitochondrial membrane!

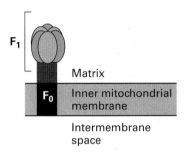

Fig. 63 ATP synthase of mitochondria.

the mitochondria, are referred to as F_1. Solubilised F_1, in the absence of a proton gradient, hydrolyses ATP. F_0 is the hydrophobic component of ATP synthase and it spans the inner membrane; this is the proton channel of the complex. The stalk between F_1 and F_0 contains several proteins, one of which is sensitive to oligomycin. This antibiotic inhibits ATP synthesis by interfering with the utilisation of the proton gradient.

Phosphorylation can be uncoupled from oxidation

Oxidation can be uncoupled from ATP synthesis by uncoupling agents, such as 2,4-dinitrophenol. These compounds are weak acids with lipid-soluble acidic and basic forms, which become protonated, traverse the inner mitochondrial membrane and thereby dissipate the proton gradient. Under these conditions, electron transport and oxygen utilisation run unchecked at their maximal rates but ATP synthesis through ATP synthase ceases.

A unique mitochondrial protein, the uncoupling protein UCP, gives brown adipose tissue (BAT) the ability of facultative heat production. BAT differs from energy-storing white adipose tissue in having an abundance of mitochondria. UCP is a proton translocator that also uncouples oxidation from ATP synthesis in BAT cells. BAT is found in mammals mainly in the interscapular, subscapular, axillary and suprasternal regions of the body. Babies have more BAT than adults do.

ATP yield

In intact, coupled mitochondria, the yield of ATP processed through oxidative phosphorylation has been calculated to be 3 ATP per NADH and 2 ATP per $FADH_2$. This can also be expressed as a P/O ratio, where P refers to the number of ATP molecules synthesised and O to an oxygen atom (one-half O_2). The actual P/O ratios are not whole numbers but 3 and 2 are universally used in texts (and exams).

ATP from glucose oxidation

Using these data and a knowledge of glucose metabolism, one can calculate that the complete oxidation of glucose can yield 38 ATP molecules, assuming handling of cytosolic NADH by the malate shuttle. 38 ATP are generated since glucose oxidation to carbon dioxide and water produces 2 NADH and 2 ATP from glycolysis, 2 NADH from PDC, and 6 NADH, 2 $FADH_2$ and 2 GTP from TCA cycle activity. If the glycerol 3-phosphate shuttle is used, the yield from glucose will be 36 ATP.

ATP from fatty acid oxidation

Beta-oxidation of an 18-carbon fatty acid involves eight complete beta-oxidation cycles in which 9 acetyl-CoA molecules are produced. Complete oxidation to CO_2 and water will then generate 146 ATP. Note that 146 ATP is significantly more than the 114 (3×38) ATP produced from the complete oxidation of three glucoses. This is a good indication of the higher energy content of the more reduced fuel!

Self-assessment: questions

Single best answer MCQs

1. Identify the correct statement or statements about the three stages of metabolism proposed by Krebs and Kornberg.
   a. Stage 1 occurs in the gastrointestinal tract for carbohydrates, proteins and fats
   b. Glycolysis is the major pathway in Stage 2 for carbohydrates
   c. Both the electron transport chain and ATP synthase are in Stage 3 of metabolism
   d. Both a and c are correct
   e. a, b and c are all correct

2. Identify the single correct explanation as to why the biochemical pathway for the catabolism of a molecule is almost never the same as the pathway for the biosynthesis of that molecule.
   a. It would be much easier to regulate the pathway if it served both functions
   b. Enzyme-catalysed reactions are always irreversible
   c. The free-energy change would be unfavourable in one direction
   d. Biochemical systems are usually at equilibrium

3. If you were studying sugar transport using various tissues derived from a rat (assume that the systems involved are identical to those found in humans), which one of the following would be inhibited by the addition of 2,4-dinitrophenol?
   a. Uptake of glucose into muscle
   b. Uptake of glucose into liver
   c. Uptake of fructose into intestinal mucosal cells
   d. Uptake of glucose into intestinal mucosal cells
   e. Uptake of glucose into neuronal cells

4. You make the diagnosis of carbohydrate malabsorption in an 18-year-old female subject. The presence of which of the following carbohydrates in high concentration in the colon will help establish that the patient cannot fully digest amylopectin?
   a. Glucose
   b. Fructose
   c. Galactose
   d. Limit dextrins
   e. Lactose

5. You are studying fuel metabolism in tissue slices prepared from a liver biopsy sample taken from a normal subject. You observe that when both glucose and palmitate are the fuels, the rate of glycolysis is much lower than when glucose only is the fuel. Identify the single statement that correctly explains this observation.
   a. Glucokinase has a higher K_m for glucose than hexokinase does
   b. Palmitate uncoupled oxidative phosphorylation
   c. An increase in [citrate], produced as a result of fatty acid beta-oxidation, has inhibited PFK-1
   d. 5'-AMP is a positive modulator of PFK-1
   e. Palmitate has inhibited glucokinase

6. A newborn infant has a very low blood pH and lactic acidosis is found to be the cause. Potential causes of the increased blood levels of lactic acid include:
   a. Low activity of the pyruvate dehydrogenase complex
   b. An inherited defect in the electron transport chain
   c. Thiamine deficiency
   d. a, b and c are all potential causes

7. During routine analysis of a urine sample from one of your patients you find high levels of ketone bodies. Blood analysis reveals ketonaemia. Potential explanations for the ketonaemia and ketonuria include:
   a. The patient has been on a starvation diet in order to lose weight
   b. The concentrations of oxaloacetate in hepatocytes and muscle are lower than normal
   c. Malonyl-CoA levels in hepatocytes are higher than normal
   d. Both a and b are correct
   e. a, b and c are all correct

8. By accident, the insecticide rotenone is added to a fish tank resulting in the death of most of the fish. Which one of the following is the target for this compound?
   a. Citrate synthase
   b. ATP synthase
   c. Cytochrome c oxidase
   d. NADH dehydrogenase
   e. Succinate dehydrogenase

9. Identify the carbohydrate or fatty acid in Column A that is NOT aligned with the correct statement about its function in the body (Column B):

	A	B
a.	Galactose	Na+-dependent transport in the gut
b.	Fructose	Product of sucrase action
c.	Oleate	Monounsaturated fatty acid
d.	Glucose	Sole product of starch digestion
e.	Sucrose	Reducing sugar

True/false questions

1. Glycogen, cellulose and starch are all polymers of glucose.
2. Maltose is a disaccharide, the monosaccharide units being glucose and fructose.
3. Hexokinase is inhibited by glucose 6-phosphate, the product of the reaction that it catalyses.
4. In most adults, the gut has a greater ability to hydrolyse lactose than it does starch.
5. Insulin action on adipocytes increases the amount of GLUT4 in the plasma membrane of these cells.
6. GLUT2 has a higher K_m for glucose than GLUT1 does.
7. Pyruvate dehydrogenase is a key enzyme in the anaerobic pathway of glucose metabolism in the body.
8. The metabolism of one glucose to pyruvate through the glycolytic pathway produces 2NADH.
9. ATP synthase is localised to the matrix of mitochondria.
10. Carbon monoxide binds to both haemoglobin and cytochrome oxidase.
11. The pyruvate dehydrogenase complex is subject to control by allosteric and covalent modification mechanisms.
12. The reaction in glycolysis catalysed by pyruvate kinase is an example of substrate-level phosphorylation.
13. Most of the oxygen used in animal tissues is used by cytochrome oxidase.
14. The respiratory chain in mitochondria contains several proteins that contain metal atoms, including copper and iron.
15. Proton transport associated with the respiratory chain in mitochondria moves protons (hydrogen ions) outwards across the inner mitochondrial membrane when the chain is functioning.
16. Cyanide reacts with cytochrome oxidase in a similar fashion to carbon monoxide.
17. 5′-AMP levels increase when ATP is being utilised at a high rate in cells.
18. Glucose utilisation per gram of tissue is higher in brain than in muscle in a subject at rest.
19. Each complete beta-oxidation cycle for fatty acid oxidation leads to the production of one molecule of NADH and one of $FADH_2$.
20. All of the enzymes of the TCA cycle are located in the mitochondrial matrix.
21. Isocitrate dehydrogenase and α-ketoglutarate dehydrogenase are important control points in the TCA cycle.

Short note questions

1. In two or three sentence discuss the role of glucose oxidation as it relates to our ability to oxidise fatty acids completely.
2. In 1861, Pasteur observed that, when yeast that had been under anaerobic conditions was switched to aerobic conditions, its glucose consumption (and ethanol production) decreased dramatically. Explain this observation using your knowledge of the control of glycolysis.
3. Explain one way in which cells that are carrying out aerobic metabolism of glucose deal with the impermeability of the inner mitochondrial membrane to NADH.
4. Discuss how the process of oxidative phosphorylation in mitochondria is affected by the presence of 2,4-dinitrophenol.
5. Prepare 'balance sheets' that explain the number of ATPs generated when (a) three molecules of glucose and (b) a molecule of an 18-carbon, saturated fatty acid are completely oxidised in cells capable of oxidative phosphorylation and utilising the malate shuttle.

Self-assessment: answers

Single best answer MCQ answers

1. a. **True**. Stage 1 involves the digestion and absorption of dietary carbohydrates, fats and proteins.
   b. **True**. Glucose is converted to pyruvate and lactate in this pathway.
   c. **True**. Both of these are components of the inner mitochondrial membrane with the former generating a 'proton gradient' and the latter utilising that gradient to synthesise ATP.
   d. **True**.
   e. **True**. This is the single best answer.

2. a. **False**. We need systems where one pathway is switched off while the opposing pathway is switched on and vice versa.
   b. **False**. This would imply that every step in a pathway has a large negative ΔG, which would make it necessary to have completely unique enzymes for every step in opposing pathways.
   c. **True**. The overall free energy change for a pathway must be negative and, clearly, that would not be possible if catabolic and anabolic pathway were the same, i.e. one of them would have an overall positive ΔG.
   d. **False**. Although many reactions in a pathway may be close to equilibrium, none of the reactions in a pathway are at equilibrium since this would mean no net flux through the pathway.

3. a. **False**. Glucose uptake into muscle occurs by facilitated diffusion involving GLUT4 and does not require ATP so would be unaffected by 2,4-dinitrophenol.
   b. **False**. Also facilitated diffusion, this time involving GLUT2.
   c. **False**. Fructose uptake from the gut involves facilitated diffusion using GLUT5.
   d. **True**. This is SGLT1 where there is cotransport of sodium and glucose with the sodium then being pumped out of the mucosal cell.
   e. **False**. Also facilitated diffusion, this time involving GLUT3.

4. a. **False**. The finding of lots of glucose implies a defect in absorption not digestion. A defect in SGLT1 is very rare.
   b. **False**. Same argument as in a. A defect in GLUT5 is very rare.
   c. **False**. Same argument as in a and b. A defect in SGLT1 is very rare.
   d. **True**. α-Dextrinase action is required to hydrolyse the α-1:6-linkages in amylopectin, the major component of starch. The limit dextrins are produced due to amylase action on amylopectin.
   e. **False**. The finding of lactose in the colon implies a defect in lactase and this occurs in patients with lactose intolerance.

5. a. **False**. Glucokinase is important in liver but doesn't explain the observation.
   b. **False**. When oxidative phosphorylation is uncoupled, the respiration rate increases.
   c. **True**. Citrate is a signal that fatty acids are being used as fuel in muscle and when that occurs less glucose need be broken down and PFK-1 is inhibited.
   d. **False**. AMP is an activator of PFK-1 and this provides the link between 'energy charge' and flux through glycolysis.
   e. **False**. There is no known inhibitory effect of palmitate on glucokinase.

6. a. **True**. Pyruvate dehydrogenase complex (PDC) deficiency will lead to an accumulation of pyruvate, resulting in increased production of lactate.
   b. **True**. With less efficient oxidative metabolism the body will turn to increased anaerobic glycolysis and the accumulation of lactate.
   c. **True**. Thiamine pyrophosphate is the coenzyme for E_1 of the PDC complex. Thiamine deficiency will result in less efficient pyruvate oxidation and therefore accumulation of lactate.
   d. **True**. Clearly, this is the single best answer.

7. a. **True**. More fatty acids are released from adipose tissue and this results in more fatty acid catabolism in the liver, with one by-product being ketone bodies.
   b. **True**. With less oxaloacetate, the entry of acetyl-CoA into the TCA cycle will be much less efficient; this will lead to more ketone bodies being formed in the liver and less efficient ketone body catabolism in muscle.
   c. **False**. High malonyl-CoA levels inhibit CPTI, thus the rate of fatty acid oxidation decreases and fewer ketone bodies would be formed.
   d. **True**. This is the single best answer.
   e. **False**. a and b are correct but c is incorrect.

8. a. **False**. There is no known effect of rotenone directly on citrate synthase.
   b. **False**. There is no known effect of rotenone directly on ATP synthase. Indirectly one would expect a decrease in ATP synthesis!
   c. **False**. There is no known effect of rotenone directly on cytochrome *c* oxidase.
   d. **True**. This is the site of action of rotenone and it seriously affects oxidative metabolism.
   e. **False**. There is no known effect of rotenone directly on succinate dehydrogenase. Also, since succinate oxidation produces $FADH_2$, NADH dehydrogenase is by-passed in the electron transport chain.

9. a. **True**. Galactose absorption involves SGLT1 and the sodium pump.
   b. **True**. The products are glucose and fructose.
   c. **True**. Oleate has 18 carbons and a double bond at the 9 position.
   d. **True**. Starch is a polymer of glucose.
   e. **False**. Sucrose has a 1–2 bond that eliminates the reducing groups of glucose and fructose, respectively.

True/false answers

1. **True**. Although cellulose is not digested by humans, like starch and glycogen it is a polymer of glucose.
2. **False**. Maltose is a disaccharide formed during the digestion of starch. It has an α-1,4-linkage between two glucoses.
3. **True**. This property distinguishes hexokinase from glucokinase.
4. **False**. Many adults from several ethnic groups show a large decrease in brush border lactase activity as they enter their teens. As a result, they have problems handling the lactose in milk.
5. **True**. Insulin action recruits GLUT4 molecules to the plasma membrane of adipocytes (and muscle), leading to greatly increased glucose uptake.
6. **True**. GLUT2 occurs in tissues that take up glucose from blood when glucose levels are high.
7. **False**. The pyruvate dehydrogenase complex catalyses a reaction that is the main determinant of aerobic metabolism of glucose in well-oxygenated tissues.
8. **True**. The glycolytic pathway has a single NAD^+-dependent dehydrogenase, 3-phosphoglyceraldehyde dehydrogenase. In effect, each glucose is converted to two molecules of 3-phosphoglyceraldehyde by the action of triosephosphate isomerase.

9. **False**. It spans the inner mitochondrial membrane, allowing it to utilise the proton gradient to drive its reversible ATPase and thus produce ATP from ADP + P_i.
10. **True**. Both are haem proteins and carbon monoxide binds to the ferrous (FeII) form, thus competing with oxygen!
11. **True**. It is E_1 of the multiple enzyme complex that is controlled by phosphorylation/dephosphorylation. The E_1 kinase and E_1 phosphatase involved are subject to allosteric control by metabolic intermediates.
12. **True**. The reaction phosphoenolpyruvate to pyruvate can be coupled to the formation of ATP from ADP. This is termed 'substrate-level' phosphorylation, contrasting it with oxidative phosphorylation.
13. **True**. Cytochrome oxidase catalyses the terminal reaction of the electron transport chain, where molecular oxygen is involved.
14. **True**. In addition to iron-containing cytochromes *b* and *c*, there is cytochrome oxidase, which contains both iron and copper. There are also iron–sulphur proteins.
15. **True**. The proton gradient generated then drives ATP synthesis using ATP synthase.
16. **False**. Cyanide reacts with the ferric (Fe^{III}) form of cytochrome oxidase (and haemoglobin), whereas carbon monoxide reacts with the ferrous (Fe^{II}) form of these haem proteins.
17. **True**. 5′-AMP is formed from ADP in the reaction catalysed by adenylate kinase: 2ADP→ATP + AMP.
18. **True**. Muscle at rest utilises significant amounts of fatty acids, whereas brain can only use glucose.
19. **True**. NAD^+- and FAD-linked dehydrogenases are involved in each beta-oxidation cycle.
20. **False**. Succinate dehydrogenase is located in the inner mitochondrial membrane.
21. **True**. Both are affected by the levels of NADH and ATP.

Short note answers

1. Fatty acids are oxidised to carbon dioxide and water in the mitochondria of tissues such as liver, skeletal muscle and cardiac muscle. The process of beta-oxidation produces many molecules of acetyl-CoA, which are then oxidised in the TCA cycle leading to the production of NADH and $FADH_2$. However, this process is very dependent upon an adequate supply of oxaloacetate to operate the first step in the TCA cycle. Without the concomitant metabolism of glucose, oxaloacetate is not maintained at adequate

levels. This is one of the reasons for excess ketone body production in type 1 diabetes mellitus. This question is covered by the old phrase 'fat burns in the flame of carbohydrate'.

2. The introduction of oxygen opens up the great potential for ATP synthesis in mitochondria. As a consequence, the amount of glucose that has to be metabolised to support the same level of work must drop by about 95% (38 ATP per glucose in aerobic metabolism versus 2 ATP per glucose in anaerobic metabolism). The point of control is the conversion of fructose 6-phosphate to fructose 1,6-bisphosphate, catalysed by phosphofructokinase-1 (PFK-1). ATP is a negative modulator of this enzyme. Therefore, when ATP production from oxidative metabolism increases, PFK-1 will be inhibited and the glycolytic rate will fall. Similar observations have been made using in vitro skeletal muscle preparations that are 'twitching' and glucose metabolism is measured under anaerobic and then aerobic conditions.

3. The glycerol 3-phosphate and malate shuttles are used to overcome this problem. In the former, dihydroxyacetone phosphate is reduced to glycerol 3-phosphate by a cytosolic glycerol-3-phosphate dehydrogenase. A similar dehydrogenase located on the inner mitochondrial membrane reforms dihydroxyacetone phosphate; $FADH_2$ is produced, which has the potential to generate ATP. Thus, NAD^+ is regenerated to maintain glycolysis and ATP is also produced. The malate shuttle is more complicated but the principle is similar. Oxaloacetate is reduced to malate in the cytosol and the opposing reaction in mitochondria regenerates oxaloacetate, producing mitochondrial NADH. The complication of this shuttle is that oxaloacetate does not cross the inner mitochondrial membrane and its equivalent amino acid, aspartate, has to be an intermediate to allow this to occur.

4. 2,4-Dinitrophenol (DNP) is a lipid-soluble compound that has acidic and basic forms. When it is added to mitochondria that are actively respiring, it becomes protonated and can pass through the inner mitochondrial membrane. The result is that the proton gradient is collapsed and this will be reflected in a sharp drop in ATP synthesis by ATP synthase (which depends upon that proton gradient!). If one is measuring both ATP synthesis and oxygen utilisation in the mitochondrial preparation, one can see the drop in ATP production accompanied by an increase in oxygen utilisation (respiration). For this reason, DNP is described as an uncoupler: it uncouples oxidation (electron transport chain activity) from phosphorylation (ATP synthesis).

5. (a) Glucose

Glycolysis→2Pyruvate + 2NADH		2ATP
2NADH	Malate shuttle	6ATP
2Pyruvate→2Acetyl-CoA + 2NADH		
2NADH		6ATP
2Acetyl-CoA	TCA cycle, electron transport chain, ATP synthase	24ATP
Total ATP for 1 glucose		38
Total ATP for 3 glucose		114

(b) Stearate

Activation of stearate		Uses equivalent of 2 ATP
8 Beta-oxidations:		
8 $FADH_2$		16 ATP
8 NADH		24 ATP
9 Acetyl-CoA	TCA cycle, electron transport chain, ATP synthase	108 ATP
Total ATP for 1 stearate		148–2 = 146

In conclusion: The complete oxidation of stearate yields more ATP per carbon than oxidation of glucose. Note that the ATP yield per oxygen is slightly greater for glucose than for stearate.

7 Other carbohydrate metabolic pathways

Overview

Glycogen is stored in significant quantities in both muscle and the liver. Muscle glycogen is used as a fuel whereas liver glycogen is used as a 'reservoir' to maintain adequate levels of glucose in blood. The pathways of glycogenesis and glycogenolysis are under control by hormones such as insulin, glucagon and adrenaline (epinephrine). Because of the requirement for glucose as a fuel by the central nervous system, gluconeogenesis occurring in the liver is another pathway vital for glucose homeostasis. Glucose metabolised by the pentose phosphate pathway provides the ribose 5-phosphate required for nucleotide synthesis throughout the body, as well as NADPH which supplies reducing power for reductive biosyntheses and defence against reactive oxygen species.

7.1 Glycogen metabolism

Learning objectives

You should be able to:

- describe the roles of muscle and liver glycogen in the body

- outline the pathways for glycogen synthesis and breakdown and how the pathways are controlled in an integrated fashion.

Glycogen is found in many cell types in the body but only in high concentration in liver and muscle. A fed man weighing 70 kg will have about 1.6 kg of liver containing about 100 g of glycogen and 35 kg of muscle containing approximately 400 g of glycogen. At a caloric value of 17 kJ/g, the stores of glycogen represent about 8500 kJ of fuel. Relative to the fat stores, this is a small reserve, yet it has great functional significance. Glycogen is stored in the fed state and utilised during fasting and exercise. Synthesis (glycogenesis) and breakdown (glycogenolysis) occur by separate but related pathways (Fig. 64) and are controlled in an integrated fashion via allosteric and covalent mechanisms; hormonal control is very critical. The enzymes of glycogen metabolism are associated with the glycogen granules in cells.

Glycogenesis

The key points about the storage of glycogen:

- A step unique to glycogenesis is the formation of UDP-glucose (UDPG) from glucose 1-phosphate (G-1-P) and the pyrimidine nucleotide UTP.
- The glucose moieties added to form glycogen come directly from UDPG.
- The hydrolysis of pyrophosphate 'pulls' the pathway towards glycogen.
- Each glycogen molecule contains a protein, *glycogenin*, which initiates the synthesis of the large glycogen molecule. Glycogenin has enzymatic activity catalysing the addition of the first 4–8 glucose moieties to a tyrosine in glycogenin, using UDPG as the source of the glucoses.
- *Glycogen synthase* transfers the glucose moiety of UDPG to the non-reducing end of the primer, giving a polymer with α-1,4-linkages.
- Glycogen is branched, the enzyme involved being a *4:6-transferase*.

Glycogenolysis

Key points about the breakdown of stored glycogen:

- *Glycogen phosphorylase* catalyses the interaction of inorganic phosphate (P_i) with terminal α-1:4-glycosidic bonds at the multiple non-reducing ends of glycogen to yield G-1-P.
- Phosphorylase contains the coenzyme pyridoxal phosphate.

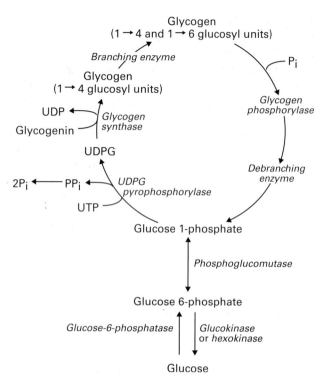

Fig. 64 Pathways of glycogenesis and glycogenolysis.

- The branching of glycogen means that there are many sites (ends) for phosphorolysis and this allows for rapid production of G-1-P, which is beneficial in both liver and muscle.
- *Debranching enzyme* has two distinct catalytic sites and is important for complete utilisation of glycogen. Phosphorylase action stops at four glucoses from branch point, then a *4:4 glucan transferase* transfers three glucoses to a different chain. This leaves a single glucose attached at the branch point and the α-1,6-linkage is hydrolysed by *α-1:6-glucosidase* to yield free glucose.
- Muscle lacks *glucose-6-phosphatase (G-6-Pase)*, so the end-products of increased muscle glycogenolysis will be pyruvate and lactate (following glycolysis); liver contains G-6-Pase, which means that the end-product there is glucose.
- Clearly the different end-products in liver compared with muscle are consistent with the role of glycogen in muscle, which is to supply that tissue with ATP, and the role of glycogen in liver to maintain blood glucose levels.

Glycogenesis and glycogenolysis are controlled in an integrated fashion

It is essential to consider the control of the synthetic and breakdown pathways together (Fig. 65) since, in general,

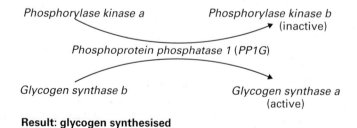

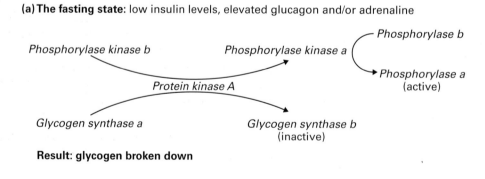

(a) The fasting state: low insulin levels, elevated glucagon and/or adrenaline

Result: glycogen broken down

(b) The fed state: high insulin levels, low glucagon levels

Result: glycogen synthesised

Fig. 65 Control of glycogenesis and glycogenolysis in the liver in the fasted (a) and fed (b) states.

when one pathway is activated, the other is switched off. Glycogen synthase and glycogen phosphorylase are the key control enzymes. They are both subject to control by allosteric and covalent modification.

Allosteric control

- ATP and G-6-P levels high: glycogen synthase active, phosphorylase inactive.
- AMP levels high: glycogen synthase inactive, phosphorylase active.

High [ATP] in muscle is indicative of high energy charge and is a signal that there is less need for glycogen breakdown. In contrast, increased [AMP] is a signal that ATP utilisation is high. Elevated [G-6-P] in both liver and muscle is associated with the fed state and increased availability of glucose (for storage).

Covalent control

- Cyclic AMP-dependent protein kinase A (PKA) active: glycogen synthase inactive, phosphorylase active.
- Phosphoprotein phosphatase active: glycogen synthase active, phosphorylase inactive.

Both enzymes exist in more active and less active states. In each case, the more active form is designated 'a', and the less active form is 'b'. Phosphorylation occurs when there is an increase in cyclic AMP. Dephosphorylation involves a phosphoprotein phosphatase.

Hormonal control

Glucagon (liver) and adrenaline (epinephrine) (muscle) action results in increased concentration of cyclic AMP within these cells and activation of PKA. This results in activation of phosphorylase and inactivation of glycogen synthase. Further description of these control mechanisms can be found in Chapters 10 and 17.

Insulin release in the fed state leads to the dephosphorylation of both phosphorylase and glycogen synthase. This results in inactivation of phosphorylase and activation of glycogen synthase (Ch. 10).

Clinical note:
Glycogen storage disease

Defects in enzymes of glycogenolysis usually result in a glycogen storage disease. Subjects with defective branching enzyme in liver have a tendency to develop hypoglycaemia, but the most severe form is seen in those with defective liver G-6-Pase. Subjects with defective muscle phosphorylase cannot support high levels of physical activity.

Effects of calcium

Phosphorylase kinase is also activated by increased concentrations of calcium (Ca^{2+}). This is explained by the fact that phosphorylase kinase has four subunits (α, β, γ, δ) and the δ-subunit is the calcium-binding polypeptide, *calmodulin*. Binding of calcium activates the enzyme, leading finally to increased phosphorylation of the α- and β-subunits of phosphorylase kinase (and thus to activation). Calcium is an important signal for muscle contraction; activation of glycogen breakdown will lead to the increased ATP formation required to support this. Adrenaline (epinephrine) action on the liver is mediated via α_1-adrenoceptors, leading to increased levels of inositol trisphosphate and Ca^{2+} (see pp 248–249).

7.2 Gluconeogenesis

Learning objectives

You should be able to:

- list the important gluconeogenic precursors
- describe the three substrate cycles and how they are controlled
- identify roles for the Cori and the glucose–alanine cycles.

This pathway is defined as 'the formation of glucose from non-carbohydrate sources'. Gluconeogenesis is vital to normal brain function in the fasting state since, despite the high concentration of glycogen in the liver, its total content would be used up by about 16–24 hours of fasting. As a result, glucose synthesis is vital. The liver is the principal site for gluconeogenesis, although the kidney also has the pathway.

Glucogenic precursors include amino acids, lactate and glycerol

Amino acids

Many amino acids are glucogenic (Ch. 8). The metabolism of their carbons results in a net increase in oxaloacetate. This means that any amino acid whose carbons enter the tricarboxylic acid cycle at any point *other than* acetyl-CoA or whose carbons are converted to pyruvate will be glucogenic (see Fig. 77, p. 116).

Lactate and glycerol

Lactate and glycerol are released during anaerobic glycolysis in muscle and fat mobilisation from adipose tissue, respectively. Lactate dehydrogenase in liver converts lactate to pyruvate. The liver contains a kinase that converts glycerol to glycerol 3-phosphate, the oxidation of which yields dihydroxyacetone phosphate, a gluconeogenesis intermediate. Glycerol is the substrate most easily converted to glucose.

The gluconeogenesis pathway

Most of the reactions of gluconeogenesis are catalysed by the enzymes of the glycolytic sequence (Fig. 66). Because glycolysis and gluconeogenesis are opposing pathways, there has to be control so that glucose formation or breakdown will occur in a physiologically sound fashion. The flux through the respective pathways is governed by:

- allosteric effectors
- covalent modification of enzymes
- enzyme concentrations.

Covalent modification of key enzymes in liver is brought about (in the main) by fluctuations in the ratio of insulin to glucagon in blood. Insulin is the principal modulator in the fed state when glycolysis should be active, glucagon in the fasting state when gluconeogenesis should be active. Three steps in glycolysis are virtually irreversible and have to be by-passed in gluconeogenesis; three *substrate cycles* are involved where control can be imposed (Fig. 67).

PEP/pyruvate substrate cycle

- The first step from pyruvate is catalysed by *pyruvate carboxylase* (PC), a biotin-requiring enzyme of mitochondria, and yields oxaloacetate. PC utilises ATP and has an *absolute requirement* for acetyl-CoA as an allosteric activator.
- The next reaction yields phosphoenolpyruvate (PEP) and is catalysed by *phosphoenolpyruvate carboxykinase* (PEPCK), which uses GTP.
- Control is through activation of PC and inhibition of PDC by an increase in the level of acetyl-CoA; the acetyl-CoA is derived from increased utilisation of fatty acids in the liver during fasting. Also involved is induction of PEPCK by glucagon action.

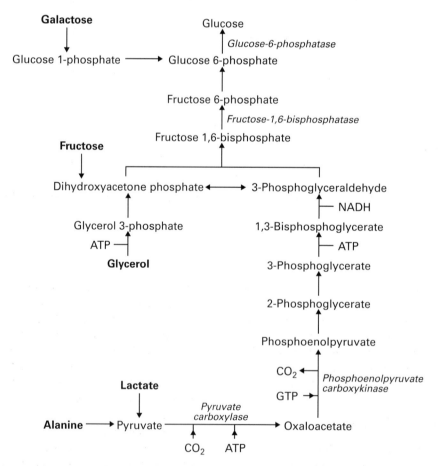

Fig. 66 The gluconeogenesis pathway. Enzymes catalysing reactions unique to gluconeogenesis are shown. The reactions are shown that are involved in the conversion of lactate, alanine, glycerol, fructose and galactose to glucose. This pathway occurs mainly in the liver.

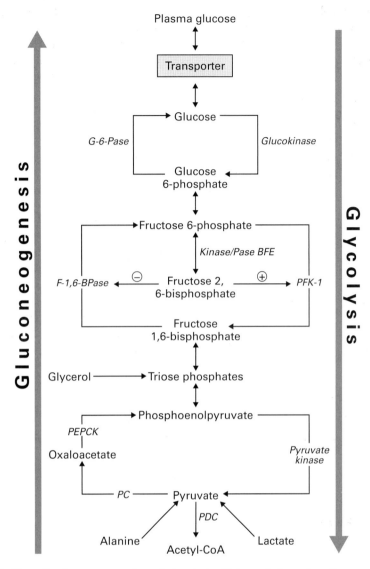

Fig. 67 Integrated control of hepatic gluconeogenesis and glycolysis. (Schematic based on Granner and O'Brien (1992) *Diabetes Care* 15: 369–395.)

- Liver-type PK is allosterically activated by fructose 1,6-bisphosphate (F-1,6-BP) and inhibited by alanine and ATP; it is also inactivated by phosphorylation. Therefore, the increase in alanine and glucagon in the fasted state results in complete inhibition of PK, avoiding a futile cycle and promoting gluconeogenesis.

F-6-P/F-1,6-BP substrate cycle

- *Fructose-1,6-bisphosphatase* (F-1,6-BPase) converts F-1,6-BP to F-6-P (fructose 6-phosphate) and inorganic phosphate (P$_i$). F-1,6-BPase is inhibited by fructose 2,6-bisphosphate (F-2,6-BP).

- [F-2,6-BP] determines the flux through this substrate cycle. F-2,6-BP is controlled by a bifunctional enzyme (BFE) which has kinase and phosphatase activities and is itself subjected to control by phosphorylation/dephosphorylation.
- Phosphorylation of BFE occurs when glucagon has increased PKA activity; the F-2,6-BPase of the BFE is activated, F-2,6-BP levels fall and gluconeogenesis is turned on.
- Dephosphorylation of BFE occurs when insulin levels are high. F-2,6-BP rises, leading to inhibition of gluconeogenesis and activation of glycolysis; the resulting increase in F-1,6-BP will activate glycolysis at the PK step.

G-6-P/glucose substrate cycle

- Glucose-6-phosphatase (G-6-Pase), located on the cisternal surface of the endoplasmic reticulum, catalyses the hydrolysis of G-6-P to give free glucose and inorganic phosphate.
- Clearly, G-6-Pase is essential for glucose production to occur from both glycogenolysis and gluconeogenesis. It is not present in muscle!
- There is no evidence as yet for short-term regulation of this cycle.

In summary. It is the PEP/pyruvate cycle that limits the rate of gluconeogenesis, since the rate of glucose synthesis is much greater for substrates that enter the pathway at the triose phosphate level (e.g. glycerol) than for substrates such as alanine and lactate that enter the pathway through pyruvate. PK is inhibited when glucose production should be favoured (i.e. in the fasted state) and is active when glucose is being processed in the fed state towards pyruvate, acetyl-CoA and fatty acid synthesis. The importance of modulating the level of F-2,6-BP is that it provides a mechanism for controlling F-1,6-BP, which is itself a major modulator of PK.

Sources of glucose

The glucose–alanine cycle connects muscle and liver metabolism

The glucose–alanine cycle (Fig. 68) describes the movement of alanine in the fasting state from muscle to the liver where it is converted to glucose. This allows for increased glucose secretion into the blood where it can be used by the central nervous system as fuel. This process also occurs during exercise and the glucose produced from alanine can return to muscle to be used as a fuel.

The Cori cycle also connects muscle and liver metabolism

The Cori cycle (Fig. 69) involves lactate leaving skeletal muscle during vigorous exercise, being converted to glucose in the liver and returning to muscle to be used as a fuel.

Galactose and fructose are glucogenic

Glucose can also be synthesised from galactose and fructose in the liver (Figs 70 and 71).

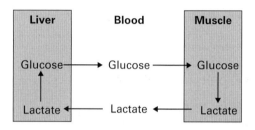

Fig. 69 The Cori cycle. In the Cori cycle, lactate released from muscle is reconverted to glucose in the liver.

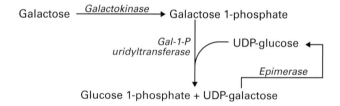

Overall: Galactose + ATP ⟶ G-1-P + ADP

Fig. 70 Glucose production from galactose.

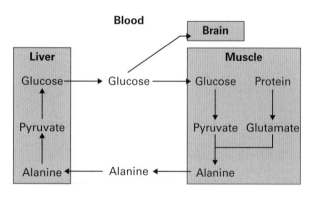

Fig. 68 The glucose–alanine cycle.

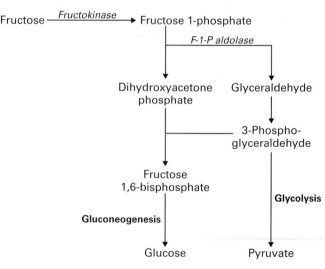

Fig. 71 Glucose production from fructose.

Newborn babies are tested to ensure that they do not have excessive levels of galactose in their blood. Galactosaemia is dangerous, especially if the defect is in *galactose-1-phosphate uridyltransferase*. In this disorder, galactose 1-phosphate accumulates, leading to depletion of phosphate in the liver. Liver failure and mental retardation are the results. Because of the serious consequences of galactosaemia and the relative ease of reducing galactose intake by restricting lactose in the diet, screening for galactosaemia is carried out routinely in samples taken from neonates and the condition has to be dealt with promptly.

7.3 Pentose phosphate pathway

Learning objectives

You should be able to:

- outline the function of the PPP in metabolism

- describe what is accomplished in the oxidative phase of the PPP

- explain how the PPP responds to the demand of cells for NADPH and ribose 5-phosphate.

The pentose phosphate pathway (PPP) is an important alternative pathway for the oxidative metabolism of G-6-P leading to the production of pentose phosphate and NADPH. In contrast to glycolysis, the PPP does not result in ATP synthesis. The PPP is important because:

- Ribose 5-phosphate production is required for the biosynthesis of purine and pyrimidine nucleotides and, therefore, for RNA and DNA and the numerous nucleotides that play key roles in intermediary metabolism, including ATP, UTP, CTP, GTP, *S*-adenosylmethionine, FAD, NAD and NADP

- Production of 'reducing power' in the form of NADPH is required for the synthesis of fatty acids, cholesterol and steroid hormones as well as for the maintenance of reduced glutathione levels which are vital for defence against reactive oxygen species.
- 3-, 4-, 5-, 6- and 7-carbon sugars are interconverted.

The overall design of the pathway

It is convenient to divide the pathway into oxidative and cycling phases (Fig. 72, p. 104).

The oxidative phase (irreversible)

- Yields pentose phosphate and NADPH.
- Consists of three reactions, two catalysed by NADP$^+$-linked dehydrogenases, including the rate-controlling step involving *G-6-P dehydrogenase* (G-6-PDH). G-6-PDH deficiency is described in Chapter 19.
- The net reaction is 6G-6-P→6 (ribulose 5-phosphate) + 12NADPH + 6CO$_2$.

The cycling phase (reversible)

- Pentose phosphates are converted to the glycolytic intermediates F-6-P and 3-phosphoglyceraldehyde through a series of reactions catalysed in sequence by *transketolase*, *transaldolase* and, again, *transketolase*.
- Transketolase has thiamine pyrophosphate (TPP) as coenzyme.
- The net reaction is 6 ribulose 5-phosphate→5G-6-P (via F-6-P).

Cells that have a high requirement for both ribose 5-phosphate and NADPH will have low activity of the 'cycling phase'. In cells that mainly require NADPH, both phases occur, which means, in effect, that six complete cycles occur for each molecule of G-6-P and 6 molecules of carbon dioxide and 12 molecules of NADPH are produced.

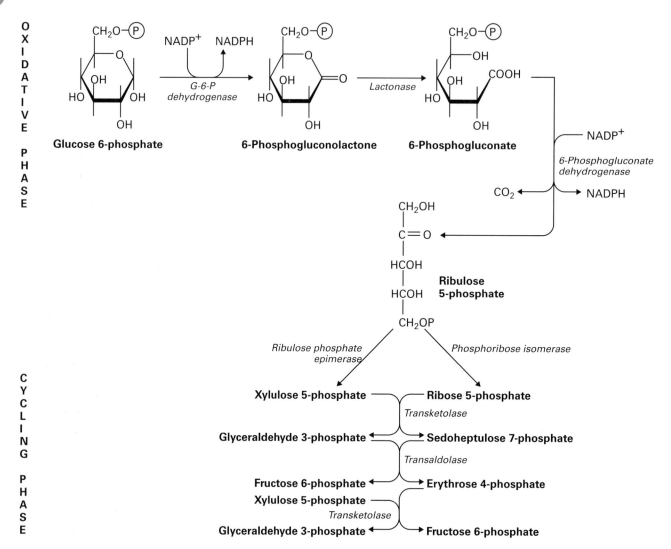

Fig. 72 The pentose phosphate pathway. The main function of this pathway is production of NADPH, used in reductive biosynthesis, and ribose 5-phosphate, needed for nucleotide synthesis.

Self-assessment: questions

Single best answer MCQs

1. Given the fact that skeletal muscle glycogenolysis can increase several hundred-fold when an athlete is a few seconds into a sprint, which of the following describes how that occurs?
   a. Activation of fatty acid oxidation
   b. Dephosphorylation of glycogen phosphorylase by phosphoprotein phosphatase-1 (PP-1)
   c. Dephosphorylation of glycogen synthase by phosphoprotein phosphatase-1 (PP-1)
   d. Allosteric activation of glycogen phosphorylase by 5'-AMP coupled with increased binding of Ca^{2+} to phosphorylase kinase
   e. Binding of glucagon to receptors in skeletal muscle

2. The activity of glycogen synthase and glycogen phosphorylase in muscle and liver are reciprocally regulated. Which of the following modulators bring this about?
   a. Fructose 1,6-bisphosphate
   b. Fructose 2,6-bisphosphate
   c. Glucose 1-phosphate
   d. Cyclic AMP
   e. UDPG

3. After noticing that his weight is no longer ideal, a 22-year-old man decides for the first time in his life to engage in exercise that includes running fast 400-metre laps. He immediately develops very painful cramps as well as noticing that his urine is red. The latter is found to be due to myoglobinuria. Further examination reveals very high muscle glycogen of normal structure and no increase in blood lactate upon exercise. The patient most likely has a deficiency of which of the following skeletal muscle enzymes.
   a. Debranching enzyme
   b. Branching enzyme
   c. Glycogen phosphorylase
   d. ATP synthase
   e. Pyruvate dehydrogenase

4. Various metabolites can be used as gluconeogenic precursors. Which of the following enzymes is required for glucose formation from alanine but not for glucose formation from glycerol?
   a. Fructose-1,6-bisphosphatase
   b. 3-Phosphoglyceraldehyde dehydrogenase
   c. Glucose-6-phosphatase
   d. Aldolase
   e. Phosphohexose isomerase

5. In the fructose 6-phosphate/fructose 1,6-bisphosphate substrate cycle, which modulator is an activator of phosphofructokinase-1 (PFK-1) and an inhibitor of F-1,6-BPase and whose concentration is increased when a bifunctional enzyme is dephosphorylated?
   a. Fructose 6-phosphate
   b. Glucose 6-phosphate
   c. 3-Phosphoglyceraldehyde
   d. Fructose 2,6-bisphosphate
   e. Phosphoenolpyruvate

6. In your paediatric practice you are asked to examine a 2-year-old child who has an enlarged liver and has had many episodes that seem to be consistent with hypoglycaemia, including sweating, tremors, pallor and hunger. You recommend a referral to a liver expert who takes a liver biopsy that has enormously high levels of glycogen with normal structure. Also noted is the inability of the patient's liver to form glucose from either glycogen or pyruvate. The most likely diagnosis is a deficiency of what?
   a. Phosphoglucomutase
   b. Glucose-6-phosphatase
   c. Phosphoenolpyruvate carboxykinase
   d. Glycogen phosphorylase
   e. Fructose-1,6-bisphosphatase

7. A mutation present in some populations and affecting millions of males causes a deficiency in glucose-6-phosphate dehydrogenase (G6PDH) in erythrocytes. Which one of the following situations results when this defect exists in mature erythrocytes?
   a. Increased ability to deal with oxidant drugs
   b. Reduced ability to synthesize ribose phosphate
   c. Haemolytic anaemia
   d. High levels of reduced glutathione in erythrocytes

8. If a cell requires ribose 5-phosphate but does not require NADPH, which of the following describes the status of the pentose phosphate pathway (PPP) at that time in that cell?
   a. Only the oxidative phase of the PPP would be operational
   b. NADPH would be destroyed by nucleotidases

   c. Glycolytic intermediates would flow into the reversible (cycling) phase of the PPP

   d. Glucose-6-phosphate dehydrogenase would be activated

True/false questions

Are the following statements true or false?

1. The gluconeogenic pathway from pyruvate requires input of both NADH and ATP.
2. Thiamine pyrophosphate is a coenzyme for transketolase of the pentose phosphate pathway.
3. Even-numbered fatty acids are glucogenic in the liver.
4. The pyruvate kinase activity in liver is inhibited by alanine and by phosphorylation.
5. In glycogenolysis, debranching produces one free glucose per branch point.
6. Glucagon activates glycogenolysis in both liver and skeletal muscle.
7. 5'-AMP is a positive modulator of glycogen phosphorylase and phosphofructokinase-1 (PFK-1).
8. Glycogenesis and glycogenolysis occur in different intracellular compartments of the liver and muscle.
9. Acetyl-CoA activates pyruvate carboxylase and thus increases gluconeogenesis.
10. The PPP produces ribose 5-phosphate required for nucleotide synthesis.
11. Both galactose and fructose are glucogenic precursors.
12. The Cori cycle is significant during exercise and the glucose-alanine cycle is significant during fasting.

Short essay questions

1. Describe the active form of the enzyme catalysing the rate-limiting step of glycogenesis and then derive from that the nature of the inactive form. Repeat for the enzyme catalysing the rate-limiting step in glycogenolysis. Describe how these changes fit logically into a system to control glycogen metabolism.
2. Describe how gluconeogenesis in the liver is controlled in order to maintain glucose homeostasis during the fasting state.

Case history

The following data were obtained from a patient.

> A liver biopsy sample when incubated in the presence of 10^{-9} M adrenaline (epinephrine) or glucagon showed increased production of pyruvate and lactate. Incubation with uniformly labelled [^{14}C]alanine showed that radioactivity could be incorporated into glycogen but not into glucose. A muscle biopsy sample when incubated with 10^{-9} M adrenaline (epinephrine) showed a large increase in lactate production. The glycogen isolated from liver and muscle had normal structure but liver glycogen concentrations were significantly above normal.

What diagnosis are these observations consistent with?

Self-assessment: answers

Single best answer MCQ answers

1. a. **False**. The rate of ATP production from fatty acid oxidation is much too slow to support sprinting. Also, it is delayed.
   b. **False**. This would lead to inactivation of phosphorylase, the opposite of what is required.
   c. **False**. This would lead to activation of glycogen synthase. We don't need glycogen synthesis, we need glycogen breakdown!
   d. **True**. 5'-AMP is an activator of phosphorylase *b*. Phosphorylase kinase is activated by the increase in Ca^{2+} that occurs when muscular contraction begins and the subsequent phosphorylation of phosphorylase gives the active form and rapid glycogen breakdown.
   e. **False**. Glucagon receptors are not present in muscle. Adrenaline (epinephrine) is the hormonal stimulator of muscle glycogenolysis.

2. a. **False**. F-1,6-BP is a glycolytic intermediate.
   b. **False**. F-2,6-BP controls PFK-1 and F-1,6-BPase. Wrong pathways.
   c. **False** An unlikely candidate since it is an intermediate in both pathways.
   d. **True**. An increase in cyclic AMP activates PKA, leading to inactivation of glycogen synthase and activation of phosphorylase.
   e. **False**. Another unlikely candidate. It is an intermediate in glycogenesis.

3. a. **False**. Although this defect would have some effect, some glycogenolysis could occur.
   b. **False**. The glycogen structure was normal.
   c. **True**. This defect would severely limit the ability to exercise vigorously. Paining cramps occur and rhabdomyolysis leads to release of myoglobin. This is glycogen storage disease type V (McArdle's syndrome).
   d. **False**. Sprinting is supported by anaerobic metabolism.
   e. **False**. Sprinting is supported by anaerobic metabolism.

4. a. **False**. This enzyme is required in both cases.
   b. **True**. Glycerol is converted to dihydroxyacetone phosphate and G-3-P, which combine to give F-1,6-BP without the dehydrogenase being involved. The dehydrogenase is required for gluconeogenesis from alanine via pyruvate.
   c. **False**. This is the critical enzyme that allows the liver to make glucose and is required for gluconeogenesis whatever the source of the carbons.
   d. **False**. This enzyme converts dihydroxyacetone phosphate and G-3-P to F-1,6-BP and is required in both cases.
   e. **False**. This enzyme converts F-6-P to G-6-P en route to glucose and clearly is required in both cases.

5. a. **False**. F-6-P is a glycolysis and gluconeogenesis intermediate. It is not directly involved in control.
   b. **False**. G-6-P is a glycolysis and gluconeogenesis intermediate. It is not directly involved in control.
   c. **False**. G-3-P is a glycolysis and gluconeogenesis intermediate. It is not directly involved in control.
   d. **True**. F-2,6-BP inhibits F-1,6-BPase (gluconeogenesis) and activates PFK-1 (glycolysis). The bifunctional enzyme (BFE) when dephosphorylated has kinase activity and converts more F-6-P to F-2,6-BP.
   e. **False**. PEP is a glycolysis and gluconeogenesis intermediate. It isn't directly involved in control.

6. a. **False**. A defect in phosphoglucomutase would not prevent the conversion of pyruvate to glucose.
   b. **True**. This enzyme is required for glucose production from both glycogen and pyruvate. Defect is glycogen storage disease type I (von Gierke's disease).
   c. **False**. This defect would not prevent glucose production from glycogen.
   d. **False**. This defect would not prevent glucose production from pyruvate.
   e. **False**. This defect would not prevent glucose production from glycogen.

7. a. **False**. These drugs generate reactive oxygen species and the defect lowers glutathione levels and the ability to respond especially in erythrocytes.
   b. **False**. Ribose 5-phosphate can be synthesised without G6PDH activity since the cycling phase of the pentose phosphate pathway is reversible.

c. **True**. Low levels of glutathione result from the deficiency, hence the defence mechanism against oxygen free radicals is impaired and erythrocytes lyse.

d. **False**. Low NADPH production lowers reduced glutathione.

8. a. **False**. NADPH would be produced and eventually the PPP would shut down.

b. **False**. The body doesn't operate in such an unsophisticated way. Metabolic control is always sensible!

c. **True**. F-6-P and G-3-P start the reverse of the cycling phase with the eventual synthesis of enough ribose 5-phosphate.

d. **False**. This would certainly lead to more NADPH being formed.

True/false answers

1. **True**. NADH is required to convert 1,3-bisphosphoglycerate to 3-phosphoglyceraldehyde and ATP (or GTP) is required at three of the steps.
2. **True**. Thiamine deficiency results in decreased activity of the pentose phosphate pathway.
3. **False**. Since they are converted entirely to acetyl-CoA, they are ketogenic rather than glucogenic.
4. **True**. These are important signals leading to inhibition of pyruvate kinase, meaning that gluconeogenesis will then proceed more effectively.
5. **True**. The debranching system includes a 1,6-glucosidase that catalyses the hydrolysis of 1,6-bonds, yielding one free glucose per bond.
6. **False**. Glucagon has no effect on muscle glycogen metabolism. Adrenaline (epinephrine) is the hormone that activates muscle glycogenolysis.
7. **True**. An increase in intracellular AMP is a signal that cells require to turn on ATP synthesis; it activates both phosphorylase *b*, the rate-controlling step in glycogen breakdown, and PFK-1, an important rate-controlling step in glycolysis.
8. **False**. The enzymes involved are found in the cytosol associated with glycogen granules.
9. **True**. This enzyme is almost inactive without bound acetyl-CoA.
10. **True**. The major function of the PPP is to make NADPH and ribose 5-phosphate.
11. **True**. Both are metabolised in the liver and can be converted to G-6-P and enter glycolysis or be converted to glycogen. Inability to handle galactose is a serious disorder!
12. **True**. The lactate produced in fast-twitch skeletal muscle during vigorous exercise can be used as a fuel by slow-twitch muscle but it can also be converted to glucose by the liver and returned to muscle as a fuel. Alanine is released from muscle in the fasting state and is converted to glucose in the liver. That glucose is then available to the brain as a fuel.

Short essay answers

1. Glycogen synthase catalyses the rate-determining step in glycogenesis and it is active when it is dephosphorylated. Logically, since it would be inefficient for glycogenolysis to be active when glycogenesis is active, the enzyme catalysing the rate-determining step in glycogenolysis, glycogen phosphorylase, must be inactive when dephosphorylated. Similarly, in glycogenolysis, phosphorylase is active when it is phosphorylated and glycogen synthase, in contrast, must be inactive when phosphorylated.

   Under conditions when glycogen should be synthesised (i.e. the fed state and when insulin and glucose levels are high), glycogen synthase and phosphorylase are both dephosphorylated, with the former then being active and the latter inactive. Under conditions when glycogenolysis should be promoted (i.e. the fasted state as far as liver glycogen is concerned and exercise as far as muscle glycogen is concerned), both control enzymes are phosphorylated, leading to activation of phosphorylase and inactivation of glycogen synthase.

2. Gluconeogenesis is controlled at the level of two of the substrate cycles that involve the opposing pathways of glycolysis and gluconeogenesis (Fig. 67).

   The pyruvate/PEP substrate cycle. Fasting conditions should lead to increased conversion of pyruvate to PEP via oxaloacetate. This is mediated largely by the action of glucagon, alanine and acetyl-CoA. Glucagon stimulates an increase in cyclic AMP, leading to activation of protein kinase A. This activity results in the phosphorylation of pyruvate kinase and to its inactivation. Alanine, which enters liver at an enhanced rate during fasting (the source is muscle protein turnover), also inhibits pyruvate kinase. Inhibition of pyruvate kinase means that any PEP formed from alanine or lactate via pyruvate and oxaloacetate will not be dissipated and futile cycling is avoided. Also, during fasting, more fatty acids are mobilised to the liver and their oxidation yields acetyl-CoA, an activator of pyruvate carboxylase, resulting in increased production of oxaloacetate from which PEP, and eventually glucose, is formed. The increase in acetyl-CoA production also inhibits the pyruvate decarboxylase and this will also increase the overall efficiency of gluconeogenesis. Glucagon increases the transcription of the PEPCK gene. This induction increases the conversion of oxaloacetate to PEP.

The F-6-P/F-1,6-BP substrate cycle. The major control of this substrate cycle is via the control of the level of F-2,6-BP, an inhibitor of F-1,6-BPase and activator of PFK-1. Under fasting conditions, increased activity of PKA leads to phosphorylation of a bifunctional enzyme (BFE), PFK-2/F-2,6-BPase, which this results in inactivation of PFK-2 and activation of the F-2,6-BPase, with the latter decreasing the levels of F-2,6-BP. The end result is relaxation of the inhibition of F-1,6-BPase and production of F-6-P, which then is converted to G-6-P and, finally, to glucose. The last reaction is catalysed by the essential G-6-Pase. This is a classic example of combined allosteric and covalent control. The BFE (and, therefore, the level of F-2,6-BP) is subjected to control by phosphorylation/dephosphorylation. The F-6-P/F-1,6-BP substrate pair is subjected to allosteric control of PFK-1 and F-1,6-BPase by the level of F-2,6-BP.

Case history answer

It is clear that both liver and muscle are able to convert their glycogen into pyruvate or lactate when stimulated: liver by glucagon or adrenaline (epinephrine), muscle by adrenaline (epinephrine). The fact that the glycogen in liver was of normal structure but was grossly elevated indicates that the glycogenesis pathway was active. The key piece of information is the ability of the liver sample to convert carbons from alanine into glycogen but not into glucose. This implies that the reaction catalysed by glucose-6-phosphatase was abnormal. This is the finding in glycogen storage disease type I, also known as von Gierke's disease. If you had such a patient, their abdomen would be abnormal owing to great liver enlargement and they would suffer from frequent occurrences of hypoglycaemia. Recall that glucose-6-phosphatase is required for glucose production by the liver from both the glycogenolytic and gluconeogenic pathways. These patients are now treated by overnight feed (by nasogastric tube) of corn starch to maintain blood glucose levels.

8 Protein and amino acid metabolism

Overview

Amino acids are required for the synthesis of proteins and many other vital body components (Fig. 73). Some can be made in the body from by-products of carbohydrate and fat metabolism but other amino acids must be obtained from the diet. The carbon skeletons of amino acids are processed by unique pathways leading to the formation of acetyl-coenzyme A (acetyl-CoA) and various tricarboxylic acid (TCA) cycle intermediates. Any excess of supply is converted to glucose and fatty acids or oxidised for generation of ATP. Amino acids present a special metabolic problem in that they have the potential to form ammonia, which is very toxic. The formation of urea from ammonia in the liver solves that problem.

8.1 General aspects

Learning objectives

You should be able to:

- describe how dietary proteins are digested
- describe how amino acids are absorbed
- explain whole body protein turnover
- define nitrogen balance.

Dietary proteins

Dietary proteins vary according to the diet of the individual. The important nutritional issue is that there should be sufficient protein in the diet to replace the amino acids that are degraded (Ch. 18).

Protein digestion involves endo- and exopeptidases

Dietary proteins are broken down to their constituent amino acids by the action of a series of proteolytic enzymes that catalyse the hydrolysis of peptide bonds. Small peptides are produced from larger peptides by the action of *endopeptidases*, which catalyse the hydrolysis of peptide bonds *within* proteins. The endopeptidases are relatively specific in the peptide bonds that they attack. *Exopeptidases* catalyse the hydrolysis of terminal peptide bonds in peptides, thus producing free amino acids. Most of the peptidases are secreted as inactive zymogens which have to be activated for them to be effective in protein digestion (see Figs 28 and 29). The logic of this arrangement must be obvious since, otherwise, these proteolytic enzymes would destroy their cells of origin!

Pepsin is the key protease in the stomach
Protein is hydrolysed by *pepsin*, an endopeptidase that has an optimum pH of about 1.0. When food enters the stomach, the production of hydrochloric acid converts pepsinogen to pepsin and creates the optimal (pH) environment for pepsin action. Hydrochloric acid also denatures dietary protein, with the result that peptide bonds that had been within globular proteins are now more accessible to proteolytic enzymes.

Trypsin and chymotrypsin from the pancreas function in the duodenum
Proteins are completely converted to small peptides in the duodenum by the action of other endopeptidases that originate in the pancreas: *trypsin*, *chymotrypsin* and *elastase*. These enzymes are also produced as inactive zymogens. Trypsinogen is activated to trypsin by the action of *enteropeptidase* secreted from mucosal cells when food enters the small intestine. Trypsin is then able to convert additional trypsinogen to trypsin (i.e. it is

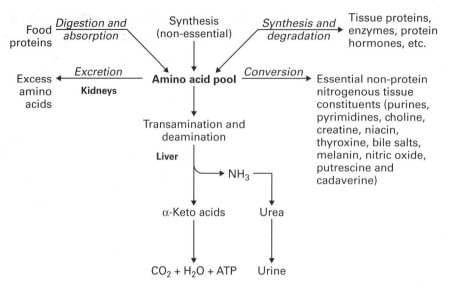

Fig. 73 General aspects of amino acid metabolism.

autocatalytic), chymotrypsinogen to chymotrypsin, proelastase to elastase and pancreatic *procarboxypeptidases A* and *B* to their active forms (Fig. 29).

Amino acids and small peptides are produced in the brush border and within intestinal mucosal cells

Exopeptidases (*dipeptidases, carboxypeptidases* and *aminopeptidases*) complete the hydrolysis of the small peptides formed by endopeptidase action. The combined effect of peptidases is to produce mainly free amino acids, but also some dipeptides and tripeptides.

Absorption of amino acids is by secondary active transport

Free amino acids plus dipeptides and tripeptides utilise a group of specific transporters that are in the brush border of mucosal cells. Both sodium-dependent and facilitated transport is involved.

Protein turnover

If one measures the nitrogen excretion from the body, one would have an inaccurate impression of the total daily turnover of protein that occurs in humans. The data shown in Figure 74 can be analysed to reveal whole body protein metabolism in a normal 70 kg adult man consuming 100 g of protein per day.

Nitrogen balance

This is calculated by measuring skin losses, faecal losses, plus the excretion of urea and ammonia in urine (conversion factor: 1 g urinary N = 6.25 g protein). Since excretion of nitrogen balances intake, the subject is in 'nitrogen balance'.

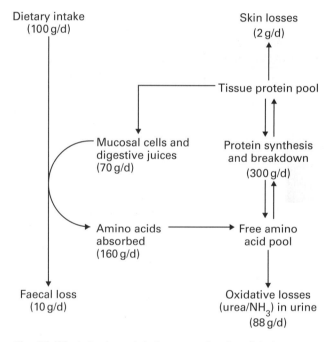

Fig. 74 Whole body protein turnover, showing data for one individual.

Whole body protein metabolism

This is calculated by using tracer amino acids. From the data given in Figure 74 it can be seen that whole body protein metabolism for one individual averages 300 g/day, which is much greater than the dietary protein intake of 100 g/day. About 23% of the protein turnover represents the production of digestive enzymes and the rapid degradation of mucosal cells in the gut. Proteolysis of these in the gut generates amino acids that are returned to the free amino acid pool. About 77% of daily protein turnover is more obscure, including turnover of muscle protein.

8.2 Protein disposal

Learning objectives

You should be able to:

- describe the pathways for protein breakdown
- explain how amino acids are deaminated
- describe the reactions of the urea cycle and their compartmentalisation
- outline the role of the TCA cycle in the metabolism of amino acid carbons and how it helps one identify ketogenic and glucogenic amino acids.

Protein catabolism involves:

- protein breakdown to amino acids (some will be reused and not degraded further)
- nitrogen removal from amino acids: transamination/deamination to give ammonia and keto acids
- urea cycle to dispose of ammonia
- keto acid metabolism via the TCA cycle.

Protein breakdown involves lysosomal and non-lysosomal pathways

The pathways for protein breakdown are shown in Figure 75.

The lysosomal pathway

Lysosomes contain an array of proteolytic enzymes that are mainly involved in the breakdown of three classes of protein: extracellular, membrane-associated and some intracellular proteins with long half-lives. This pathway is ATP independent and is inhibited by insulin and amino acids. Coupled with the action of insulin and amino acids to increase protein synthesis, this explains the positive nitrogen balance that can occur in the fed state, especially in growing children.

The non-lysosomal pathway

The major non-lysosomal pathway involves *ubiquitin*, is ATP-dependent and processes abnormal proteins and normal proteins with short half-lives, as well as the proteins of the muscular apparatus (actin and myosin). Ubiquitin is a small, highly conserved protein that is found in all cells. In the ubiquitin pathway, proteins are covalently linked to ubiquitin. Corticosteroids and the cytokine interleukin 1 activate the ubiquitin pathway.

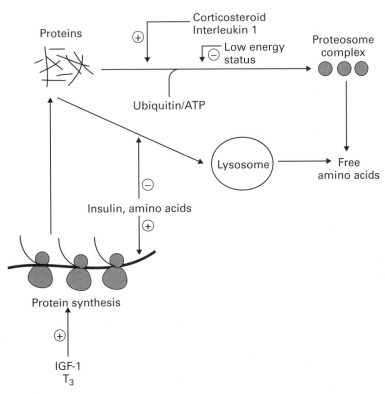

Fig. 75 Control of protein turnover. IGF-1, insulin growth factor-1; T_3, thyroid hormone.

Nitrogen disposal from amino acids

For the majority of the amino acids found in the body (exceptions are threonine, serine, histidine and lysine) the amino group is transferred to α-ketoglutarate, forming glutamate and the keto acid corresponding to the amino acid (Fig. 76). The biological advantage of such an arrangement is that the subsequent steps are common, since it is only the glutamate nitrogen that has to be handled. Glutamate is deaminated and the ammonia produced is converted to urea.

Transamination

The enzymes catalysing the transamination reactions are *aminotransferases* (transaminases), which have pyridoxal phosphate (PLP) as coenzyme. Liver, kidney, muscle and brain contain appreciable amounts of these enzymes.

Deamination

The glutamate formed is then subjected to oxidative deamination by *glutamate dehydrogenase*, with ammonium as a product and α-ketoglutarate regenerated (Fig. 76).

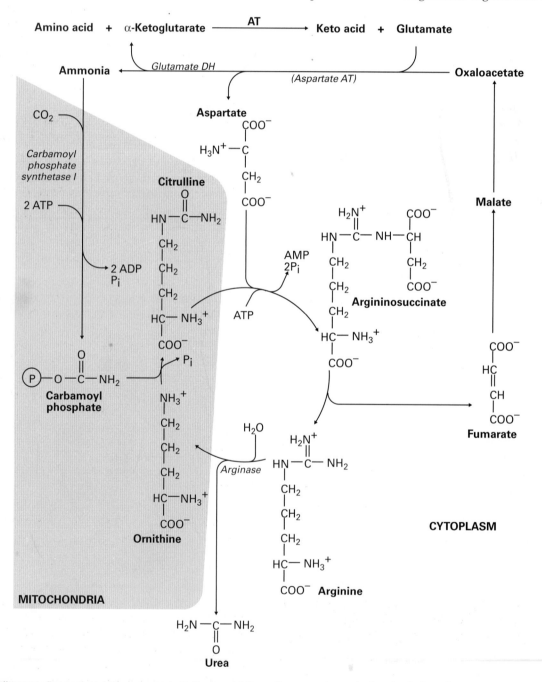

Fig. 76 Nitrogen disposal and the urea cycle (mitochondrial reactions are shown in the shaded area). DH = dehydrogenase; AT = aminotransferase

Glutamate dehydrogenase activity will affect the rate of ammonia production as well as the availability of carbon skeletons for the TCA cycle. GDP and ADP are allosteric activators. Hence, a lower energy charge accelerates the entry of carbon skeletons into the TCA cycle for conversion to substrates that can be oxidised to carbon dioxide, with the eventual production of ATP.

The urea cycle detoxifies ammonia

Ammonia is toxic if the concentration in blood goes above 4×10^{-5} M. Therefore, it is vital to deal efficiently with the ammonia generated.

Extrahepatic tissues

Ammonia generated is converted to glutamine by *glutamine synthetase*:

$$\text{Glutamate} + NH_3 + ATP \rightarrow \text{Glutamine} + ADP + P_i$$

The glutamine formed is transported to the gut, kidney and liver.

Liver

The liver has a high capacity to catabolise amino acids. Ammonia is disposed of by conversion to urea; this is a non-toxic compound that can be transported in the blood to the kidneys and excreted in the urine. The pathway used is the urea cycle (Fig. 76), also discovered by Krebs.

Carbamoyl phosphate is synthesised from ammonia and carbon dioxide in a reaction catalysed by *carbamoyl phosphate synthetase I* (CPSI). CPSI is stimulated by N-acetylglutamate and NH_4^+ (formed from glutamine by the action of glutaminase). Both of these are positively correlated with amino acid turnover in the body. The interaction of carbamoyl phosphate and ornithine generates citrulline, which then acquires a second nitrogen from aspartate to form argininosuccinate, which is then converted to arginine and a molecule of fumarate. Cytosolic fumarase and malate dehydrogenase regenerate oxaloacetate from the fumarate, and the oxaloacetate is used once more to form the required aspartate. The hydrolysis of arginine, catalysed by arginase, yields urea plus ornithine. Urea has two nitrogen atoms: one arises from ammonia and the other is derived from aspartate.

Other important points include the following:

- In order to ensure that ammonia is removed efficiently, there is high expenditure of ATP in the formation of carbamoyl phosphate and in the synthesis of argininosuccinate.
- The first two reactions are mitochondrial in location, the other reactions are in the cytosol. The localisation of CPSI to the mitochondria in hepatocytes is important since a second enzyme (CPSII) is involved in carbamoyl phosphate synthesis required for pyrimidine nucleotide biosynthesis (Ch. 11) and is localised to the cytosol.
- Ornithine is used in the first reaction, where ammonia enters the cycle as carbamoyl phosphate, and is regenerated in the last reaction of the cycle.
- Entry of ornithine and exit of citrulline (across the inner mitochondrial membrane) utilise transport systems.

The metabolism of amino acid carbons

Following the removal of amino acid nitrogen, the resultant keto acids are metabolised to TCA cycle intermediates. Thus, carbons from amino acids can all eventually be converted to acetyl-CoA, which can undergo complete oxidation in the TCA cycle or serve as a precursor for fatty acid biosynthesis. Although many of the amino acids share common types of reaction in terms of their catabolism, more often than not each of the amino acids undergoes a complicated series of unique steps. This can be simplified to some extent as the carbon skeletons appear in six major metabolites (Fig. 77).

The entry points for amino acid carbons into the TCA cycle are:

- oxaloacetate
- fumarate
- succinyl-CoA
- α-ketoglutarate
- acetyl-CoA.

Other keto acids produce pyruvate, which is readily converted to oxaloacetate.

Glucogenic amino acids

Amino acids for which the carbon atoms are metabolised to intermediates of the TCA cycle other than acetyl-CoA are glucogenic. To determine whether or not an amino acid is glucogenic, observe from Figure 77 whether or not the metabolism of the amino acid metabolite will result in an increase in the level of oxaloacetate or malate. If the answer is yes, the amino acid is glucogenic. If the answer is no, the amino acid is ketogenic.

Clinical note:
Liver damage

Ammonia toxicity in adults usually results from severe liver damage, caused by alcohol, other poisons or viral infection.

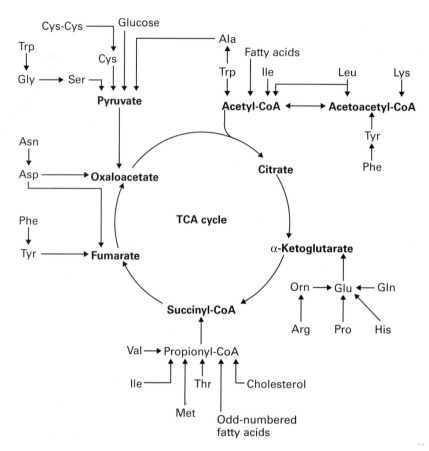

Fig. 77 Entry points for amino acid carbons in the TCA cycle.

Ketogenic amino acids

Those amino acids that are metabolised to acetyl-CoA are ketogenic. Some amino acids are both glucogenic and ketogenic (e.g. phenylalanine, tyrosine and isoleucine). Only lysine and leucine are purely ketogenic!

8.3 Essential and non-essential amino acids and their roles

Learning objectives

You should be able to:

- list the essential and conditionally essential amino acids
- outline the key roles of the 20 amino acids.

Those amino acids that cannot be synthesised in the body are termed *essential amino acids* (Table 6). The requirement for amino acids varies with species and with the state of the organism. For example, eight of the 20 amino acids used for protein synthesis are essential for adults, with an additional two (histidine and arginine) being essential in growing children.

Specific amino acids

Because of the unique pathways for the metabolism of the 20 common amino acids, this is a huge topic; we will concentrate on the truly important information for each. Several of the amino acids are involved in the synthesis of vital body constituents.

Small amino acids

Glycine

- δ-aminolaevulinic acid, a key intermediate in haem synthesis, is made from glycine and succinyl-CoA
- required for detoxification reactions in the liver
- principal inhibitory transmitter in the brain stem and spinal cord
- occurs at every third amino acid residue in collagen.

Alanine

- most important glucogenic amino acid; it is exported from muscle during fasting and exercise.

Table 6 Amino acid requirements for an adult

Essential amino acids	Non-essential amino acids	Conditionally essential amino acids[a]
Phe[b]	Gly	Cys (synthesised from Met)
Trp	Ser	Tyr (synthesised from Phe)
Val	Ala	Gln (synthesised from Glu, for which requirements are high in illness)
Ile	Tyr	His (synthesised from Glu; required in diet in babies)
Leu	Asp	Arg (formed in urea cycle; required in growing children)
Met[c]	Asn	
Lys	Glu	
Thr	Gln	
	Cys	
	Pro	
	Arg	
	His	

[a]Amino acids that can be synthesised in the body, but this may at times be inadequate, leading to a dietary requirement.
[b]Tyr in diet spares the requirement for Phe.
[c]Cys in diet spares the requirement for Met.

Proline

- an imino acid; common in collagen.

Aromatic amino acids: phenylalanine, tyrosine, tryptophan, histidine

Phenylalanine

- precursor of tyrosine; the enzyme catalysing the reaction, *phenylalanine hydroxylase*, is defective in phenylketonuria (Ch. 20).

Tyrosine

- precursor of melanin in melanocytes
- precursor of thyroid hormones in the thyroid gland
- precursor of catecholamines such as *adrenaline (epinephrine), noradrenaline (norepinephrine)* and *dopamine* (important neurotransmitters)
- phosphorylation of tyrosine in some proteins by tyrosine kinases controls metabolic reactions
- insulin receptor has tyrosine kinase activity.

Tryptophan

- precursor of the neurotransmitter serotonin (5-hydroxytryptamine)
- precursor of nicotinamide (Ch. 18).

Histidine

- precursor of one-carbon unit (formimino-FH_4)
- is decarboxylated to *histamine*, a biological amine that stimulates gastric acid secretion by effects on H_2 receptors and also causes contraction of smooth muscle through actions on H_1 receptors.

Branched-chain amino acids: valine, isoleucine, leucine

All branched-chain amino acids

- catabolised via a branched-chain keto acid dehydrogenase (BCKADH) complex, which is similar to the pyruvate dehydrogenase complex (Ch. 6).
- BCKADH is the enzyme defective in maple syrup urine disease.

Leucine

- metabolism requires biotin.

Basic amino acids: arginine, lysine

Arginine

- precursor of creatine
- synthesised in urea cycle from ornithine
- precursor of nitric oxide (Ch. 17)
- synthesis of polyamines (e.g. spermine).

Lysine

- lysine residue interacts with a glutamine when factor XIIIa converts a low tensile strength fibrin polymer into a high tensile strength clot (Ch. 19).

Sulphur-containing amino acids: cysteine, methionine

Cysteine

- provides the functional SH group of glutathione, acyl carrier protein and coenzyme A.

Methionine

- when activated as *S*-adenosylmethionine is a methyl donor in methylation reactions (e.g. noradrenaline (norepinephrine) to adrenaline (epinephrine))
- provides sulphur for cysteine biosynthesis.

Hydroxy amino acids: serine, threonine

Serine

- provides carbons for cysteine synthesis
- part of phospholipid (phosphatidylserine)
- required for synthesis of sphingolipids
- principal source of one-carbon units in the body
- phosphorylation of serine residues in some proteins by protein kinases controls the function of the proteins.

Threonine

- phosphorylation of threonine residues in some proteins by protein kinases controls the function of the proteins.

Acidic amino acids and their amides: glutamate and glutamine, aspartate and asparagine

Glutamate

- participates in transamination reactions in nitrogen disposal
- component of *glutathione* and *tetrahydrofolate*
- most abundant excitatory neurotransmitter in brain
- decarboxylated to γ-aminobutyric acid (GABA) in neurons.

Glutamine

- transports ammonia from extrahepatic tissues to the liver and splanchnic bed
- participates in de novo purine nucleotide biosynthesis and in GMP biosynthesis
- participates in pyrimidine nucleotide biosynthesis
- generates ammonium ions through action of glutaminase in the renal response to acidosis
- detoxification reactions in the liver
- precursor for glutamate in neurons
- fuel for enterocytes.

Aspartate

- biosynthesis of urea
- AMP biosynthesis
- pyrimidine nucleotide biosynthesis
- acts as a neurotransmitter.

Asparagine

- *N*-Linked di-oligosaccharide synthesis.

8.4 One-carbon metabolism

Learning objectives

You should be able to:

- list the 'one-carbon' compounds and their sources
- describe the roles of folic acid and vitamin B_{12} in one-carbon metabolism
- explain the solution to the 'folate trap'
- describe the importance of S-adenosylmethionine in transmethylation reactions.

The utilisation or formation of carbon dioxide by carboxylation and decarboxylation reactions is common and requires cofactors:

- carboxylation: biotin
- decarboxylations: thiamine pyrophosphate (TPP), pyridoxal phosphate.

'One-carbon metabolism' refers to sources of carbon in a more reduced form than carbon dioxide. These one-carbon units participate in several reactions related to the biosynthesis of key components of cells. They are carried on two carriers: *tetrahydrofolate* (FH_4; a derivative of folic acid) and *S*-adenosylmethionine (SAM; methionine, activated by the adenosyl moiety).

Sources of one-carbon units

- carried by FH_4: serine, glycine, histidine
- carried by SAM: methyl-FH_4.

Uses of one-carbon units

- carried by FH_4: purine and pyrimidine nucleotide synthesis
- carried by SAM: biosynthesis of creatine, adrenaline (epinephrine) and phosphatidylcholine; methylation of DNA and myelin basic protein.

Tetrahydrofolate carries one-carbon units

FH_4 is a reduced pteridine (Fig. 78), which is derived from folate, a water-soluble vitamin present in the diet. Animals and humans depend on plants for their principal supply. FH_4 is formed in the intestinal mucosa and is converted at that site to N^5-methyl-FH_4. This 'traps' the FH_4, making it unavailable for the production of the

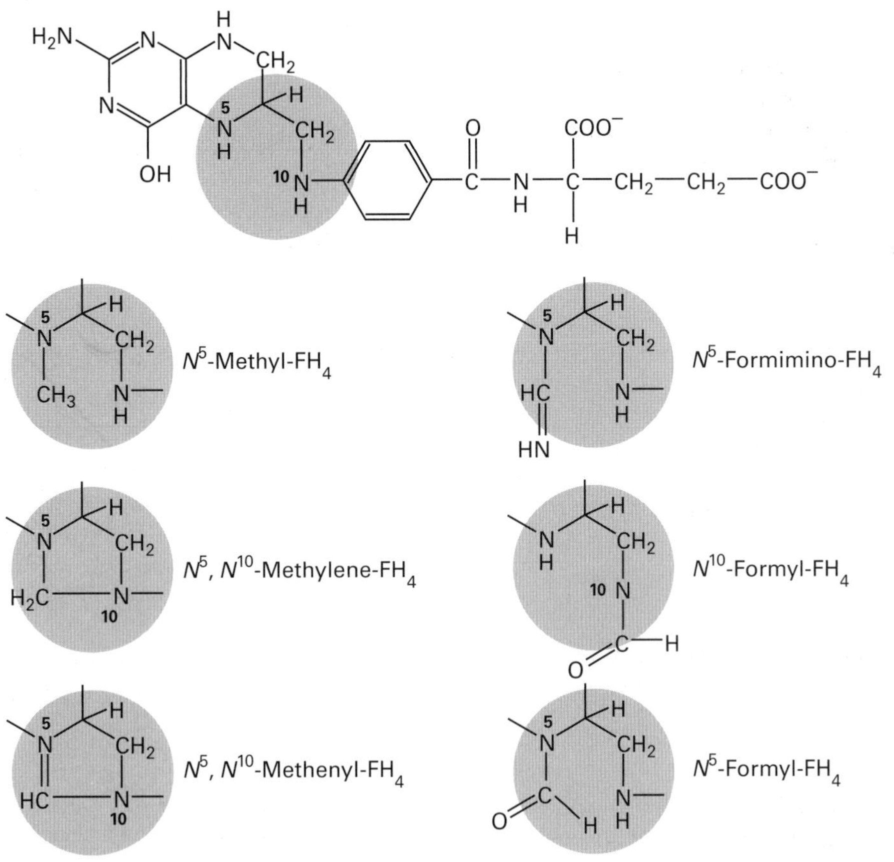

Fig. 78 Derivatives of tetrahydrofolate (FH$_4$). Various one-carbon units can be attached to N^6 and/or N^{10} of FH$_4$.

critical one-carbon derivatives used for purine and pyrimidine nucleotide synthesis. The solution to this problem is the reaction in which methionine is regenerated from homocysteine, catalysed by *homocysteine-N^5-methyl-FH$_4$ transferase (methionine synthase)*:

$$N^5\text{-methyl-FH}_4 + \text{homocysteine} \rightarrow \text{Methionine} + \text{FH}_4$$

This reaction involves a vitamin B$_{12}$ coenzyme, methylcobalamin, which participates in the reaction. Obviously, the regeneration of methionine has two biological advantages. One is to produce more methionine. The other is to untrap FH$_4$. The reduction of N^5,N^{10}-methylene FH$_4$ is irreversible! In an individual with a B$_{12}$ deficiency, the reaction is defective and N^5-methyl-FH$_4$ accumulates. In addition, there is increased excretion of formiminoglutamate, formate and 4(5)-amino-5(4)-imidazole carboximide, an intermediate in the synthesis of purine nucleotide. These metabolites all require folate cofactors for further conversion.

The one-carbon units carried by FH$_4$ are described in Figure 78 and can be interconverted as shown schematically in Figure 79. Serine is the primary source of one-carbon units derived in the reaction catalysed by *serine hydroxymethyltransferase*.

S-Adenosylmethionine is a source of methyl groups

Methionine contains a methyl group that can be transferred to other molecules after the methionine has been 'activated' by interaction with ATP to form SAM. SAM then interacts with acceptor molecules by a process known as *transmethylation*. Examples of transmethylation using SAM include:

- adrenaline (epinephrine) from noradrenaline (norepinephrine) (Ch. 17)
- phosphatidylcholine from phosphatidylethanolamine (see Ch. 9, p. 136)
- creatine synthesis; the last step is an *N*-methylation:

    Glycine + arginine→Guanidinoacetate→Creatine

- methylation of myelin basic protein and DNA.

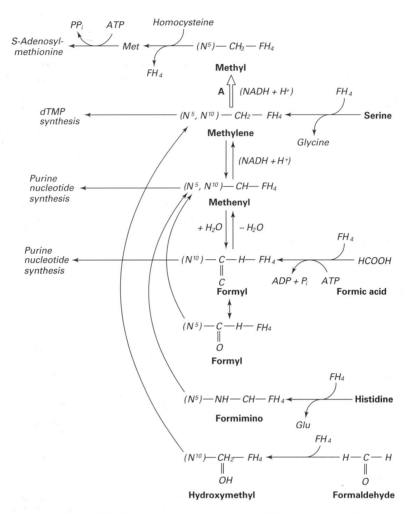

Fig. 79 Metabolism of tetrahydrofolate (FH$_4$). The methylated derivative of FH$_4$ is a 'trap' for FH$_4$ because Reaction A is irreversible.

8.5 Haem synthesis

Learning objectives

You should be able to:

- outline the pathway for haem synthesis
- describe how haem synthesis is regulated in liver and bone marrow
- explain the pathogenesis of acute intermittent porphyria.

Haem proteins such as haemoglobin and the cytochromes have critical functions in the body in oxygen transport and biological oxidation, respectively. Other haem proteins include myoglobin, catalase and tryptophan pyrrolase. Cytochrome oxidase is the terminal carrier of the electron transport chain. Cytochromes P-450 are involved in xenobiotic metabolism in the liver and also in steroid hormone biosynthesis. The liver and bone marrow are the major sites for haem synthesis. In bone marrow most of the haem is used for haemoglobin synthesis. In the liver, about 65% of the haem is used for cytochromes P-450 synthesis. The structure of haem is shown in Figure 80.

Haem synthesis starts with glycine and succinyl-CoA

The initial and last three steps of haem synthesis occur in the mitochondria, the others in the cytosol. The reaction of succinyl-CoA with glycine is the starting point

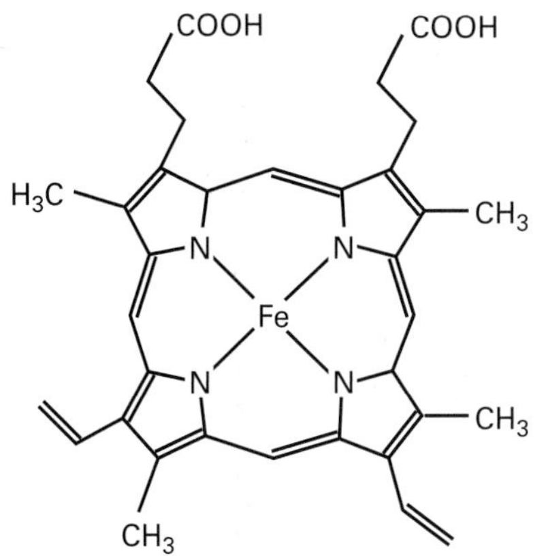

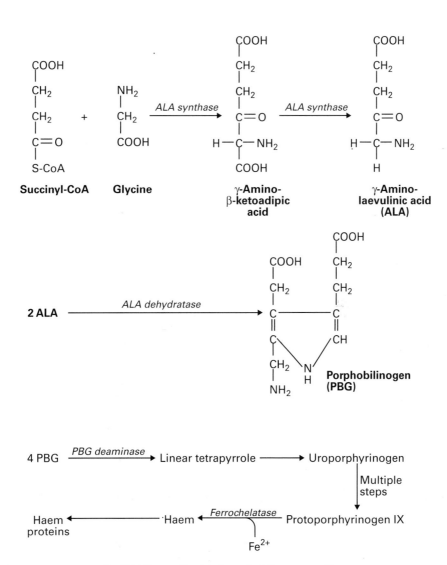

Fig. 80 The structure of haem. Haem consists of a porphyrin ring that is coordinated with an atom of iron. The porphyrin ring has four pyrrole rings. There are two side chains on each of the pyrroles: propionyl (P; CH_2CH_2COOH), methyl (M; CH_3) and vinyl (V; $CH=CH_2$). The clockwise order of these groups is M, V, M, V, M, P, P, M.

for the synthesis of the porphyrin ring. Condensation of these two compounds yields δ-aminolaevulinic acid (ALA), catalysed by *ALA synthase* (Fig. 81), an enzyme that requires pyridoxal phosphate. ALA is exclusively committed to haem synthesis. Condensation of two ALA molecules gives a pyrrole, porphobilinogen (PBG); this reaction is catalysed by *ALA dehydratase*, an enzyme that contains zinc and is inactivated by lead. The association of four PBG molecules, catalysed by *PBG deaminase (uroporphyrinogen I synthase)*, gives a straight-chain tetrapyrrole, which is cyclised to form a porphyrinogen. Multiple steps yield the precursor of haem, protoporphyrin IX, which incorporates ferrous iron, catalysed by *ferrochelatase*, to yield haem. Ferrochelatase also contains zinc and is inactivated by lead.

Fig. 81 The synthesis of porphobilinogen and haem.

Regulation of haem synthesis

Haem regulates its formation by several actions on ALA synthase. They include feedback inhibition, interference with the transport of the enzyme into mitochondria (its site of action) and repression of transcription of the ALA synthase gene. The last effect is profound given the short half-life of about 60 minutes of ALA synthase (this is unusually short for a mitochondrial enzyme). In summary, in the liver, haem synthesis increases when haem levels are low and vice versa. In contrast, erythrocyte haem synthesis in bone marrow is an 'all or none' phenomenon that follows inevitably erythroid cell differentiation.

Clinical note:
Porphyrias

Porphyrias are disorders in which there are partial deficiencies in haem biosynthetic pathway enzymes, leading to the accumulation of haem precursors. Acute intermittent porphyria is the most common hepatic porphyria; the defect here is in PBG deaminase. Neurological symptoms are present (e.g. the periodic madness of George III of Britain). Several drugs (e.g. barbiturates) when administered to patients increase the synthesis of cytochromes P-450; this places demands upon the haem pool and more haem is synthesised through induction of ALA synthase. If a patient has a deficiency in PBG deaminase, this will lead to even greater accumulation of intermediates and exacerbation of symptoms. Interestingly, exacerbation of symptoms also occurs in patients who reduce their calorie intake (diet) and, in contrast, a high glucose intake suppresses haem synthesis and relieves symptoms.

Self-assessment: questions

Single best answer MCQs

1. One of your patients, a 6-month-old female child is found to have a lack of enteropeptidase. The processing of which of the following zymogens is directly affected by this defect?
   a. Proelastase
   b. Trypsinogen
   c. Procarboxypeptidase A
   d. Pepsinogen
   e. Chymotrypsinogen

2. You investigate a 40-year-old male patient who tells you that he had been diagnosed with some form of porphyria many years ago. He had come to your attention because he had been reported by his wife to have recently started to act rather oddly. A careful history reveals that he had found a bottle of barbiturates and had started taking them as a sedative. You recognize that the episode of porphyria is due to barbiturates stimulating cytochrome P-450 synthesis in the liver, leading to induction of what?
   a. Ferrochetalase
   b. PBG deaminase
   c. Cytochrome *c*
   d. ALA synthase –
   e. Biliverdin reductase

3. The 'folate trap' is overcome by activity of what?
   a. Methylmalonyl-CoA mutase
   b. Serine hydroxymethyltransferase
   c. Methionine synthase
   d. Intrinsic factor

4. A very ill neonate is found to have hyperammonaemia. Further studies lead to a diagnosis of ornithine transcarbamylase (OTC) deficiency. Which of the following findings would be important in making that diagnosis?
   a. Hypercitrullinaemia
   b. Orotic aciduria
   c. Hyperargininaemia
   d. Argininosuccinic aciduria

5. Which combination of amino acids if removed from the diet in an adult would result in negative nitrogen balance?
   a. Ala, Pro, Glu
   b. Gly, Asp, Glu
   c. Arg, Asn, Cys
   d. Phe, Ala, Ser
   e. Tyr, Glu, His

6. The conversion of noradrenaline (norepinephrine) to adrenaline (epinephrine), phosphatidylethanolamine to phosphatidylcholine and guanidinoacetate to creatine each involves transmethylations. Which of the following is the (direct) donor of the methyl groups in every case?
   a. Methionine
   b. Malonyl-CoA
   c. Homocysteine
   d. *S*-Adenosylmethionine (SAM)
   e. β-Hydroxy-β-methylglutaryl-CoA (HMG-CoA)

7. Identify the amino acid in Column A that is NOT aligned with the correct statement about its function in the body (Column B):

A	B
a. Arginine	Precursor of nitric oxide
b. Serine	Source of one-carbon units
c. Tryptophan	Precursor of adrenaline (epinephrine)
d. Glutamate	Excitatory neurotransmitter
e. Aspartate	Biosynthesis of urea

8. Identify the single correct statement about the aromatic amino acids.
   a. Some of our requirement for nicotinamide comes from the metabolism of tyrosine
   b. Tyrosine in the diet spares the requirement for phenylalanine
   c. All of the aromatic amino acids are purely ketogenic
   d. Tryptophan is the precursor of melanin in melanocytes
   e. Subjects with a deficiency of phenylalanine hydroxylase always have sufficient tyrosine for normal nutritional health

9. The carbons of all amino acids eventually end up in the TCA cycle. Identify the single entry point for these carbons that cannot result in net synthesis of glucose in the liver.
   a. Acetyl-CoA
   b. Oxaloacetate
   c. Fumarate
   d. Succinyl-CoA
   e. α-Ketoglutarate

10. The liver is a major site for haem synthesis in the body, and knowledge of its synthesis and control are important for the practice of medicine. Which one of the following is correct?
    a. All of the reactions of haem synthesis occur in the mitochondria of hepatocytes
    b. The starting substrates for haem synthesis are alanine and acetyl-CoA
    c. ALA dehydratase, the enzyme catalysing the formation of porphobilinogen from δ-aminolaevulinic acid (ALA), contains zinc and the zinc can be displaced by lead
    d. In a subject with acute intermittent porphyria, she or he will benefit from a change in diet that leads to more cytochrome P-450 being synthesised in her/his liver

True/false questions

Are the following statements true or false?
1. Ferrochelatase is inhibited by lead.
2. Serine is the principal source of one-carbon units in the body.
3. Our dietary protein contains only essential amino acids, with the non-essential amino acids being formed from them in the body.
4. Glutamine formation and secretion from muscle has an important role to play in nitrogen disposal from muscle.
5. Leucine is the principal glucogenic amino acid in the body.
6. Amino acids with carbons that are converted to succinyl-CoA are potentially glucogenic.
7. Tyrosine is the precursor of adrenaline (epinephrine), noradrenaline (norepinephrine) and thyroid hormones.
8. Alanine is the principal ketogenic amino acid in the body.

Short essay questions

1. If 100 mmoles of valine are being catabolised in the liver, describe how the nitrogens in the valine are handled.
2. By a careful search through this textbook and others, give examples of the use of amino acids in the biosynthesis of key compounds in the body.
3. Explain the term 'conditionally essential amino acid' and give as many examples as you can.

Self-assessment: answers

Single best answer MCQ answers

1. a. **False**. Enteropeptidase does not directly activate proelastase. Trypsin does!
    b. **True**. Processing would be impaired since enteropeptidase catalyses the conversion of trypsinogen to trypsin.
    c. **False**. Enteropeptidase does not directly activate procarboxypeptidase A. Trypsin does!
    d. **False**. The activation of pepsinogen to pepsin is due to hydrochloric acid in the stomach.
    e. **False**. Enteropeptidase does not directly activate chymotrypsinogen. Trypsin does!

2. a. **False**. This is not a rate-controlling step.
    b. **False**. This enzyme is defective in this form of porphyria.
    c. **False**. This is a haem protein of the electron transport chain.
    d. **True**. This is a rate-controlling enzyme. The demand for P-450 will induce ALA synthase in an attempt to make haem. Because of the defect, intermediates accumulate.
    e. **False**. This is an enzyme of haem catabolism.

3. a. **False**. This is the enzyme that requires adenosyl-B_{12} as a coenzyme and completes the conversion of propionyl-CoA to succinyl-CoA.
    b. **False**. This is an enzyme that requires FH_4 and is one reason why the 'trap' must be solved.
    c. **True**. The conversion of homocysteine to methionine utilizes N^5-methyl-FH_4, liberating FH_4 for reactions in which essential one-carbon units are attached to FH_4.
    d. **False**. Intrinsic factor is not directly involved in solving the folate trap. However, indirectly it is important since B_{12} absorption requires that intrinsic factor be produced in the stomach (see Ch. 18, p. 266) and methyl-B_{12} is required for the reaction catalysed by methionine synthase.

4. a. **False**. With OTC deficiency citrulline synthesis is defective.
    b. **True**. Due to OTC deficiency, carbamoyl phosphate accumulates in liver mitochondria, leaks out of these organelles and then pyrimidine nucleotide synthesis is stimulated (see Ch. 11), resulting in the accumulation of orotic acid.
    c. **False**. Arginine levels will be low.
    d. **False**. Since citrulline synthesis is defective, the next step in the urea cycle will also be defective due to lack of substrate.

5. a. **False**. They are all non-essential in adults.
    b. **False**. They are all non-essential in adults.
    c. **False**. They are all non-essential in adults.
    d. **True**. Phenylalanine is an essential amino acid.
    e. **False**. They are all non-essential in adults.

6. a. **False**. Methionine needs to be 'activated' in order to donate its methyl group.
    b. **False**. Malonyl-CoA is a key intermediate in fatty acid synthesis.
    c. **False**. Homocysteine does not have a methyl group to transfer!
    d. **True**. Methionine is activated by interacting with ATP to give SAM.
    e. **False**. HMG-CoA is a key intermediate in ketone body and cholesterol biosynthesis.

7. a. *Nitric oxide synthase* is the enzyme catalysing the reaction.
    b. Serine is the source of $N^{5,10}$-FH_4.
    c. Tyrosine is the precursor of adrenaline (epinephrine). This is the answer to the question.
    d. Glutamate is responsible for about 75% of the excitatory neurotransmission in the brain.
    e. Aspartate and citrulline form argininosuccinate in the urea cycle.

8. a. **False**. Tryptophan is the precursor of nicotinamide.
    b. **True**. Tyrosine is required for protein synthesis and several other purposes. It is formed from phenylalanine by hydroxylation. Clearly, tyrosine in the diet reduces the need for phenylalanine.
    c. **False**. They are all *both* ketogenic and glucogenic.
    d. **False**. The pathway involves tyrosine and an enzyme, *tyrosinase*.
    e. **False**. This is discussed under b. Important in phenylketonuria to supplement the diet with tyrosine!

9. a. There can be no net synthesis of glucose from acetyl-CoA since oxaloacetate is required to get acetyl-CoA into the TCA cycle. Correct answer to question!
    b, c, d, e. All are convertible to malate which exits the mitochondrion to enter the gluconeogenic pathway via phosphoenolpyruvate.

10. a. **False**. The initial and final steps occur there but the rest are in the cytosol.
    b. **False**. The starting substrates are glycine and succinyl-CoA.
    c. **True**. The fact that its zinc prosthetic group can be displaced by lead helps explain the toxicity of lead.
    d. **False**. If more cytochrome P-450 has to be synthesised, this stimulates haem synthesis, with the attendant accumulation of toxic intermediates in AIP.

True/false answers

1. **True**. This is part of the known toxicity of lead (e.g. for children).
2. **True**. It generates the important one-carbon intermediate $N^{5,10}$-methylene-FH$_4$ in a reaction that also produces glycine.
3. **False**. Both types of amino acid are present in the diet. The key point is that one has to have sufficient essential amino acids in our diet, whereas deficiencies in the non-essential amino acids can be made good by metabolic processes.
4. **True**. Glutamine is formed by the amidation of glutamate; this allows for nitrogen disposal.
5. **False**. HMG-CoA is an intermediate in the catabolism of leucine. Also, HMG-CoA is the precursor of ketone bodies.
6. **True**. The succinyl-CoA is converted to malate via the TCA cycle and malate is glucogenic.
7. **True**. Tyrosine has a very important role in the biosynthesis of several biologically active molecules.
8. **False**. Alanine is converted to pyruvate and hence is glucogenic. It is a major source of glucose in the fasted state.

Short essay answers

1. It is important to recognise that only one of the two nitrogens in the urea formed by the urea cycle is derived directly from ammonia and the other directly from aspartate. Therefore, if 100 mmoles of valine are being catabolised, we need to end up with equal amounts of both ammonia and aspartate. The series of reactions will be as follows:

100 valine + 100 α-ketoglutarate→100 α-ketoisovalerate + 100 glutamate

This reaction is catalysed by an *aminotransferase*.

50 glutamate→50 α-ketoglutarate + 50 NH$_3$

This reaction is catalysed by *glutamate dehydrogenase*.

50 glutamate + 50 oxaloacetate→50 aspartate + 50 α-ketoglutarate

This reaction is catalysed by an *aminotransferase*. These reactions give the necessary equimolar amounts of ammonia and aspartate.

2. a. Serine is the precursor of one-carbon units necessary for purine and pyrimidine nucleotide synthesis.
   b. Glycine is required for the first step in haem synthesis.
   c. Glycine and arginine are required for synthesis of guanidinoacetate, the precursor of creatine.
   d. Glutamine is used in purine and pyrimidine nucleotide synthesis as a donator of nitrogen.
   e. Glycine and glutamine are used extensively in the formation of polar metabolites of drugs (which can then be eliminated from the body).
   f. Glycine is required for bile salt synthesis.
   g. Serine is required for sphingolipid synthesis.
   h. Aspartate is required for urea synthesis.

3. Conditionally essential amino acids are those that are non-essential under some circumstances but become essential under other situations. The body has the ability to make them, but in some cases the ability is not developed, is insufficient or is lost. This can be the situation in the neonate and in individuals with specific inborn errors of metabolism affecting amino acids.

   Cysteine is one such amino acid. It is obtained from many dietary proteins but can also be synthesised by a pathway where the sulphur is derived from methionine and the carbons from serine. If this pathway has low activity, as occurs in neonates, then cysteine becomes essential and it is important to ensure that there are adequate levels in dietary protein.

   Tyrosine is non-essential in that it is in many dietary proteins, but most of our requirements come from its production from phenylalanine, catalysed by phenylalanine hydroxylase. In individuals with phenylketonuria, where the phenylalanine hydroxylase system is defective, tyrosine becomes an essential amino acid.

   Other examples are glutamine, the requirements for which are increased in severe illness, histidine, required to be sufficient in the diet of babies, and arginine, required in increased amounts in growing children.

9 Lipid synthesis and transport

Overview

Lipids have multiple roles in the body. Fatty acids are the major components of our largest energy store, triacylglycerols (TAG), found mainly in adipose tissue. Fatty acids can be synthesised de novo from carbohydrates or amino acids and stored in adipose tissue as TAG. The control of these processes is fundamental to an understanding of the control of metabolism in the fed state. Phospholipids, cholesterol and other complex lipids are important components of membranes, and their synthesis is of great interest and of clinical significance. Essential fatty acids are the precursors of eicosanoids such as prostaglandins and thromboxanes which are vasoactive, regulate platelet function and modulate ion transport.

9.1 Fatty acid and triacylglycerol biosynthesis

Learning objectives

You should be able to:

- outline the pathways for fatty acid and TAG synthesis

- explain how fatty acid synthesis is controlled.

Fatty acid biosynthesis

In outline, the fatty acid synthesis pathway utilises 8 acetyl-CoA molecules and ends with the synthesis of palmitic acid (C_{16}) (Fig. 82). The process requires that 7 malonyl-CoA be formed from 7 acetyl-CoA (for each palmitate synthesised) and this is the principal rate-controlling step. A fatty acid synthase (FAS) multiple enzyme protein catalyses fatty acid chain growth by two carbons each cycle. Palmitic acid can be elongated to give larger fatty acids such as stearate (C_{18}). Fatty acids can also be unsaturated in the body to produce, for example, oleate ($C_{18:1}$). Odd-numbered fatty acids can also be synthesised.

Important features of fatty acid biosynthesis include the following:

- Acetyl-CoA for fatty acid synthesis needs to be transferred to the cytosol from mitochondria but it cannot cross the inner mitochondrial membrane. This problem is overcome by synthesising citrate from acetyl-CoA and the citrate can then exit the mitochondria (Fig. 83).

- Malonyl-CoA formation is catalysed by *acetyl-CoA carboxylase* (ACC). The enzyme contains biotin to act as a CO_2 carrier. Bicarbonate stimulates fatty acid synthesis!

$$CH_3COSCoA + HCO_3^- + ATP \rightarrow$$
$$HOOCCH_2COSCoA + ADP + P_i$$

- *Short-term regulation* of ACC is achieved by allosteric and covalent mechanisms. ACC is activated by dephosphorylation and switched off by phosphorylation. Phosphorylation can be due to an AMP-dependent kinase or protein kinase A. The former is active when [AMP] is high, i.e. when the energy charge in a cell is low. The rationale is that low ACC activity will lower malonyl-CoA levels and allow carnitine palmitoyltransferase I (CPTI) to be active and therefore fatty oxidation will proceed (see Ch. 6, pp 83–84). Glucagon and adrenaline (epinephrine) via protein kinase A lead to inactivation of ACC, the rationale being that these are also signals for fatty acid catabolism. Citrate activates

ACC by causing the enzyme to polymerise. Palmitoyl-CoA, the end-product of FAS, is an effective inhibitor of the enzyme.

- *Long-term regulation* of ACC is at the level of gene transcription. Fasting followed by a high carbohydrate diet leads to increased synthesis of both ACC and FAS.

- The synthesis of palmitate from 1 acetyl-CoA and 7 malonyl-CoA molecules involves FAS, which is a multifunctional enzyme complex with seven enzyme activities and an acyl carrier protein (ACP)

in a *single polypeptide chain*. Acyl groups are attached to ACP during the reactions catalysed by FAS. The FAS monomer cannot carry out the condensation reaction that initiates the production of palmitate since the ketosynthetase and ACP are too far apart. Hence the requirement for the dimeric form of the enzyme complex arranged head to tail. Two important sulphydryl (SH) groups are involved in fatty acid synthesis. One on ketosynthetase can carry an acyl group and the other is on ACP, which initially carries a malonyl group (Fig. 84). When

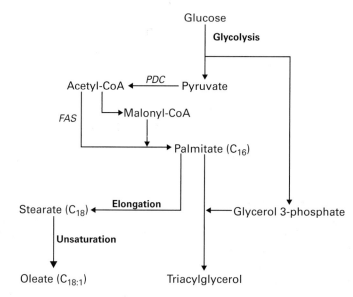

Fig. 82 The conversion of glucose to fatty acids and triacylglycerols.

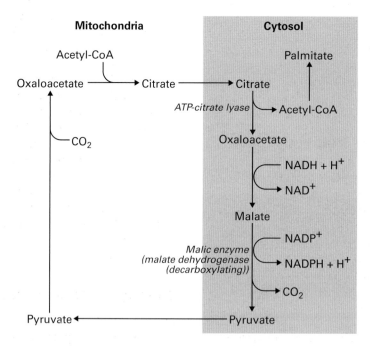

Fig. 83 The citrate–malate–pyruvate cycle.

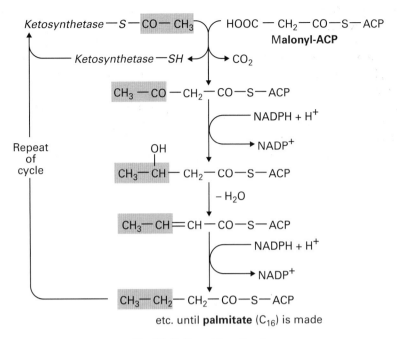

Fig. 84 Fatty acid synthesis.

both SH sites are charged, condensation occurs leaving a larger ketoacyl group on the ACP. Reduction, dehydration followed by reduction produces an acyl group now two carbons longer (this sequence is the opposite of that found in fatty acid beta-oxidation). The carbon dioxide incorporated into malonyl-CoA is lost at the condensation step. The cycle shown in Figure 84 is repeated until the acyl group has 16 carbons. A *thioesterase* (deacylase) removes the completed fatty acid from the ACP. Highest activity of the thioesterase is exhibited with palmitoyl-CoA, and to a lesser extent with stearoyl-CoA (C_{18}) and myristoyl-CoA (C_{14}). In the lactating mammary gland, a different thioesterase is present, *thioesterase II*. This enzyme preferentially hydrolyses fatty acyl-CoA derivatives of chain length C_8 and C_{12} and plays a role in determining the fatty acid content of TAG in milk.

- *Synthesis of odd-numbered fatty acids* uses the same pathway as that for even-numbered, except that the primer molecule is propionyl-CoA (with a three-carbon acyl group) rather than acetyl-CoA with its two-carbon acyl group.

- *Synthesis of unsaturated fatty acids* requires *fatty acid desaturases* located in the endoplasmic reticulum. *Cis* double bonds are introduced no farther in the fatty acid chain than the C_9 to C_{10} position of palmitic acid, i.e. must be seven or more carbon atoms from the ω end. Mammalian systems can desaturate various chain lengths at Δ^4, Δ^5, Δ^6 and Δ^9 positions. The desaturase complex contains cytochrome b_5, NADH–cytochrome b_5 reductase and the desaturase. The overall reaction is:

Palmityl-CoA (C_{16}) + NADH + H$^+$ + O$_2$ →
$$\text{Palmitoleyl-CoA } (C_{16:1}) + NAD^+ + 2H_2O$$

- The body is capable of synthesising many unsaturated fatty acids and these have a special role in the lipids found in membranes. It is important to note, however, that the eicosanoid precursors linoleic acid (18:2 *cis*-Δ^9,Δ^{12}) and γ-linolenic acid (18:3 *cis*-Δ^9,Δ^{12},Δ^{15}) are essential fatty acids since they cannot be synthesised in the body.

- *Fatty acid elongation* enzymes are located in mitochondria and on the endoplasmic reticulum. Elongases on the endoplasmic reticulum add (to fatty acyl-CoAs) two carbon units via malonyl-CoA, whereas elongases present in the mitochondrion add two carbon units via acetyl-CoA. The sequence of reactions is the same as those outlined for the synthesis of palmitate except the intermediates are CoA derivatives rather than ACP derivatives. NADPH is the reductant in a reverse of beta-oxidation, with the exception that the final reduction is carried out with NADPH.

Triacylglycerol biosynthesis

Free fatty acids are not found in significant quantities in tissues but are present largely as esters. Synthesis of TAG occurs primarily in adipose tissue and liver.

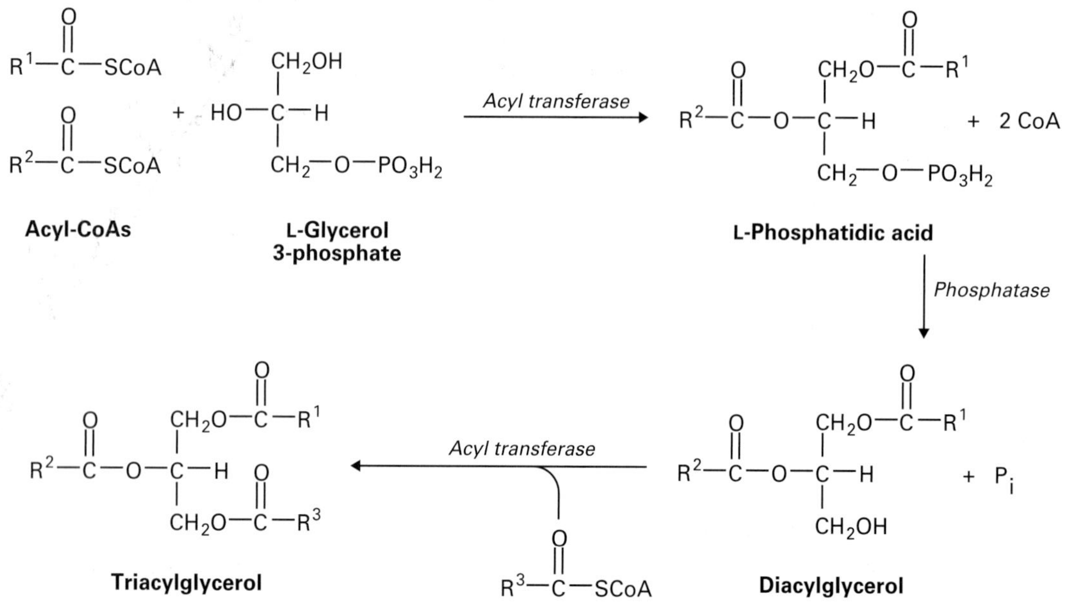

Fig. 85 Triacylglycerol (triglyceride) biosynthesis. This is the pathway that is used in adipose tissue and the liver.

Two fatty acyl-CoA molecules interact with glycerol 3-phosphate to produce phosphatidic acid (Fig. 85). The reaction proceeds preferentially with C_{16} and C_{18} saturated and unsaturated fatty acyl-CoA derivatives. The glycerol 3-phosphate is derived from the glycolytic intermediate dihydroxyacetone phosphate. Phosphatidic acid is dephosphorylated to yield diacylglycerol, which is then acylated to form a TAG.

In the liver, TAG are incorporated into very low density lipoproteins (VLDL) for transport to adipose tissue where fat is stored (Fig. 100, p. 151).

9.2 Triacylglycerol transport

Learning objectives

You should be able to:

* describe the roles of chylomicrons and VLDL in triacylglycerol transport
* understand the role of lipoprotein lipase and how it is controlled.

The important issues vis-à-vis fat transport are:

* How is fat transported from the gut to storage sites?
* How is fat transported from the liver to storage sites?

Since fats are hydrophobic, they have to be packaged in a way that allows them to be transported in an aqueous medium. The packaging involves the formation of lipoproteins consisting of aggregates of apolipoproteins, TAG, cholesteryl esters and phospholipids in various proportions. The core of the particle contains hydrophobic lipids and the apolipoproteins; the phospholipid head groups are on the outside. The major classes of lipoprotein are shown in Table 7 and their functions are given in Table 8.

Fat is transported as chylomicrons from the gut to storage sites

During digestion, dietary TAG are hydrolysed to fatty acids and monoglycerides, which are absorbed into the intestinal mucosal cells in micelles (Ch. 6, p. 78). TAG are reformed in mucosal cells using a pathway that involves monoacylglycerols (Fig. 86); they are then incorporated into chylomicrons along with apoprotein B-48. The chylomicrons are secreted into the lymphatic system, entering blood at the level of the thoracic duct. In blood, other apoproteins are transferred from HDL to chylomicrons; these include the apoproteins Apo-E and Apo-CII.

Fat is transported as VLDL from the liver to storage sites

Fatty acids synthesised in the liver, or delivered to the liver from chylomicrons, are converted to TAG using a pathway that involves phosphatidate; they are incorporated into VLDL (Fig. 86) and also acquire Apo-CII from circulating HDL along with apoprotein B-100.

Table 7 Composition of plasma lipoproteins

	Chylomicrons	VLDL	LDL	HDL
Density	<0.95	0.95–1.006	1.019–1.063	1.063–1.21
Protein (%)	1–2	10	25	45–55
Triacylglycerol (%)	80–95	55–65	10	3
Phospholipid (%)	3–6	15–20	22	30
Cholesterol (%)	1–3	10	8	33
Cholesteryl ester (%)	2–4	5	37	15

Table 8 Major functions of lipoproteins

	Apoprotein	Functions
Chylomicrons	Apo-As, Apo-B48, Apo-CII, Apo-E	Transport of triacylglycerols from gut
VLDL	Apo-B100, Apo-CII, Apo-E	Transport of triacylglycerols from liver to adipose tissue
LDL	Apo-B100	Enriched in cholesteryl ester; deliver cholesterol to extrahepatic tissues
HDL	Apo-As, Apo-Cs, Apo-E	Scavenges for cholesterol as it circulates in blood

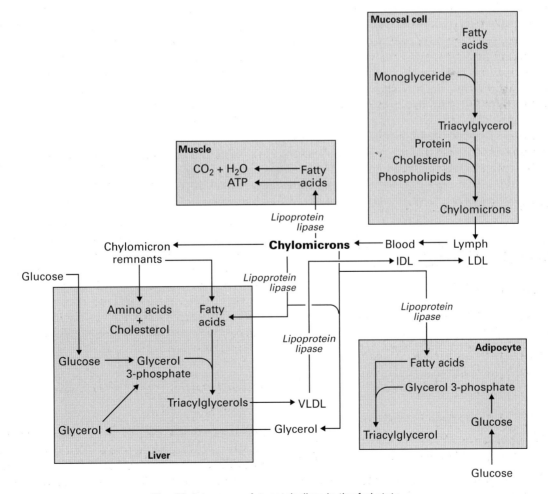

Fig. 86 Inter-organ fat metabolism in the fed state.

Lipoprotein lipase clears fatty acids from chylomicrons and VLDL

Chylomicrons and VLDL are cleared of their TAG by the action of *lipoprotein lipase* (LPL), an enzyme that is attached to endothelial cells lining capillary walls. LPL is produced in adipocytes, cardiac muscle, other muscle cells and also in the mammary gland. Its level is increased by insulin action. The Apo-CII component of chylomicrons and VLDL activates LPL. The products of LPL action on the lipoprotein-associated TAG are glycerol and fatty acids.

> **Clinical note:**
> Defective LPL
>
> Subjects with defective LPL will have hypertriglyceridaemia after a meal because of their impaired ability to clear chylomicrons. High-speed centrifugation of their blood will show chylomicrons floating on the surface.

Adipose tissue

Fatty acids taken up into adipocytes are converted to and stored as triacylglycerols by the pathways described above.

Muscle

In muscle cells, the fatty acids serve as fuels, being completely oxidised for ATP synthesis. Some TAG are stored here too.

LPL depletes chylomicrons of their TAG, resulting in *chylomicron remnant* particles that are metabolised by the liver since receptors in that tissue recognise their Apo-E component. LPL action on VLDL leaves intermediate density lipoproteins (IDL); these are also cleared by the liver, in this case by LDL receptors. IDLs are also the precursors of LDL.

9.3 Cholesterol and bile acids

> ### Learning objectives
>
> You should be able to:
>
> - describe in outline the cholesterol biosynthetic pathway
> - explain how HMG-CoA reductase is controlled
> - describe how cholesterol is delivered to extrahepatic tissues
> - explain how statin drugs act to reduce serum cholesterol levels
> - describe key reactions in bile acid synthesis.

Cholesterol

Cholesterol is the most commonly occurring steroid: it is present in nearly all living organisms but not in bacteria. It contains the common steroid ring system (Fig. 87). Cholesterol has a number of roles:

- structural component of membranes
- an important component of plasma lipoproteins
- the precursor of bile acids
- the precursor of steroid hormones.

There is great interest in cholesterol metabolism because of its association with cardiovascular disease. In Western societies, the cholesterol intake in the diet per day is 600–1200 mg, of which 300–400 mg are absorbed. Above average levels can be found in skin and egg yolk. Cholesterol and cholesteryl esters in the diet are absorbed along with other fats.

Cholesterol is synthesised from acetyl-CoA

In addition to dietary sources, cholesterol can be synthesised in the body, with the liver and the intestinal mucosal cells being the principal sites. Cholesterol in the diet controls to some extent the amount of cholesterol synthesised in that there is feedback inhibition of liver cholesterol synthesis (but not of synthesis in mucosal cells). Mucosal cell synthesis of cholesterol is directly affected by bile acids, with high levels being inhibitory. The biosynthetic pathway is outlined in Figure 88.

The key points are:

- All of the carbons are derived from acetate (acetyl-CoA).
- HMG-CoA is an intermediate; its conversion to mevalonate is the key rate-controlling step.
- From mevalonate, active C_5 compounds are formed and these condense to yield intermediates with 10, 15 and, finally, 30 carbons; the last compound is *squalene*.

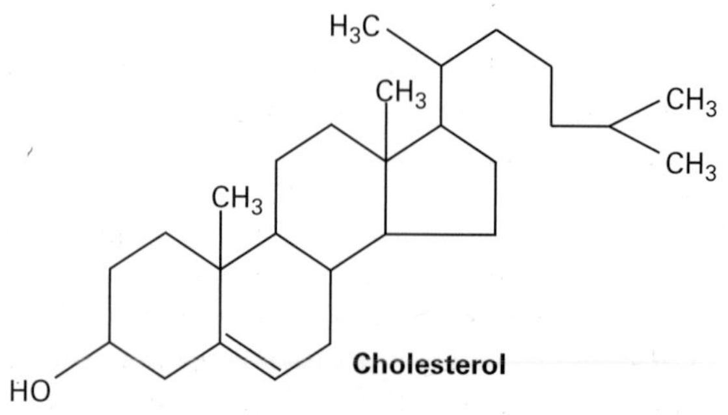

Fig. 87 The structure of cholesterol.

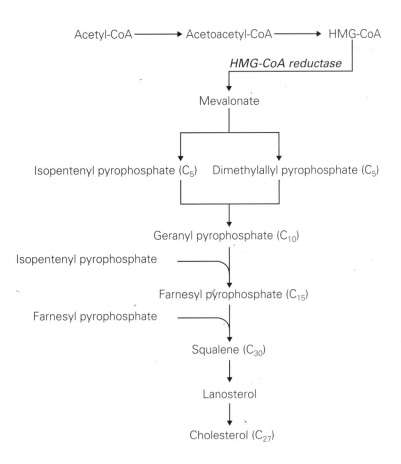

Acetyl-CoA ⟶ Acetoacetyl-CoA ⟶ HMG-CoA

HMG-CoA reductase

Mevalonate

Isopentenyl pyrophosphate (C_5)   Dimethylallyl pyrophosphate (C_5)

Geranyl pyrophosphate (C_{10})

Isopentenyl pyrophosphate

Farnesyl pyrophosphate (C_{15})

Farnesyl pyrophosphate

Squalene (C_{30})

Lanosterol

Cholesterol (C_{27})

Fig. 88 Cholesterol biosynthesis.

- Cyclisation yields the parent steroid *lanosterol*, from which cholesterol is formed.
- This pathway occurs in the cytosol and requires NADPH.

HMG-CoA reductase is the important control step in cholesterol biosynthesis

There is a circadian (diurnal) variation in *HMG-CoA reductase* (HMGCoAR) activity in humans, with maximum activity between midnight and 4:00 a.m. HMGCoAR activity changes in response to dietary cholesterol and hormonal status. Regulation includes inhibition of HMGCoAR gene expression by cholesterol as well as phosphorylation of the enzyme. The expression of HMGCoAR is only inhibited 90% by treatment with statin drugs, but there is also feedback inhibition by cholesterol itself on the enzyme catalysing squalene synthesis. This means that when HMGCoAR inhibitors are used clinically there is enough farnesyl pyrophosphate to allow for the synthesis of important non-sterol isoprenoids such as ubiquinone and farnesylated pro-

teins. The control of HMGCoAR and LDL receptor transcription (see Fig. 89) involves the interaction between a sterol regulatory element (SRE) and an SRE binding protein. High cholesterol inhibits the formation of SRE binding protein.

Clinical note:
Inhibitors of HMG-CoA reductase in the treatment of hypercholesterolaemia

Compactin, isolated from cultures of a species of *Penicillium*, and mevinolin, isolated from *Aspergillus*, are competitive inhibitors of HMG-CoA reductase and they therefore lower plasma cholesterol through this inhibition of HMG-CoA, and especially because of the associated increase in LDL receptor levels in the liver. This is an important therapy for some patients with elevated cholesterol levels.

Cholesterol is transported to extrahepatic tissues as LDL

Most extrahepatic tissues, although having a requirement for cholesterol, have low activity of the cholesterol biosynthetic pathway. Their cholesterol requirements are supplied by LDL, which is internalised by receptor-mediated endocytosis. This process is depicted in Figure 89.

The key features are:

1. 'High-affinity' LDL receptors are present to which the Apo-B100 of LDL binds; there is then internalisation of the receptor–LDL complex and processing of this complex leads to the provision of cholesterol for the cell in question.
2. Internalisation occurs at special parts of the plasma membrane surface called *coated pits*; these are depressions in the cell surface with a specific protein, *clathrin*, bound to the cytoplasmic surface giving it a 'coated' appearance (Fig. 37).
3. Coated pits then 'pinch' off from the surface to form coated vesicles.

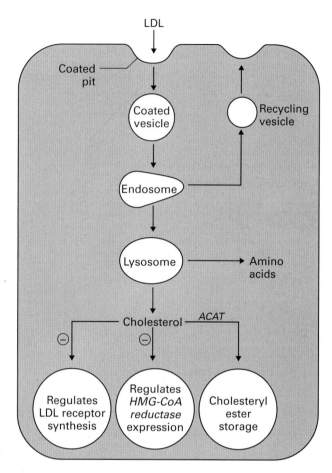

Fig. 89 Receptor-mediated endocytosis for cholesterol delivery to cells. ACAT, acyl-CoA:cholesterol acyltransferase.

4. Coated vesicles lose their coat after endocytosis to become endosomes (smooth surface vesicles).
5. The receptors in the endosome then return to the cell surface and the LDL in the endosomes fuses with lysosomes where the LDL proteins and cholesteryl esters are hydrolysed.
6. The free cholesterol formed down-regulates LDL receptor synthesis in the cell and also controls endogenous cholesterol synthesis by repression of HMGCoAR.
7. Cholesterol is stored as cholesteryl esters, formed by the action of *acyl-CoA:cholesterol acyltransferase* (ACAT).

Bile acids

Compared to other steroids of biological significance, bile acids have an hydroxyl group at position 7 in the B ring (Fig. 90). Two series of bile acids are synthesised: one yields cholic acid and the other chenodeoxycholic acid. In the cholic acid series, there are hydroxyl groups at positions 3, 7 and 12 in the steroid nucleus. In the chenodeoxycholic acid series, the hydroxyls are only at

---

Clinical note:
Defective LDL receptors

Defects in the LDL receptor system results in *hypercholesterolaemia* and *arteriosclerosis*. There are numerous disorders of lipoprotein metabolism but *familial hypercholesterolaemia* (FH) has been the most studied. FH is inherited as an autosomal dominant trait with a gene dosage effect, i.e. homozygotes are more severely affected than are heterozygotes. Heterozygotes number about 1 in 500 persons. They have twofold elevations in plasma cholesterol (range 7.8–12 mmol/litre). Homozygotes number 1 in 1 million persons. They have severe hypercholesterolaemia (as high as 20 mmol/litre). Coronary heart disease begins in childhood and frequently causes death before age 20. The primary defect in FH is a mutation in the receptor for plasma LDL. FH heterozygotes have one normal allele and one mutant allele at the LDL receptor locus; as a result, their cells are able to bind and take up LDL at approximately half the normal rate. Phenotypic homozygotes possess two mutant alleles at the LDL receptor locus; their cells show a total or near-total inability to bind or take up LDL. Subjects with defective LDL receptors have absent or reduced receptor-mediated endocytosis in the liver and extra-hepatic tissues. This results in increased cholesterol biosynthesis in extra-hepatic tissues but, more important, IDL clearance by the liver is impaired and more LDL will then be formed. Treatment for heterozygotes and homozygotes involves lowering the plasma level of LDL. In heterozygotes, the best strategy is to stimulate the single normal gene to produce more LDL receptor mRNA.

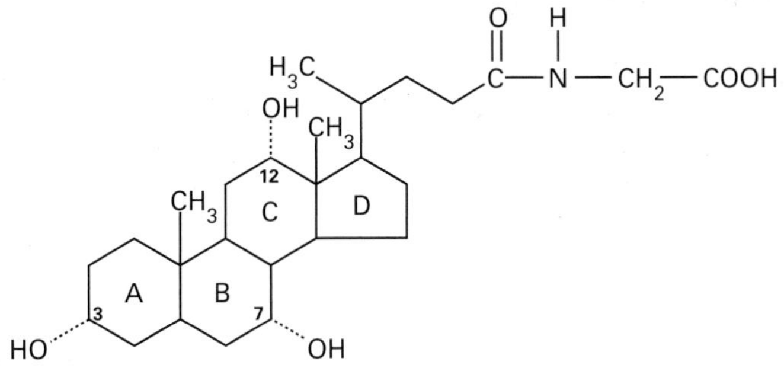

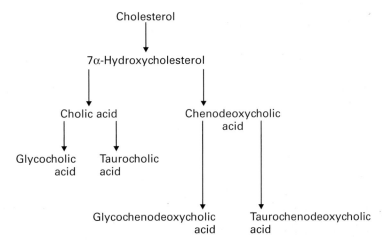

Fig. 90 Structure of the bile acid glycocholic acid.

Cholesterol

↓

7α-Hydroxycholesterol

Cholic acid   Chenodeoxycholic
                          acid

Glycocholic   Taurocholic
acid   acid

Glycochenodeoxycholic   Taurochenodeoxycholic
acid   acid

Fig. 91 Bile acid synthesis.

the 3 and 7 positions. Both function in fat digestion and absorption (Ch. 6, pp 77–78). Bile salts are conjugates of the bile acids and are very effective as detergents since they are amphiphiles containing a polar region (in the side chain) and a non-polar region, the steroid nucleus.

Bile acids are synthesised from cholesterol

Bile acids are produced in the liver (Fig. 91). The initial step involves 7α-hydroxylation of cholesterol; then there are further hydroxylations and limited side chain cleavage to yield a C_{24} steroid with a carboxyl at carbon-24 in the side chain. 7α-Hydroxylation is controlled. Cholic acid can form an amide with the amino groups of taurine ($H_2NCH_2CH_2SO_3H$) or glycine (H_2NCH_2COOH) to form *taurocholic acid* and *glycocholic acid*, respectively. It is these two compounds that are the major bile salts secreted in the bile. Similar conjugates are formed with chenodeoxycholic acid.

Bile acids secreted by liver hepatocytes are stored in the gallbladder until fats in the duodenum (via cholecystokinin) signal its contraction. After bile acids facilitate intestinal fat digestion and absorption, they are

Clinical note:
Bile acid binders in treatment of hypercholesterolaemia

Cholestyramine, an anion exchange resin, binds bile acids in the gut and prevents their reabsorption. Cholestyramine has been utilised therapeutically, along with inhibitors of HMG-CoA reductase, to control cholesterol levels in hypercholesterolaemic subjects.

absorbed in the distal ileum and return to the liver via the portal circulation. Hepatocytes extract the bile acids from portal blood. The overall process is amazingly efficient: 98% of secreted bile acids return to the liver to be re-secreted into bile, with the bile acids lost in faeces being replaced by synthesis from cholesterol in the liver.

Steroid hormones are derived from cholesterol

In the adrenal cortex, gonads and placenta, cholesterol is the precursor of active steroid hormones made by these tissues, including cortisol, aldosterone, testosterone, oestradiol and progesterone (Ch. 17, p. 238). 7-Dehydrocholesterol is the precursor of vitamin D, which can be made in skin under the influence of ultraviolet light (Ch. 17, p. 245).

9.4 Complex lipids

Learning objectives

You should be able to:

- describe in outline how phospholipids are synthesised and the role of CTP

- outline the pathways for sphingolipid synthesis

- summarise the major types of sphingolipidoses and their pathogenesis.

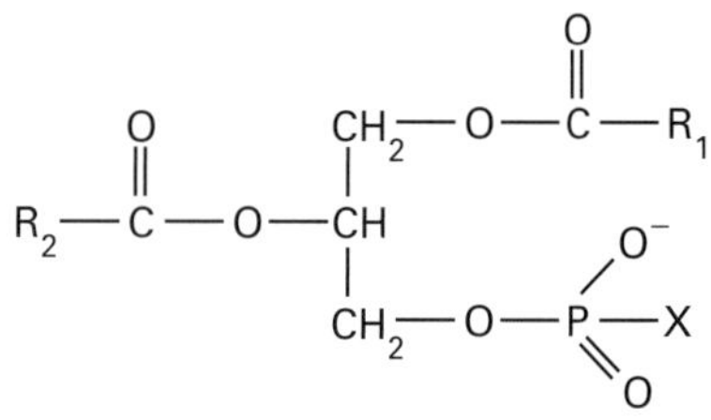

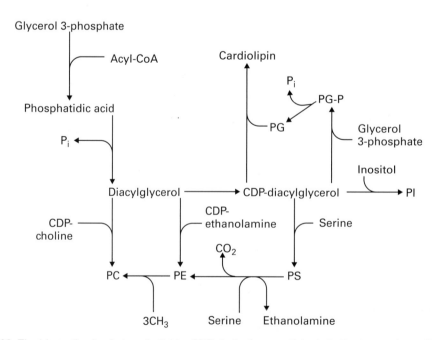

Fig. 92 General formula for a glycerophospholipid. 'X' represents choline (PC), ethanolamine (PE), serine (PS), glycerol (PG) or inositol (PI).

Phospholipids

Phosphoglycerides are amphiphiles having both polar and non-polar groups. Some, such as phosphatidylcholine (PC), are dipolar ions. They are all important constituents of cell membranes (see Ch. 4, p. 48). This class of complex lipids includes PC, phosphatidylethanolamine (PE), phosphatidylglycerol (PG), phosphatidylinositol (PI) and phosphatidylserine (PS). The general formula for the phosphoglycerides is given in Figure 92.

CTP is involved in phospholipid biosynthesis

The major pathways involved in phospholipid biosynthesis are outlined in Figure 93. Phosphatidate (diacylglycerol 3-phosphate) is an intermediate in the synthesis of phospholipids as it is in the synthesis of triacylglycerols. Depending upon the particular phospholipid, activated intermediates are formed using the pyrimidine nucleotide CTP:

- CDP-diacylglycerol is an intermediate in the major pathways for PS, PI and PG formation.
- CDP-choline and CDP-ethanolamine are intermediates in PC and PE synthesis with phosphorylcholine and phosphorylethanolamine being precursors.

In another important pathway, decarboxylation of PS yields PE, which can then be converted to PC by three successive methylations involving SAM (*S*-adenosylmethionine). In the liver, PS can be formed from PE by the

Fig. 93 The biosynthesis of phospholipids. CDP derivatives participate in the two major pathways.

enzyme-catalysed transfer of serine for the ethanolamine moiety of the phospholipid. Cardiolipin (diphospha-tidylglycerol), a phospholipid found mainly in mito-chondria, is formed from PG by interacting with CDP-diacylglycerol.

Sphingolipids

Sphingolipids are important in the nervous system, and abnormal levels are found in several diseases affecting that system. Gangliosides play a special role in plasma membrane receptors for hormones, viruses, etc. They contain, in addition to sugar residues, the compound *N-acetylneuraminic acid* (NANA), also known as *sialic acid*.

Ceramide is a key intermediate in sphingolipid synthesis

Sphingolipid biosynthesis is outlined in Figure 94. All sphingolipids are based on sphinganine, which is formed from serine and palmitoyl-CoA. The addition of choline to ceramide gives *sphingomyelin*; the addition of sugars gives *cerebrosides* and *globosides*. The addition of NANA to globosides gives gangliosides.

The sphingolipidoses

The sphingolipidoses are inherited disorders of sphin-golipid metabolism and most of them are autosomal recessive. In several of these disorders, homozygotes show progressive mental and motor deterioration, with onset in childhood and fatal outcomes. One current interest in the sphingolipidoses stems from the finding that these diseases are amenable to heterozygote detec-tion and prenatal diagnosis, since most are autosomal recessive. The sphingolipidoses are lipid storage diseases and in each of them the defect is in an enzyme of the degradative pathway occurring in lysosomes.

Sphingolipidoses include:

- Tay–Sachs disease, where ganglioside GM_2 accumulates
- Niemann–Pick disease, where sphingomyelin accumulates

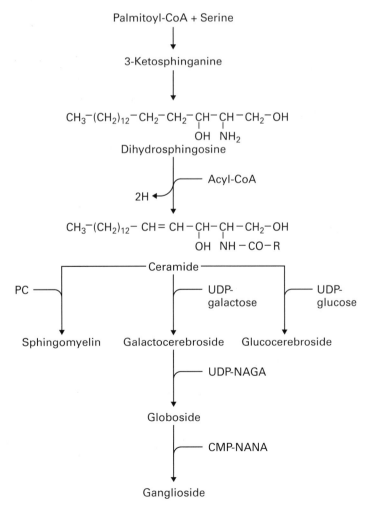

Fig. 94 The biosynthesis of sphingolipids. NANA, *N*-acetylneuraminic acid (sialic acid); NAGA, *N*-acetylgalactosamine.

Clinical note:
Tay–Sachs disease

Tay–Sachs disease (TSD) is the most common ganglioside storage disease. The heterozygote frequency for TSD mutation among Ashkenazi Jews is 1 in 27, whereas it is 1 in 125 for non-Jews. Heterozygotes can be reliably determined by a serum assay of the deficient enzyme *hexosaminidase A*. This was the first example of a genetic disease where mass screening for heterozygotes was conducted in at-risk populations.

- Gaucher's disease, where glucocerebroside accumulates
- Fabry's disease (X-linked inheritance), where a globoside accumulates
- Krabbe's disease, affecting galactocerebroside metabolism.

9.5 Eicosanoids

Learning objectives

You should be able to:

- outline prostaglandin synthesis and the mechanisms by which aspirin and glucocorticoids affect the biosynthetic pathways.

The eicosanoids form a group of 'local' hormones and are produced in most tissues of the body. They are participants in the inflammatory response that follows injury or infection. They include *prostaglandins, thromboxanes, prostacyclin* and *leukotrienes* and are derived from *arachidonate*, a polyunsaturated fatty acid that is synthesised from the essential fatty acid linoleate. Eicosanoids act through receptors in the plasma membranes of target cells, where they influence either protein kinase A or intracellular calcium levels.

Biosynthesis

Arachidonate is normally found at the *sn*-2 position of phospholipids and is released when *phospholipase A_2* is activated by various stimuli (Fig. 95). This activation occurs when a variety of agonists, such as histamine and cytokines, interact with a specific receptor on the target cell plasma membrane.

The cyclo-oxygenase pathway
This pathway forms prostaglandins (including PGE_2, $PGF_{2\alpha}$ and PGD_2), prostacyclin (PGI_2) and thromboxane

A_2 (TXA_2). Arachidonate is converted by the *cyclo-oxygenase* (COX) complex to PGG_2, which contains a five-membered ring and an hydroperoxy group. The latter is reduced to an hydroxyl in the formation of PGH_2. PGI_2 is derived from PGH_2 by the action of PGI synthase in endothelial cells. TXA_2 is formed from PGH_2 by the action of thromboxane synthase, an enzyme present in platelets.

The lipoxygenase pathway
This pathway forms leukotrienes in mast cells and leucocytes. *Lipoxygenases* catalyse hydroperoxidations at various positions in arachidonate to give 5-, 12- and 15-HPETEs (hydroperoxyeicosatetraenoic acids) from which a variety of HETEs (hydroeicosatetranoic acids) are formed. 5-HPETE is also the precursor of leukotriene LTA_4, which in turn is converted to LTB_4 and LTC_4. LTC_4 is formed from LTA_4 by the addition of reduced glutathione and is then processed to yield in turn LTD_4 and LTE_4. Leukotrienes have many biological actions, including increasing vascular permeability and being potent bronchoconstrictors.

Aspirin acts as an anti-inflammatory agent by inhibiting cyclo-oxygenase

Aspirin (acetylsalicylate) acetylates and irreversibly inactivates COX. Levels of the active enzyme in platelets are especially susceptible because these cells do not have nuclei and cannot regenerate COX. COX in endothelial cells is also affected but the enzyme at that site is restored to normal within a few hours. If subjects are treated with low-dose aspirin, there is a large fall in thromboxane A_2 relative to PGI_2 and platelet aggregation is inhibited. Low-dose aspirin therapy is used effectively to prevent myocardial infarction and is also used in patients to prevent recurrence of a heart attack. Other non-steroidal anti-inflammatory drugs (NSAIDs) such as ibuprofen and acetaminophen are reversible inhibitors of COX. COX exists in two isoforms: COX-1 (constitutive) and COX-2 (inducible). Most of aspirin's therapeutic effects are due to acetylation of COX-2. Its ulcerogenic effects are due to acetylation of COX-1. Aspirin is more potent against COX-1 than against COX-2.

Glucocorticoids act as anti-inflammatory agents by inhibiting phospholipase A_2

Glucocorticoids are potent anti-inflammatory agents that are used extensively in clinical practice for conditions such as chronic obstructive lung disease. They increase the production of proteins called *lipocortins*, which inhibit phospholipase A_2. As can be seen from Figure 95, inhibition of phospholipase A_2 will reduce the synthesis of prostaglandins, leukotrienes and thromboxane.

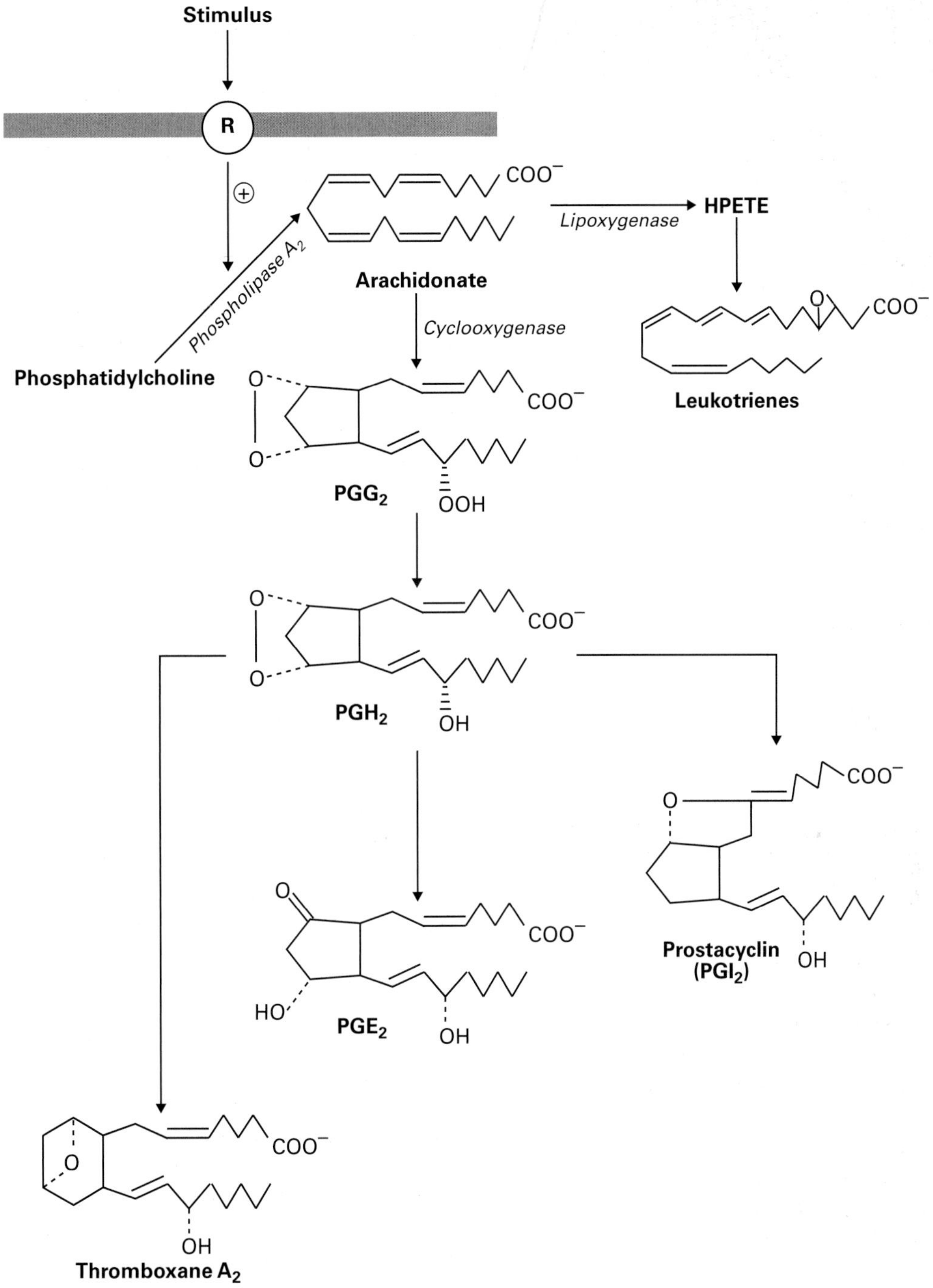

Fig. 95 Conversion of arachidonate to prostaglandins, leukotrienes and thromboxanes. HPETE, hydroperoxyeicosatetraenoic acid.

Self-assessment: questions

Single best answer MCQs

1. As a practising doctor you will be required to evaluate lipid profiles on your patients; this will require that you know basic aspects of lipid metabolism. Illustrate this knowledge by identifying the single correct statement below about lipid transport in the body.
   a. The rate of production of apolipoprotein Apo-B48 in intestinal mucosal cells determines the rate of synthesis of chylomicrons (CM) in these cells
   b. CM secreted into lymph acquire Apo-E and Apo-CII from LDL after they enter the blood
   c. The major function of both VLDL and CM is to transport cholesterol in blood
   d. After clearing of TAG from CM, the remnants are taken up by the liver, mediated by the LDL receptor in hepatocytes
   e. HDL has the lowest proportion of protein (relative to lipid) of all the circulating lipoproteins

2. Identify the single correct statement about lipoprotein lipase (LPL).
   a. LPL is synthesised in adipocytes and is then stored in fat globules of adipocytes
   b. Apo-CII is an activator of LPL and is present in both CM and VLDL
   c. LPL action brings about partial hydrolysis of a TAG (triacylglycerol) to monoacylglycerol and two fatty acids
   d. LPL activity in adipocytes is least active in the postprandial period following increased secretion of insulin in response to a meal that contains fat
   e. LPL activity in skeletal muscle tissue is inhibited during long-term exercise

3. Treatment of hypercholesterolaemia requires knowledge of the control of HMG-CoA reductase activity and LDL receptor (LDLR) levels. Which one of the following statements is correct concerning HMG-CoA reductase and LDLR?
   a. Their production (synthesis) in the liver is increased following a meal containing lots of cholesterol and cholesteryl esters
   b. They both contain coenzyme A (CoA)
   c. LDLR when active in extrahepatic tissues eventually leads to increased HMG-CoA activity in these tissues

   d. If LDLR is defective in extrahepatic tissues, then these tissues can compensate by synthesising cholesterol by the de novo pathway that involves HMG-CoA reductase

4. High-carbohydrate diets are known to promote fatty acid biosynthesis, contributing to obesity. Identify the correct statement that explains this observation.
   a. Formation of the polymeric state of acetyl-CoA carboxylase (ACC) is stimulated by palmitoyl-CoA
   b. ACC is activated by adenosine monophosphate (AMP)
   c. Fatty acid synthase (FAS) is allosterically activated by citrate
   d. FAS is activated by protein kinase A mediated phosphorylation
   e. ACC is allosterically activated by citrate

5. Identify the enzyme from Column A that is correctly matched with the statement in Column B.

A	B
a. FAS	Contains coenzyme A
b. Cytosolic 'malic enzyme'	Generates NADH for fatty acid synthesis
c. Citrate synthase	Transference of acetyl-CoA from mitochondria to cytosol
d. ATP-citrate lyase	Catalyses production of malonyl-CoA
e. Ketosynthetase of FAS	Contains glutathione

6. Tay–Sachs disease is caused by an inherited mutation in the gene encoding the α-subunit of a lysosomal enzyme called hexosaminidase A (Hex A), which catalyses the removal of an N-acetylgalactosamine residue from ganglioside G_{M2}, an acidic sphingoglycolipid. What enzyme reaction is mediated by Hex A?
   a. Converts ganglioside G_{M2} into ganglioside G_{M3}
   b. Generates a reaction product which is less acidic than ganglioside G_{M2}
   c. Is utilised clinically to screen potential carriers of this disease by a simple serum or amniotic fluid assay
   d. Both a and c are correct
   e. Both b and c are correct

7. Which of the following statements is a function, feature or property of phosphatidylcholine (PC)?
   a. PC is required for the production of sphingomyelins in the body
   b. PC is a major component of the lung surfactant
   c. PC can be produced by the methylation of phosphatidylethanolamine
   d. Both a and c are correct
   e. a, b and c are all correct

8. Identify from the following list the enzyme catalysing the rate-controlling step in bile acid synthesis from cholesterol in the liver.
   a. Cholesterol side chain cleavage cytochrome P-450
   b. Cholesterol 7α-hydroxylase
   c. Steroid 11β-hydroxylase
   d. Steroid 17α-hydroxylase
   e. Steroid 21-hydroxylase

9. Glucose metabolism in adipocytes in humans is critical for triacylglycerol (TAG) production because it is the source of what?
   a. Glycogen
   b. Polyunsaturated fatty acids (PUFA)
   c. Saturated fatty acids
   d. Glycerol 3-phosphate
   e. Glycerol

True/false questions

Are the following statements true or false?
1. Clathrin is concentrated in the Golgi apparatus in extrahepatic tissues.
2. The LDL receptor recognises Apo-B48 in LDL.
3. Atheromatous plaques recovered from a patient who has died from a coronary contain high concentrations of cholesterol and its esters.
4. CM and VLDL both contain Apo-CII.
5. Extrahepatic tissues derive cholesterol from a circulating lipoprotein by a process that involves receptor-mediated endocytosis.
6. Cholesterol 7α-hydroxylase is a rate-controlling step in bile acid synthesis in the liver.
7. The synthesis of PC from PE requires S-adenosylmethionine.
8. Gangliosides are unique from other sphingolipids in their content of N-acetylgalactosamine.
9. The action of acetyl-CoA carboxylase generates an intermediate in fatty acid biosynthesis that is also an inhibitor of fatty acid utilisation.
10. Mammalian FAS is active as a dimer.
11. Dipalmitoylphosphatidylcholine is the principal phospholipid in surfactant.

Short essay questions

1. Discuss cholesterol metabolism in the body in the context of the pathogenesis of familial hypercholesterolaemia.
2. Compare and contrast the roles of pancreatic lipase, lipoprotein lipase (LPL) and 'hormone-sensitive' lipase in the body
3. Construct a table that contrasts fatty acid oxidation with fatty acid synthesis.
4. Compare and contrast the action of aspirin and glucocorticoids on prostaglandin synthesis.

Self-assessment: answers

Single best answer MCQ answers

1. a. **True**. This is easily established by studying patients who have defective Apo-B production.
   b. **False**. Apo-E and Apo-CII are acquired from HDL.
   c. **False**. Their role is to transport TAG in blood.
   d. **False**. CM remnants are cleared by the liver using the Apo-E receptor.
   e. **False**. HDL is high density because of its high content of protein.

2. a. **False**. This lipase is synthesised in adipocytes and then transported to endothelial cells.
   b. **True**. Apo-CII is present in both VLDL and CM.
   c. **False**. LPL action on TAG yields glycerol and three fatty acids.
   d. **False**. Insulin increases LPL expression and this is consistent with the fed state where more fat is being stored.
   e. **False**. LPL is activated by adrenaline (epinephrine) and the fatty acids produced are used as fuels.

3. a. **False**. It should be obvious that, when cholesterol is abundant, both HMG-CoA reductase and LDLR should be less active.
   b. **False**. Neither contain coenzyme A.
   c. **False**. If LDLR is active, more cholesterol is delivered and thus HMG-CoA reductase activity should fall.
   d. **True**. This is all consistent with ensuring adequate supply of cholesterol in cells to be used for membrane synthesis.

4. a. **False**. Given the principle of 'product inhibition' (negative feedback), it should be obvious that palmitoyl-CoA (the product) should, if anything, inhibit the formation of the active form of the rate-controlling enzyme.
   b. **False**. AMP is a signal for fuel oxidation and it thus inhibits ACC, lowers malonyl-CoA levels and this promotes fatty acid catabolism by relieving inhibition of CPTI (carnitine palmitoyltransferase I).
   c. **False**. FAS activity is controlled by the supply of substrate (acetyl-CoA).
   d. **False**. Phosphorylation of ACC causes inhibition.
   e. **True**. Citrate transports acetyl groups from mitochondria to the cytosol; also the increase in citrate activates the rate-controlling enzyme, ACC.

5. a. **False**. FAS contains acyl carrier protein (ACP) not coenzyme A.
   b. **False**. It is NADPH that is generated.
   c. **True**. The inner mitochondrial membrane is impermeable to acetyl-CoA. Citrate is used to shuttle acetyl units to the cytosol and FAS.
   d. **False**. This enzyme produces acetyl-CoA from citrate.
   e. **False**. Both FAS and glutathione contain important SH groups, but glutathione is a tripeptide not contained in FAS.

6. a. **True**. The nomenclature is a bit weird and it means that, with one less carbohydrate unit, G_{M2} is converted to G_{M3}. The number when subtracted from 5 tells us the number of carbohydrate units!
   b. **False**. Hexosaminidase A removes an N-acetylgalactosamine, so the product is, if anything, more acidic than G_{M2}.
   c. **True**. The assay can be used to find carriers in that they will have about half the normal level.
   d. **True**. a and c are both correct. This is the single best answer.
   e. **False**. b is incorrect.

7. a. **True**. PC interacts with ceramide to produce sphingomyelin.
   b. **True**. Note that PC is not the only component. Certain proteins are needed as 'positioning factors'.
   c. **True**. Three methylations are involved. SAM (S-adenosylmethionine) is the methyl donor.
   d. **False**. b is also correct
   e. **True**. This is the single best answer.

8. a. **False**. This is a rate-controlling in steroid hormone biosynthesis.
   b. **True**. The 7α-hydroxyl distinguishes bile acids from other steroids.
   c. **False**. This enzyme is critical for cortisol synthesis.
   d. **False**. This enzyme is critical for cortisol, androgen and oestrogen biosynthesis.
   e. **False**. This enzyme is critical for cortisol and aldosterone biosynthesis.

9. a. **False**. Glycogen in adipocytes (very low!) has nothing to do with TAG synthesis.
   b. **False**. PUFA are not synthesised in the body and certainly not from glucose.

c. **False**. Although fatty acids can be made from glucose, that is not the critical role of glucose given the fact that most fatty acids are delivered to adipose tissue by VLDL or chylomicrons.

d. **True**. Glycerol cannot be phosphorylated in adipocytes, so glycerol 3-phosphate has to be made via glycolysis from dihydroxyacetone phosphate. Insulin stimulates glucose uptake and therefore efficient TAG synthesis.

e. **False**. See d.

True/false answers

1. **False**. It is concentrated in 'coated pits'.
2. **False**. It is Apo-B100 that binds to the LDL receptor.
3. **True**. This is part of the evidence relating cholesterol with coronary artery disease.
4. **True**. They are both acted upon by LPL and Apo-CII activates that enzyme.
5. **True**. The lipoprotein is LDL.
6. **True**. Following 7α-hydroxylation, other hydroxyls are added and side chain cleavage occurs to give the C_{24} bile acids.
7. **True**. *S*-Adenosylmethionine provides the methyl groups for many important methylations involved in the synthesis of key compounds in the body.
8. **False**. Gangliosides differ from other sphingolipids in containing sialic acid, also called *N*-acetylneuraminic acid.
9. **True**. Malonyl-CoA is required for fatty acid biosynthesis, but it is also an inhibitor of carnitine acyltransferase I, the rate-limiting step in fatty acid utilisation.
10. **True**. It is the monomer that is inactive.
11. **True**. It is not the only component but it is very important.

Short essay answers

1. Here are the key points that should be in your response.
   - It is now clear that there is a correlation between elevated levels of circulating cholesterol and the pathogenesis of coronary heart disease (CHD). However, CHD is multifactorial.
   - There is a very clear relationship between elevated cholesterol and CHD in the case of familial hypercholesterolaemia (FH), an autosomal dominant disorder affecting the receptor-mediated endocytosis pathway for LDL metabolism in the body.
   - Homozygotes for FH have defective or absent LDL receptor (LDLR) in the liver and extrahepatic tissues. The consequence is that the handling of both IDL and LDL is grossly impaired.
   - The defective LDLR-mediated endocytosis pathway in extrahepatic tissues results in these tissues turning on their endogenous cholesterol biosynthetic pathways.
   - Unless treated heroically to reduce their cholesterol levels (or given a liver transplant), FH homozygotes die in their teens or early twenties. Heterozygotes also have very high cholesterol levels and they die in their thirties or forties.

2. It is important to recognise that these three lipases function in three different anatomical sites.
   - Pancreatic lipase is secreted from the pancreas, ending up in the small intestine where it catalyses the hydrolysis of triacylglycerol derived from the diet. The products are 2-monoacylglycerol plus two fatty acid molecules (partial hydrolysis).
   - Lipoprotein lipase (LPL) is an enzyme attached to endothelial cells that catalyses the hydrolysis of triacylglycerols carried in chylomicrons and VLDL. The fatty acids released can either be stored in adipose tissue or used as fuels in, for example, muscle. LPL is activated by Apo-CII, which is a component of both VLDL and chylomicrons. LPL is synthesised in adipose tissue cells stimulated by insulin and is then translocated to the endothelial cells. The fact that insulin has this action is consistent with its role in fuel storage.
   - Hormone-sensitive lipase (HSL) is a triacylglycerol lipase found within adipocytes. It catalyses the first step in the complete hydrolysis of stored triacylglycerols to glycerol and three fatty acid molecules. It is the key enzyme in lipid mobilisation and is activated by a series of regulatory hormones that counteract the inhibitory action of insulin. Lipid mobilisation is increased in the fasting state to provide an alternative fuel to glucose for tissues such as muscle and liver. Activation of HSL by hormones such as glucagon involves phosphorylation, brought about by cyclic AMP dependent protein kinase.

3. Table 9 contrasts fatty acid oxidation and synthesis.

4. Both aspirin and glucocorticoids affect prostaglandin synthesis. Aspirin is more selective in that it inhibits cyclo-oxygenase 1 (COX-1), thus affecting prostacyclin (PGI_2), PGE_2 and thromboxane A_2 (TXA_2) synthesis. If low doses of aspirin are taken,

Table 9 A comparison of fatty acid oxidation and synthesis

Parameter	Fatty acid oxidation	Fatty acid synthesis
Location in cells	Mitochondria	Cytosol
Transport	Carnitine	Acetate as citrate
Carrier	Coenzyme A	Acyl carrier protein
Addition or removal of two-carbon units	Acetyl-CoA	Malonyl-CoA
Oxidation/reduction of keto $\rightleftharpoons$ hydroxyl	$NAD^+/NADH + H^+$	$NADPH + H^+/NADP^+$
Oxidation/reduction of crotonyl $\rightleftharpoons$ butyryl	$FAD/FADH_2$	$NADPH + H^+/NADP^+$

there can be a beneficial effect on platelet aggregation. The mechanism of this effect is related to the fact that aspirin is a 'suicide' inhibitor of COX-1, the inhibition occurring in both platelets, where TXA_2 is synthesised, and endothelial cells, where PGI_2 is synthesised. Endothelial cells recover their COX-1 activity within a few hours since they are capable of protein synthesis. In contrast,

platelets do not have the ability to synthesise more COX-1; the ratio of PGI_2 to TXA_2 is therefore greatly increased and platelet aggregation leading to clot formation is suppressed. Glucocorticoids inhibit phospholipase A_2 thus reducing arachidonic acid production and therefore both the lipoxygenase and cyclo-oxygenase pathways of inflammatory mediators.

10 Integration of metabolism

Overview

Many individuals are able to maintain exquisite control of their metabolism, as evidenced by the fact that over periods of many years they show quite small fluctuations in body weight despite consuming a staggering number of calories in the form of carbohydrates, protein and fat. The overall strategy of metabolism is to store fuel when food is available and to mobilise these stores when necessary. Hormonal control is the key to fuel homeostasis, with insulin and glucagon being the main regulators.

10.1 The fed and fasted states

Learning objectives

You should be able to:

- describe the role of food intake, exercise, leptin and other factors in controlling body weight

- list fuels stored in the body and their relative amounts

- explain how metabolism is controlled in the fed state

- outline key aspects of insulin and glucagon secretion and sites of action

- explain how metabolism is controlled in the fasted state

- outline key aspects concerning the sites of action of the counter-regulatory hormones

- describe the body's response to starvation and the key role of ketone bodies.

Regulation of body weight

Despite the recognition that obesity is a major disease in modern society, many individuals are able to maintain exquisite control of their metabolism. In contrast, when individuals achieve weight loss through dieting they usually regain the weight over time. This is suggestive of regulatory mechanisms being involved to control the amount of energy (triacylglycerols) stored in adipose tissue. From studies on obese mice, it has been shown that adipose tissue produces a polypeptide hormone, *leptin*, which is involved in controlling food intake. Leptin deficiency and/or leptin resistance leads to obesity. Insulin, the hormone of the fed state, also appears to act in the negative feedback control of adiposity. It is thought that both insulin and leptin control food intake and energy expenditure through interactions in the hypothalamus.

What follows is an account of how *the storage of fuels* is achieved and *how fuels are mobilised* for the various tissues of the body. Familiarity with the contents of Chapters 6–9 will assist the reader in understanding the control of metabolism.

The key hormones are insulin and glucagon and we will deal here with their secretion and actions. Other aspects will be covered in Chapter 17.

The fed state

It is interesting to examine the amount of the various fuels that are stored in normal subjects (Table 10). Many people tend to believe that glucose and glycogen are the most significant fuels in humans, but it is quite clear that, in terms of total stored fuel, triacylglycerols are prodigious by comparison.

Table 10 Distribution of stored fuels in a 70 kg man

Storage fuel	Weight (kg)	Energy (kJ)
Glucose: extracellular	0.02	334
Glycogen: liver	0.07	1 170
muscle	0.12	2 000
Triacylglycerol: adipose	9	564 000
Protein: muscle	6	100 300

How does one measure control of metabolism in the fed state?

This is done routinely using a *glucose tolerance test* in which a subject fasts overnight, a fasting blood sample is taken and a glucose drink is then swallowed. Blood glucose is measured at 30 minute intervals for up to 150 minutes. On average, normal subjects show a blood glucose concentration rise from 90 mg/100 ml (5 mM) to about 140 mg/100 ml (7.8 mM). The effectiveness of glucose homeostasis is illustrated by considering the fate of 50 g of glucose that is completely absorbed into a person with a 5 litre blood volume or a 15 litre extracellular fluid (ECF) volume. The glucose concentration would rise by 1000 mg/100 ml if the glucose was confined to the blood and by 333 mg/100 ml if confined to the ECF, yet in normal individuals blood levels rarely exceed 180 mg/100 ml after a carbohydrate meal. The important question is: Why does the blood glucose not reach very high (non-physiological) values? An answer is revealed by the study of subjects with diabetes mellitus. Their blood glucose levels reach much higher levels (greater than 10 mM) following a challenge with oral glucose. These patients either make little or no insulin or they have insulin resistance. Clearly, insulin is vital to the ability to control blood glucose in the fed state.

Insulin

Insulin is the hormone of the fed state and is made in pancreatic beta cells. Important points about insulin are the following:

- *Insulin chemistry.* It is a small protein hormone with 51 amino acid residues comprising two peptide chains (A and B) linked by two disulphide bonds.
- *Control of insulin secretion.* Insulin secretagogues are factors that increase insulin secretion. The principal one is glucose. High blood glucose levels lead to increased glucose uptake into beta cells via GLUT2. Glucokinase (also with a high K_m for glucose) catalyses the entry of glucose into glycolysis and subsequent oxidative metabolism, generating ATP. The ATP blocks an ATP-sensitive K^+ channel, leading to depolarisation of the cell, calcium entry and subsequent insulin release (Fig. 96). Drugs called sulphonylureas (e.g. tolbutamide), which are used to treat type 2 diabetes, block the ATP-sensitive K^+ channel, cause depolarisation of the beta cell and thus increase insulin secretion.
- *Mechanism of action.* The major sites for insulin action in the body are the liver, muscle and adipose tissue (Fig. 97 and Table 11). Clearly, the pathways affected are numerous and the effects include both activation of key enzymes and the induction of

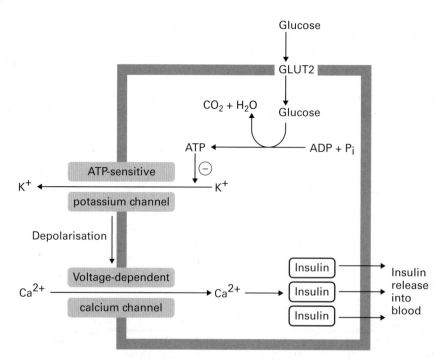

Fig. 96 Control of insulin secretion by glucose.

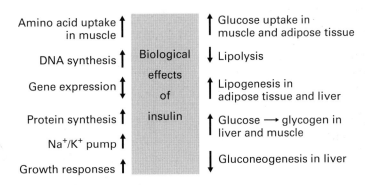

Fig. 97 Multiple actions of insulin.

Table 11 Effect of insulin in target tissues

Tissue	Activation	Inhibition
Liver	Glycogenesis	Gluconeogenesis
	Lipogenesis	Ketogenesis
Adipose tissue	Glucose uptake	Lipolysis
	Lipogenesis	
Muscle	Glycogenesis	Protein degradation
	Glucose uptake	
	Amino acid uptake	

enzyme synthesis. The insulin receptor structure and signal transduction pathway are shown in Figure 98. The insulin receptor is a plasma membrane receptor tyrosine kinase. It has two identical alpha chains and two identical beta chains joined by disulphide linkages. The alpha chains are extracellular; the beta chains have an extracellular portion as well as membrane spanning and intracellular portions. The activation of tyrosine kinase activity in the receptor that results from binding of insulin is followed by phosphorylation of several insulin receptor substrates (IRS 1, 2, 3 and 4). This allows for linkage to several complex signalling pathways. Some involve phosphatidylinositol-3-kinase (PI3K) which activates protein kinase B (PKB). PKB regulates the translocation of GLUT4 into the plasma membranes of adipocytes and muscle cells. They also are part of the pathway that results in activation of phosphoprotein phosphatase-1 (PP-1) and subsequent activation of glycogen synthase (Ch. 7, p. 99) in liver and muscle. Other pathways lead to increased synthesis of the key enzymes of fat synthesis. In cardiac muscle, the important action is activation of PFK-1 and, therefore, increased ATP production. Binding of insulin to the insulin receptor can also activate the Ras pathway and the MAP (mitogen-activated protein) kinase pathway, leading to increased DNA/RNA/protein synthesis.

- **Diabetes mellitus.** Diabetes is the most common endocrine disorder in a global sense. There are two major forms of diabetes mellitus: insulin-dependent diabetes mellitus (IDDM; type 1 diabetes) and non-insulin-dependent diabetes mellitus (NIDDM; type 2 diabetes). The most common findings in diabetes mellitus are hyperglycaemia, glucosuria, decreased glycogenesis, decreased fatty acid synthesis, increased lipolysis, increased fatty acids in blood, ketonaemia, ketonuria, metabolic acidosis and negative nitrogen balance. All of these are easily explained given our knowledge of the actions of insulin on target tissues. There is a switch from utilisation of glucose to utilisation of fat. Low levels of oxaloacetate (OAA) in liver means that ketone body production will be greater. Greater output coupled with less efficient utilisation of ketone bodies in muscle (low [OAA] again!) explains the development of dangerous ketonaemia. Ketonaemia is usually restricted to type 1 diabetics but can also occur in type 2 diabetics with insulinopenia.

The fasted state

The regulation of blood glucose concentration in the fasted state is of prime importance to those tissues in the body (e.g. brain) that cannot utilise other fuels such as fatty acids. The liver plays the major role, but muscle protein turnover also contributes inasmuch as alanine and glutamine, the amino acids leaving muscle in the fasted state, are glucogenic. Hormone-stimulated enzyme induction may also play an important role. The key hormone of the fasted state is *glucagon*, with several others, including growth hormone (hGH), adrenocorticotrophic hormone (ACTH), cortisol, adrenaline (epinephrine) and thyroid hormone, having important roles; as a group they are referred to as *counter-regulatory hormones*.

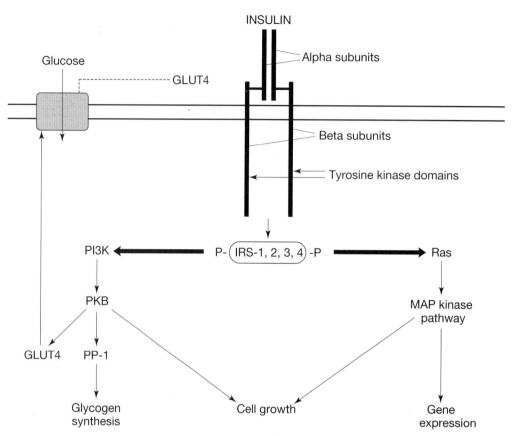

Fig. 98 Insulin receptor structure and signal transduction pathways. IRS, insulin receptor substrate; PPP-1, phosphoprotein phosphatase-1.

How does one measure a subject's response to hypoglycaemia?

The subject fasts overnight, a fasting blood sample is taken and insulin is administered; the amount of insulin injected depends upon weight of the subject. Blood samples are taken and glucose is measured to determine that hypoglycaemia was produced (usually within 30 minutes). In normal subjects, glucagon, hGH, cortisol and ACTH levels will be high at the 90 minute time period and fasting glucose levels restored.

Glucagon

Glucagon is the hormone of the fasted state and is made in pancreatic alpha cells. Important points about glucagon are:

- *Chemistry.* Small polypeptide with 29 amino acid residues.
- *Control of secretion.* Its secretion is increased when the blood glucose falls to less than 5 mM. Glucagon secretion is also increased following a protein meal and in response to prolonged exercise.

Table 12 Effect of glucagon in target tissues

Tissue	Activation
Liver	Glycogenolysis
	Gluconeogenesis
	Ketogenesis
	Amino acid catabolism
	Urea synthesis
Adipose tissue	Lipolysis
Muscle	No effect

- *Mechanism of action.* Glucagon binding to its receptor results in activation of protein kinase A (see Ch. 17, p. 246), leading to phosphorylation of liver glycogen phosphorylase and adipocyte hormone-sensitive lipase. Glucose and fatty acids are mobilised. Gluconeogenesis in liver is activated at several sites. The main sites for glucagon action are listed in Table 12.

Other counter-regulatory hormones

Growth hormone (hGH)

Although mainly of interest because of its role in growth, this hormone plays a dynamic role in glucose homeostasis. *Direct actions* of hGH include increasing fatty acid release from adipose tissue and serving as an insulin antagonist.

Adrenocorticotrophic hormone (ACTH, corticotrophin)

The principal role of ACTH is to control cortisol production by the adrenal cortex (Ch. 17, p. 241). However, it has effects on whole body metabolism including stimulation of adipocyte triacylglycerol lipase and release of fatty acids into blood.

Cortisol

Cortisol increases protein turnover and gluconeogenesis. Long-term treatment with high doses of glucocorticoid can cause diabetes mellitus.

Thyroxine

Thyroxine (T_4) has effects on almost every cell in the body. It is a prohormone that is de-iodinated in target tissues to the active hormone T_3 (Ch. 17, p. 243). T_4 and T_3 enhance cellular intermediary metabolism (they increase the basal metabolic rate), sustain brain growth and development and are required for normal hGH secretion to occur. They also increase lipid mobilisation from adipose tissue and uncouple oxidative phosphorylation.

Adrenaline (Epinephrine)

Adrenaline (epinephrine) stimulates liver and muscle glycogenolysis and lipid mobilisation from adipose tissue. Also, consistent with its role as a counter-regulatory hormone, adrenaline (epinephrine) inhibits insulin release from the pancreas; this action contributes to the normalisation of blood glucose during hypoglycaemia.

In summary

The response to hypoglycaemia involves several hormones, with glucagon and adrenaline (epinephrine) having major roles. Patients with defects in hGH and ACTH secretion exhibit hypoglycaemia, and this potential has to be recognised, especially in children.

Starvation is a special situation

During the first week or so of starvation, the individual makes glucose from protein in order to satisfy the fuel needs of the brain. This is the *gluconeogenic phase*. If starvation is prolonged, the individual enters the *protein conservation phase* (or he/she will die!). There is increased ketone body production coupled with decreased utilisation of ketone bodies in muscle (probably because of decreased [OAA]). The result is a large increase in circulating ketone bodies, which achieve concentrations that enable them to compete with glucose as the fuel for the brain. The individual develops a significant metabolic acidosis but survives for a longer period. Fatty acids per se cannot be utilised directly as fuels by the brain because they cannot cross the blood–brain barrier.

10.2 Metabolic support and control in tissues

Learning objectives

You should be able to:

- explain the key role of glucose as the fuel for the brain and how this 'directs' glucose homeostasis

- describe the major metabolic pathways and their control in the fed state in liver, muscle and adipose tissue

- describe the major metabolic pathways and their control in the fasted state in liver, muscle and adipose tissue

- outline the fuels used by heart, kidney, intestine and skin.

The major tissues of the body work together in order to maintain a constant supply of oxidisable fuels to all cells. In this chapter we focus on the major metabolic pathways related to fuel metabolism in brain, liver, muscle and adipose tissue. What is presented is a very general treatment of the subject, but if you review the major points that follow on these tissues and consult Figures 99–105, you should have a clear picture of the important concepts of integrated metabolism in the body.

The brain uses glucose as its fuel and cannot use fatty acids

Much of the ATP production in the brain is used to generate and maintain the concentration gradients of Na^+, K^+ and Ca^{2+} across the plasma membrane of neurons and of H^+ across vesicular membranes. Na^+/K^+-ATPase is the major user of ATP. Under non-starving conditions, glucose is the fuel used by the brain (Fig. 99). The brain requires a steady supply of glucose (from blood) in order to function normally. Levels of blood glucose less than 2.5 mM lead to brain dysfunction. The brain has

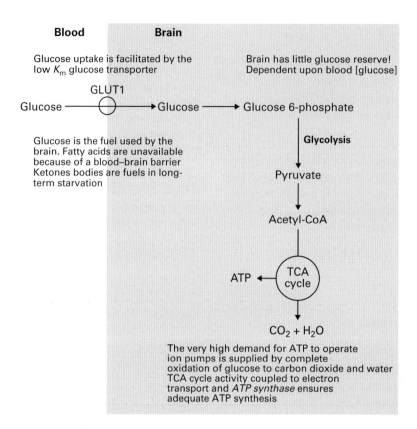

Blood **Brain**

Glucose uptake is facilitated by the low K_m glucose transporter

Brain has little glucose reserve! Dependent upon blood [glucose]

GLUT1

Glucose ───○──→ Glucose ──→ Glucose 6-phosphate

Glucose is the fuel used by the brain. Fatty acids are unavailable because of a blood–brain barrier Ketones bodies are fuels in long-term starvation

Glycolysis

Pyruvate

Acetyl-CoA

ATP ← TCA cycle

$CO_2 + H_2O$

The very high demand for ATP to operate ion pumps is supplied by complete oxidation of glucose to carbon dioxide and water TCA cycle activity coupled to electron transport and *ATP synthase* ensures adequate ATP synthesis

Fig. 99 Control of metabolism in the brain in the fed or fasted state.

low levels of stored glycogen (about 1% of the concentration found in the liver) and so temporary anaerobic metabolism is very limited. It is important to recognise that the brain cannot utilise fatty acids as fuel because they cannot cross the blood–brain barrier. Also, the brain seems unable to use as fuels the high concentrations of glutamate and aspartate present.

Normal conditions

Although the brain constitutes only 2% of the body weight of adults, 20% of the total resting oxygen consumption of the body occurs there.

Starvation

The brain uses ketone bodies as an exceptional fuel to conserve body protein during prolonged starvation (see above).

Liver stores glycogen in the fed state and releases it in the fasted state

The liver is ideally placed in the body to serve as a metabolic clearing house. It has the major role to play in con-

trolling the levels of blood glucose in that it responds to insulin and glucagon, the principal hormones of the fed and fasted states, respectively. The critical functions possessed by the liver that relate to fuel metabolism are as follows:

- *In the fed state* (Fig. 100). Liver takes up large quantities of glucose, most of which is converted to glycogen. A limited amount of triacylglycerol (TAG) is also formed. Insulin controls these processes. Glucose metabolism provides the glycerol 3-phosphate required for TAG synthesis. Fatty acids are converted to TAGs, which are exported as very low density lipoproteins (VLDL) for storage as fat elsewhere in the body.
- *In the fasted state* (Fig. 101). Liver glycogen serves as a reservoir of glucose. Glycogenolysis ensures that the blood glucose concentration is sufficient to supply fuel to the brain and other glucose-dependent tissues. Glucose can also be produced by gluconeogenesis. Glucagon controls these processes. Oxidation of fatty acids in liver in the fasted state provides the ATP required for gluconeogenesis and for the other biosynthetic

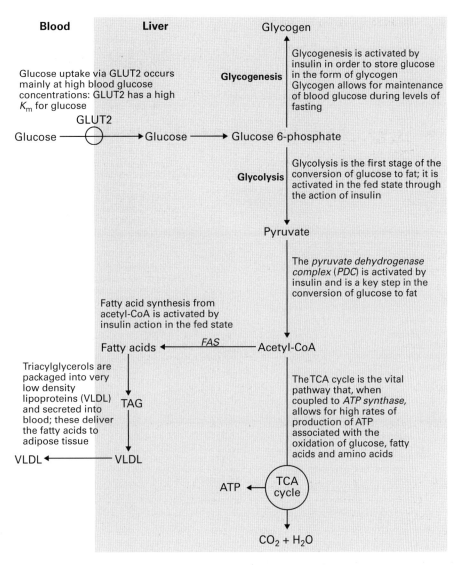

Fig. 100 Liver metabolism in the fed state.

reactions occurring there. Some of the fatty acids are converted to ketone bodies, which are exported for use by muscles.

Adipose tissue stores triacylglycerols in the fed state and releases fatty acids and glycerol in the fasted state

As can be seen from Table 9, adipose tissue contains by far the major store of energy in the body, in the form of TAGs. It is a 'fuel buffer', which the body can call upon during lengthy periods of fasting or exercise. Healthy fat individuals survive starvation for a longer period than non-obese subjects do. The major points related to fuel metabolism are as follows:

- *In the fed state* (Fig. 102). Fatty acids and glucose are taken up by adipose tissue. The fatty acids come from VLDL and chylomicrons by the action of endothelial lipoprotein lipase (LPL) (Ch. 9). Glucose metabolism provides the glycerol 3-phosphate required for TAG synthesis. Insulin is the key hormone of storage in that it increases glucose uptake through recruitment of GLUT4 to the plasma membrane. It also induces LPL synthesis and translocation to endothelial cells and inhibits hormone-sensitive lipase (HSL). Apo-CII in chylomicrons and VLDL activate LPL.
- *In the fasted state and during exercise* (Fig. 103). Insulin levels fall, counter-regulatory hormones rise and HSL is activated, leading to fatty acid production from TAGs. HSL action produces free

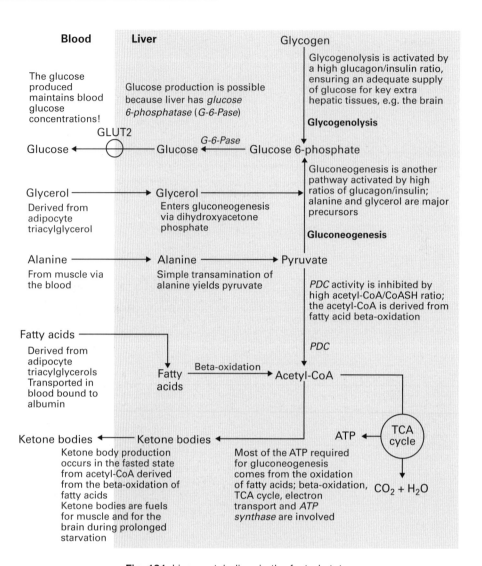

Blood **Liver**

Glycogen

Glycogenolysis is activated by a high glucagon/insulin ratio, ensuring an adequate supply of glucose for key extra hepatic tissues, e.g. the brain

The glucose produced maintains blood glucose concentrations!

Glucose production is possible because liver has *glucose 6-phosphatase* (*G-6-Pase*)

Glycogenolysis

GLUT2

Glucose ← Glucose ← *G-6-Pase* Glucose 6-phosphate

Gluconeogenesis is another pathway activated by high ratios of glucagon/insulin; alanine and glycerol are major precursors

Glycerol → Glycerol →

Derived from adipocyte triacylglycerol

Enters gluconeogenesis via dihydroxyacetone phosphate

Gluconeogenesis

Alanine → Alanine → Pyruvate

From muscle via the blood

Simple transamination of alanine yields pyruvate

PDC activity is inhibited by high acetyl-CoA/CoASH ratio; the acetyl-CoA is derived from fatty acid beta-oxidation

Fatty acids

Derived from adipocyte triacylglycerols Transported in blood bound to albumin

PDC

Fatty acids

Beta-oxidation

Acetyl-CoA

TCA cycle

Ketone bodies ← Ketone bodies ←

ATP ←

Ketone body production occurs in the fasted state from acetyl-CoA derived from the beta-oxidation of fatty acids
Ketone bodies are fuels for muscle and for the brain during prolonged starvation

Most of the ATP required for gluconeogenesis comes from the oxidation of fatty acids; beta-oxidation, TCA cycle, electron transport and *ATP synthase* are involved

$CO_2 + H_2O$

Fig. 101 Liver metabolism in the fasted state.

fatty acids, which are released into blood, bound to albumin and transported to liver, skeletal and cardiac muscle etc. to serve as fuel. Glycerol is also produced and it goes to the liver where it can be converted into glucose.

Muscle also stores glycogen in the fed state and can utilise fatty acids

Muscle can use a variety of different fuels, including glucose (glycogen), fatty acids and ketone bodies. These fuels can be completely oxidised to carbon dioxide and water. The initial pathway of glucose metabolism in muscle is glycolysis. Phosphofructokinase-1 is the key control step of glycolysis (Ch. 6, p. 81). A potential end-point of glycolysis is lactic acid, the formation of which allows for increased ATP production by fast-twitch muscle fibres during high-intensity physical exercise.

Muscle contains stores of glycogen that are metabolised to provide ATP; this is very important in support of short bursts of activity. Long-term exercise requires fatty acid use by slow-twitch muscle fibres.

- *In the fed state* (Fig. 104). Glucose uptake and glycogen storage are stimulated by insulin.
- *In the fasted state* (Fig. 105). Under fasted conditions (e.g. overnight) the respiratory quotient (RQ) of muscle is approximately 0.7. This indicates that the fuel being used is long-chain fatty acids (the RQ for glucose is 1.0). Muscle cannot export glucose to contribute to glucose homeostasis in the fasted state since it does not contain glucose-6-phosphatase. For the same reason, muscle does not participate in gluconeogenesis. However, in the fasted state, muscle degrades some of its protein to alanine, which is a glucogenic substrate in the liver; thus, indirectly, muscle contributes to glucose homeostasis.

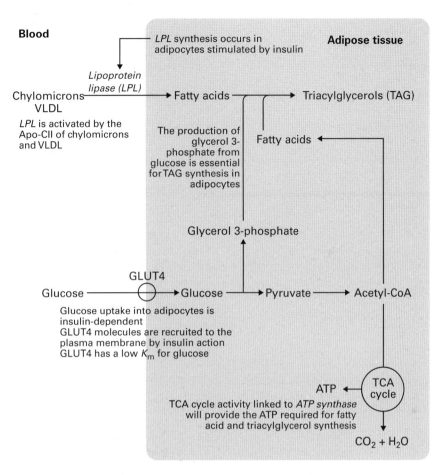

Fig. 102 Adipose tissue metabolism in the fed state.

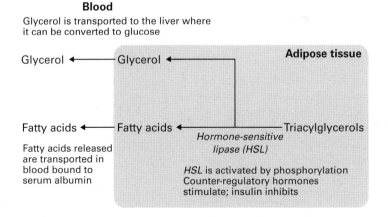

Fig. 103 Adipose tissue metabolism in the fasted state.

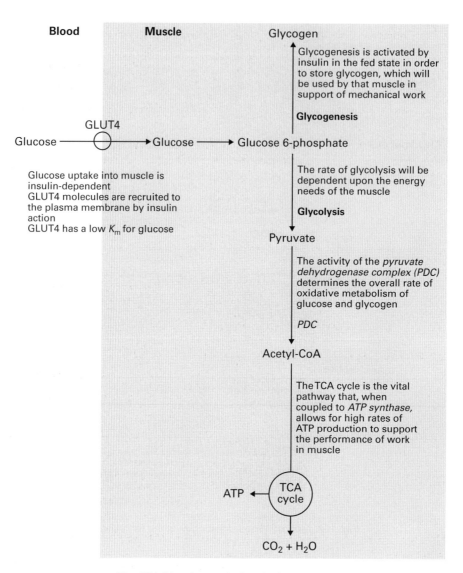

Fig. 104 Muscle metabolism in the fed state.

Cardiac muscle utilises all fuels, especially fatty acids

The heart needs to produce ATP constantly and at a high rate. In order to accomplish this it has the ability to oxidise all fuels and has a higher content of mitochondria than most other tissues. At rest, the heart has a much higher rate of oxygen consumption per kilogram compared with skeletal muscle. Heart is one of the major contributors to the basal metabolic rate, again much more important than skeletal muscle. Fuels used by heart muscle include the following:

- *Glycogen* is stored in the heart in the fed state but is not a major contributor to the fuel needs of the heart. It is available for use when oxygen supply to heart muscle is impaired.

- *Glucose* is transported via (insulin-dependent) GLUT4. Its utilisation is greatest immediately following meals containing carbohydrate. Insulin action activates cardiac muscle PFK-1.
- *Lactate* produced by anaerobic glucose metabolism in skeletal muscle (during vigorous exercise) can be readily used by heart muscle because its high oxidative capacity results in lactate/pyruvate and $NAD^+/NADH$ ratios that favour the oxidation of lactate to pyruvate. The major form of lactate dehydrogenase in heart is LD_1 (H_4).
- *Fatty acids* are quantitatively the most important fuels for heart muscle. This is consistent with their role as the major storage form of energy in the body (as TAG) and the fact that they have higher potential (per carbon) to generate ATP compared

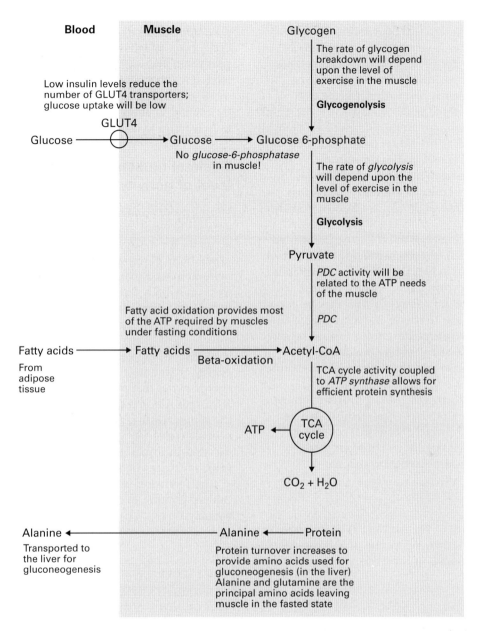

Fig. 105 Muscle metabolism in the fasted state.

with glucose. Exercise increases fatty acid release from adipose tissue, providing more fuel to support the increased work required to increase cardiac output. The heart preferentially uses fatty acids over glucose.

- *Ketone bodies* are very well catabolised in the heart. Consistent with this ability, the heart has a high level of β-hydroxybutyrate dehydrogenase.

Creatine kinase
The heart has a high content of creatine kinase, the enzyme catalysing the formation of ATP from creatine phosphate plus ADP. The major isoforms of creatine kinase in heart muscle are MM and MB, the amount of the latter being 30 times higher than in skeletal muscle.

The kidney

The renal medulla is apparently restricted to glucose as the fuel that it uses to generate ATP. The renal cortex utilises glucose, fatty acids and ketone bodies as fuels.

The intestine

The small intestine and colon have different fuel preferences.

- Glucose, glutamine, glutamate, asparagine and aspartate are metabolised by *enterocytes* to provide ATP. Enterocytes have very active glutaminases and use glutamine derived from the circulation. The amino acids are oxidised to carbon dioxide or converted to alanine and lactate. During an overnight fast, these amino acids are in short supply in the lumen and most of the glutamine is obtained from the bloodstream. Under these conditions, glutamine and ketone bodies provide almost all of the fuel for the small intestine. In critically ill patients, most of the glutamine for enterocytes arises from increased protein breakdown in skeletal muscle.

- Bacteria in the lumen of the colon use undigested starch and non-starch polysaccharides (also known as dietary fibre) as fuel. One of their fermentation products is butyrate, a short-chain fatty acid, which is the major fuel for *colonocytes*. This may be part of the explanation as to why diets high in starch and non-starch polysaccharides protect against colonic cancer. They cause colonocyte proliferation and stimulate mucosal growth. Butyrate is beta-oxidised to yield acetyl-CoA, which enters the TCA (tricarboxylic acid) cycle leading to ATP synthesis. Butyrate is not a product of metabolism in other cells of the body, which means that colonocyte function can be impaired by antibiotic therapy, resulting in mucosal barrier breakdown.

The skin

Skin derives most of the required ATP by anaerobic glycolysis, with lactate being one of the constituents of sweat. Lactic acid in sweat is considered to be bactericidal.

10.3 Use of fuels during exercise

Learning objectives

You should be able to:

- describe the utilisation of fuels during severe, moderate and long-term exercise

- explain the importance of the creatine phosphate shuttle in muscle.

Metabolic pathways of muscle include oxidative metabolism of carbohydrate, fats and amino acids and formation of lactate from carbohydrate. Under certain circumstances, muscular work is also supported by protein catabolism. Oxidative capacity is limited by mitochondrial numbers as these contain the enzymes of the TCA cycle, beta-oxidation of fatty acids, the electron transport chain and ATP synthase. Fast-twitch muscle cells have few mitochondria; slow-twitch muscle cells have many mitochondria and the number can be increased by training. Training increases the ability for slow-twitch muscle fibres to use lactate as fuel.

Skeletal muscle fuel use depends on level of activity

During exercise, energy expenditure in muscle increases greatly. Skeletal muscle, because of its large mass, accounts for a large proportion of the body's energy expenditure at rest despite having a low metabolic rate per unit mass. What is special about muscle cells is that their metabolic rate can vary over a wide range, increasing more than 200–1000 times from rest to maximal exercise. The immediate available substrates are in muscle itself. They are creatine phosphate (CP) and glycogen, which can be utilised without delay when energy output must increase. The 'CP shuttle' acts as an energy buffer that maintains ATP levels in muscle cells (Fig. 106). CP and glycogen are in close contact with the contractile machinery within muscle. CP is spontaneously converted to creatinine in muscle. Creatinine is excreted in urine; its production is relatively constant from day to day in normal individuals.

The following sections summarise fuel metabolism during sprinting, middle-distance running and marathon running.

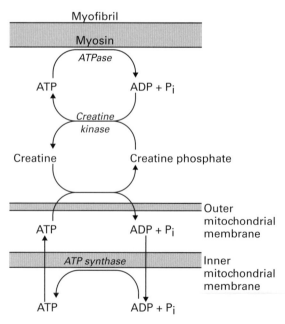

Fig. 106 The creatine phosphate (CP) shuttle.

High-power exertion (e.g. sprinting) is supported by anaerobic glycolysis

The controlling event in a working muscle is the hydrolysis of ATP to ADP + P_i by muscular contraction. The resultant increase in ADP concentration will cause CP to be used to reform ATP (catalysed by *creatine kinase*) in order to support continued muscular contraction. For continued high exertion, metabolism of glycogen to lactate has to be switched on (and is). In summary, for a 100 metre sprint, muscles are using:

- available ATP
- ATP formed from CP: generates ATP at a very high rate
- ATP formed by anaerobic metabolism of glycogen: generates ATP at a high rate (oxidative metabolism is too slow!).

For a 1000 metre run oxidative metabolism can be used

A longer exercise is powered by anaerobic glycolysis plus oxidative metabolism, mainly of glycogen and glucose. The rate is slower, so overall velocity is slower. The increase in glycogen metabolism is controlled by:

- AMP levels, which increase and activate glycogen phosphorylase and PFK-1

- adrenaline (epinephrine) secretion, which activates glycogen phosphorylase via activation of cyclic AMP dependent protein kinase A (Ch. 17, p. 246).

Marathon running requires use of increasing amounts of fatty acids

The runner must use lots of fat since there are not enough glycogen stores, even if 'carbohydrate loading' is attempted to increase the stores.

- Overall velocity will be lower since fat oxidation is slower.
- In a run lasting several hours, stored TAG and glycogen are used for 98% of the energy production; only 2% comes from use of protein.
- The evidence for a switch to the utilisation of fat comes from the observation that the respiratory quotient ($RQ = CO_2/O_2$) declines throughout.
- Blood glucose falls significantly during a marathon and about 90% of the total liver glycogen is used.
- Blood insulin levels gradually fall and there is an increase in glucagon levels.
- The increase in glucagon coupled with the fall in insulin allows for efficient fat mobilisation from adipose tissue since HSL will be active.

Self-assessment: questions

Single best answer MCQs

Answer questions 1–3 using the following scenario:

> A normal adult male is scheduled for a physical examination. In order to obtain a fasting blood sample, his physician tells him not to eat after 8 p.m. the previous night. The blood is drawn at 10 a.m. next day.

1. After the overnight fast, one would expect a *decrease* in what?
    a. Phosphorylated PFK-2
    b. Alanine aminotransferase
    c. Pyruvate carboxylase activity
    d. Aldolase activity
    e. Phosphoenolpyruvate carboxykinase (PEPCK) activity

2. After the overnight fast, one would expect increased activity of what?
    a. Pancreatic lipase
    b. Hepatic acetyl-CoA carboxylase
    c. Hepatic pyruvate dehydrogenase complex
    d. Adipocyte hormone-sensitive lipase
    e. Hepatic glycogen synthase

3. After the overnight fast one would expect glucose transporter activity to be what?
    a. decreased in brain cells
    b. decreased in hepatocytes
    c. enhanced in adipocytes
    d. decreased in red blood cells
    e. decreased in muscle cells

4. During prolonged (8 weeks) starvation, the adaptations in whole body metabolism are geared to extend the survival period. To achieve this goal, different tissues adapt differently. Which one of the following statements is correct for metabolism during prolonged starvation compared to day 7 of a starve?
    a. Oxaloacetate levels are higher in muscle in week 8 than at day 7
    b. The rate of gluconeogenesis in the liver decreases because there is a reduced demand for glucose oxidation at 8 weeks compared to day 7 of the starve.
    c. The degradation of proteins is increased in skeletal muscle due to an increased demand for amino acids for gluconeogenesis
    d. Gluconeogenesis stops in the kidneys in week 8

    e. Heart generates more of its energy from oxidising glucose

5. After a 48-hour fast, amino acid metabolism is altered in the body compared to amino acid metabolism during the absorptive state. Which one of the following statements is correct for amino acid metabolism during the fasting state compared to the fed state?
    a. Less alanine and less glutamine are released into blood by skeletal muscle
    b. Skeletal muscle uses blood glucose as its preferred fuel
    c. Glutamine is preferentially taken up by cells of the small intestine
    d. Alanine is utilised by the liver for glycogen synthesis
    e. Ammonia generated from glutamine by the kidneys is released into urine

6. Which of the following occurs in cardiac muscle but not in the brain, even in the fasted state?
    a. Glucose uptake via a glucose transporter
    b. Fatty acid oxidation
    c. Glycolysis
    d. The reaction in which glucose is converted to glucose 6-phosphate
    e. The TCA cycle

7. A normal adult male is scheduled for a physical examination. In order to obtain a fasting blood sample, his physician tells him not to eat after 8 p.m. the previous night. The blood is drawn at 10 a.m. next day. Afterwards the patient has a modest mixed meal containing carbohydrate, fat and protein. Identify the enzyme or system in adipocytes that would be less active 1 hour later.
    a. Lipoprotein lipase (LPL)
    b. GLUT4
    c. Hormone-sensitive lipase (HSL)
    d. Glycolysis
    e. Triacylglycerol synthesis

8. Identify the single correct statement concerning insulin action.
    a. Insulin action on adipocytes and skeletal muscle cells results in recruitment of GLUT4 molecules to the plasma membrane of these cells
    b. Insulin action on the liver leads to inhibition of glycogenesis

c. Insulin activation of gluconeogenesis would be consistent with the normal response to the fed state

d. Insulin stimulates (activates) 'hormone-sensitive' lipase (HSL) in adipose tissue

e. Type 2 diabetics are more sensitive than normal subjects to the effects of insulin

9. Which one of the following statements accurately describes events critical for insulin secretion by pancreatic beta cells?

a. Adrenaline (epinephrine) action (directly) on the pancreatic beta cell, via interaction with the α_2-adrenoceptor, results in increased insulin secretion

b. Hypoglycaemia is the major stimulus for increased insulin secretion

c. Glucose metabolism in beta cells causes a decrease in ATP levels

d. Inhibition of a potassium channel by ATP in beta cells leads to depolarisation of the cells, calcium entry and increased insulin secretion

e. GLUT4 is the glucose transporter most important for glucose uptake into beta cells in the fed state

10. Identify the single correct match between Column A and Column B as they relate to metabolic support and control in tissues of the body.

A	B
a. Glutamine	Major fuel for colonocytes
b. Fatty acids	Fuel for the renal medulla
c. Skin	ATP synthesis by aerobic metabolism
d. Glucose	Quantitatively the major fuel for the heart
e. Ketone bodies	Fuels for cardiac muscle and the brain

11. A fit long-distance runner is running a marathon. His overall metabolism is monitored. Which one of the following is a correct finding?

a. His overall respiratory quotient (RQ) gradually rose during the run

b. His leg muscle RQ gradually fell during the race

c. His skeletal muscle glycogen levels rose during the race

d. The output of glucose by his liver would be lower than in the rested state

e. The output of fatty acids by his adipose tissue would be lower than in the rested fed state

True/false questions

Are the following statements true or false?

1. Both glucose and fatty acids are efficient fuels for muscle, with the latter requiring an active carnitine palmitoyltransferase-I (CPTI) system.

2. Blood glucose levels greater than 20 mM following a carbohydrate load are consistent with a subject making insufficient insulin.

3. In brain ATP production is mainly through anaerobic glycolysis.

4. An RQ (respiratory quotient) of 1.0 in skeletal muscle indicates that the major fuels being oxidised are fatty acids.

5. Muscle is not able to produce and release glucose.

6. Hormones made in corticotrophs, chromaffin cells and the zona fasciculata are all 'counter-regulatory' hormones.

7. Glucose is the principal fuel of colonocytes.

8. Growth hormone is one of the counter-regulatory hormones directly inhibiting the action on insulin on glucose utilisation

9. Tolbutamide stimulates insulin secretion by depolarising the beta cells.

Short essay questions

1. Prepare a table that summarises the mechanisms that are involved in preventing hyperglycaemia in the fed state and allows for lipid storage. You are not required to differentiate between enzyme activation and enzyme induction.

2. Prepare a table that summarises the mechanisms that are involved in preventing hypoglycaemia in the fasted state and allows for lipid mobilisation. You are not required to differentiate between enzyme activation and enzyme induction.

3. Prepare a table that indicates the fuels used by the intestine, renal medulla, renal cortex, cardiac muscle, liver and the skeletal and nervous systems.

4. Compare and contrast fuel metabolism in skeletal muscles during (a) a 100 metre sprint and (b) a marathon.

Self-assessment: answers

Single best answer MCQ answers

1. a. **True**. The decrease in PFK-2 leads to lower levels of fructose 2,6-bisphosphate and this allows for efficient gluconeogenesis.
   b. **False**. More alanine is being taken up by the liver for gluconeogenesis so the aminotransferases activity is high.
   c. **False**. Pyruvate carboxylase activity is required for efficient gluconeogenesis and occurs mainly due to stimulation by acetyl-CoA (derived from increased fatty acid oxidation).
   d. **False**. Aldolase is a key enzyme in gluconeogenesis.
   e. **False**. PEPCK catalyses one of the rate-controlling steps in gluconeogenesis and is induced by glucagon.

2. a. **False**. By 10 a.m. any fat in the previous meal will have been completely digested and absorbed.
   b. **False**. Fatty acid synthesis is not activated in the fasting state so malonyl-CoA formation is not turned on.
   c. **False**. The pyruvate dehydrogenase complex (PDC) needs to be turned off if gluconeogenesis is to be productive. If pyruvate is converted to acetyl-CoA by the PDC, glucose formation is prevented. E_1 of the PDC is phosphorylated, stimulated by high acetyl-CoA/CoA, NADH/NAD$^+$ and ATP/ADP ratios, all due to increased fatty acid oxidation.
   d. **True**. Adipocytes are the source of fatty acids which are then catabolised in the liver, providing signals that turn on gluconeogenesis. Also, the fatty acids are fuels for muscle and this conserves glucose for the brain.
   e. **False**. Hepatic glycogenolysis will be active, not glycogen synthesis.

3. a. **False**. No change since the brain continues to use glucose as its fuel.
   b. **False**. GLUT2 continues to be important since glucose is being transported out of the liver to maintain blood glucose levels.
   c. **False**. GLUT4 levels will be low since insulin levels are low in the fasting state.
   d. **False**. Glucose continues to be the fuel of erythrocytes and GLUT1 is the transporter.
   e. **True**. GLUT4 is low due to the low insulin level. Less glucose is taken up by muscle, preserving the glucose for the brain.

4. a. **False**. Oxaloacetate is derived from glucose and that pathway is less active in severe starvation. This allows ketone body levels to become very high.
   b. **True**. Protein has to be conserved if the subject is to survive, so less protein is turned over and gluconeogenesis falls. Ketone bodies increase, so less glucose need be produced.
   c. **False**. Protein conservation must occur in order to maintain life.
   d. **False**. The high levels of ketone bodies cause a metabolic acidosis. Part of the response to the ketoacidosis is ammonia production from glutamine in the kidney with concomitant increased gluconeogenesis.
   e. **False**. The heart uses fatty acids and ketones as its major fuels.

5. a. **False**. Glutamine and alanine are released in increased amounts, with both being gluconeogenic.
   b. **False**. Glucose is preserved for the brain. Fatty acids replace glucose as fuels for muscle.
   c. **False**. Preference is given to the kidney where the glutamine is important for acid–base balance.
   d. **False**. Any alanine metabolised in the liver is for glucose production and release.
   e. **True**. The production of ammonia from glutamine in the kidney enables more H$^+$ to be excreted in urine and more HCO$_3^-$ to be produced and used to replace HCO$_3^-$ used in buffering organic acids.

6. a. **False**. Glucose is taken up by both using GLUTs.
   b. **True**. There is a blood–brain barrier for fatty acids but they are major fuels of heart muscle.
   c. **False**. Glycolysis is important in both since glucose is being used as a fuel in both locations.
   d. **False**. This is the first step in glycolysis and occurs in both.
   e. **False**. Oxidative metabolism occurs in both sites.

7. a. **False**. LPL will be active to clear fatty acids from chylomicrons.
   b. **False**. GLUT4 will be present in higher levels in the plasma membrane of adipocytes due to insulin action. Glucose is the source of glycerol 3-phosphate!

c. **True**. HSL activity is very low due to the action of insulin, the hormone of the fed state.
d. **False**. The rate of glycolysis will be high, with most of the product being glycerol 3-phosphate required for TAG synthesis (see Ch. 9).
e. **False**. TAG is synthesised at a high rate, with the fatty acids released from chylomicrons being stored in adipocytes.

8. a. **True**. Glucose metabolism is required in adipocytes in the fed state (to supply glycerol 3-phosphate) and glucose is stored in skeletal muscle as glycogen in the fed state.
b. **False**. Glycogen synthesis is stimulated by insulin.
c. **False**. Gluconeogenesis is not required when one has taken a meal which usually has some carbohydrate. Insulin inhibits gluconeogenesis.
d. **False**. Insulin is the hormone of the fed state and HSL is active when insulin is low in the fasted state.
e. **False**. Type 2 diabetics show 'insulin resistance'.

9. a. **False**. In keeping with its role as a counter-regulatory hormone, adrenaline (epinephrine) inhibits insulin release.
b. **False**. Hyperglycaemia is the major stimulus.
c. **False**. Glucose is catabolised leading to increased [ATP].
d. **True**. The increase [ATP] affects an ATP-sensitive K^+ channel and the beta cells are depolarised, leading to Ca^{2+} entry and insulin secretion.
e. **False**. GLUT has a low K_m for glucose and would not be suitable. GLUT2 is the logical glucose transporter since it can respond to high glucose levels.

10. a. **False**. It is the fuel for enterocytes. Butyrate is a major fuel for colonocytes!
b. **False**. Glucose is the fuel for renal medulla.
c. **False**. Anaerobic metabolism of glucose is the source of ATP.
d. **False**. Given the enormous requirement for energy metabolism in cardiac muscle it is logical that the major storage fuel, fat, is the major fuel for cardiac muscle.
e. **True**. Ketone bodies are fuels used by the heart every day and by the brain during starvation.

11. a. **False**. The increased use of fatty acids later in the run means that the overall RQ falls.
b. **True**. This is due to the greater proportion of fatty acids being used. There is a limited supply of glycogen and glucose!

c. **False**. Glycogen levels are gradually depleted during the race.
d. **False**. Glucose output by the liver increases since gluconeogenesis from glycerol and alanine increases due to the higher ratio of glucagon to insulin.
e. **False**. The high ratio of glucagon to insulin activates HSL.

True/false answers

1. **True**. Other than in short sprints, muscle uses fatty acids and glycogen (or glucose) as fuels.
2. **True**. This is an abnormally high glucose level and consistent with diabetes mellitus. Insufficient insulin means that glucose is less efficiently stored in liver and muscle.
3. **False**. The fact that under quiescent (non-exercise) conditions the brain uses about 20% of the total oxygen being used by an individual, points to the fact that aerobic metabolism (of glucose) is what is happening.
4. **False**. An RQ of 1.0 indicates that glucose (or glycogen) is the fuel being used. With long-chain fatty acids as fuel, the RQ is close to 0.7.
5. **True**. This is because muscle does not contain glucose-6-phosphatase.
6. **True**. They are ACTH, adrenaline (epinephrine) and cortisol.
7. **False**. Short-chain fatty acids such as butyrate produced by colonic bacterial action on non-digestible dietary carbohydrates are the fuels for colonocytes.
8. **True**. The decrease in insulin allows fat mobilisation to increase from adipose tissue. The greater use of fatty acids as fuel is reflected in a significant decrease in RQ in muscle.
9. **True**. Hypoglycaemic sulphonylureas used in the treatment of type 2 diabetes mellitus inhibit the ATP-sensitive K^+ channel in beta cells.

Short essay answers

1. Table 13 summarises the mechanisms that prevent hyperglycaemia in the fed state and allow storage of energy as lipid.
2. Table 14 summarises the mechanisms that prevent hypoglycaemia in the fasted state and allow mobilisation of energy stored as lipids.
3. Table 15 lists the fuels used by the tissues in question and the relevant pathways.
4. High-power exertion (e.g. sprinting): ATP, creatine phosphate and then anaerobic metabolism of glycogen (glucose) occur. Control of glucose metabolism occurs through activation of

glycogenolysis and glycolysis at the level of phosphorylase and PFK-1.

In a marathon: Fatty acids and glucose are utilised, with the proportion of fatty acids used increasing the longer the run (RQ gradually falls).

Fatty acids are released in increasing amounts from adipose tissue through activation of hormone-sensitive lipase, brought about by a decrease in insulin and an increase in glucagon.

Table 13 Glucose homeotasis in the fed state

Organ	Pathway activated	System activated	Pathway inhibited	System inhibited
Liver	Glycogenesis	Glycogen synthase	Glycogenolysis	Phosphorylase
	Glycolysis	PFK-1, pyruvate kinase	Gluconeogenesis	F-1,6-Bpase, PEPCK
Skeletal muscle	Glycogenesis	Glycogen synthase	Glycogenolysis	Phosphorylase
	Glucose uptake	GLUT4		
	Glycolysis	PFK-1, pyruvate kinase		
Adipose tissue	Glucose uptake	GLUT4	Fat mobilisation	HSL
	Glycolysis	PFK-1		
	Fat storage	LPL		

F-1,6-BPase, fructose-1,6-bisphosphatase.
See text for other abbreviations.

Table 14 Glucose homeostasis in the fasted state

Organ	Pathway activated	System activated	Pathway inhibited	System inhibited
Liver	Glycogenolysis	Phosphorylase	Glycogenesis	Glycogen synthase
	Gluconeogenesis	F-1,6-Bpase, PEPCK, pyruvate carboxylase	Glycolysis	PFK-1, pyruvate kinase
Skeletal muscle	Protein degradation	Ubiquitin pathway	Glycogenesis	Glycogen synthase
Adipose tissue	Fat mobilisation	HSL	Fat storage	LPL
			Glucose uptake	GLUT4
			Glycolysis	PFK-1

F-1,6-BPase, fructose-1,6-bisphosphatase.
See text for other abbreviations.

Table 15 The fuels used by various tissues

Tissue	Fuel used	Pathway
Intestine		
Enterocytes	Glutamine	TCA cycle
Colonocytes	Short-chain fatty acids	Beta-oxidation plus TCA cycle
Kidney		
Medulla	Glucose	Glycolysis
Cortex	Glucose, fatty acids	Oxidative metabolism, TCA cycle, etc.
Muscle		
Cardiac muscle	Fatty acids, glucose, lactate, ketone bodies	Oxidative metabolism, TCA cycle, etc.
Skeletal muscle	Glycogen, ketone bodies, fatty acids, glucose	Glycolysis, oxidative metabolism, TCA cycle, etc.
Liver	Fatty acids, glucose, lactate, amino acids	Oxidative metabolism, TCA cycle, etc.

11 Purine and pyrimidine nucleotides

Overview

It is easy to forget just how important purine and pyrimidine nucleotides are in the body. However, when told that ATP, NAD, UTP and FAD are such nucleotides and that, in addition, DNA and RNA are polynucleotides, one can see the importance of understanding how purine and pyrimidine nucleotides are synthesised and metabolised. It is obvious that, for DNA and RNA synthesis, the production of purine and pyrimidine nucleotides must be balanced. The dTMP biosynthetic pathway is a target for anti-cancer drugs.

11.1 Synthesis of purine and pyrimidine nucleotides

Learning objectives

You should be able to:

- give multiple examples of roles for purine and pyrimidine nucleotides

- describe in outline the de novo and salvage pathways for purine and pyrimidine nucleotide synthesis and how they are controlled.

The general structures of nucleotides and nucleosides are shown in Figure 107 and the nomenclature in Table 16. A nucleotide consists of a purine or pyrimidine base, a sugar (D-ribose or 2-deoxy-D-ribose) and one or more phosphates. Nucleosides lack the phosphates. Note that purine (smaller name) bases are larger molecules than pyrimidine (larger name) bases. Nucleoside triphosphates (NTP) are required for RNA synthesis and dNTP for DNA synthesis (Chs 12 and 13).

As shown in Table 17, purine and pyrimidine nucleotides have a wide variety of metabolic roles in addition to being constituents of DNA and RNA.

Purine nucleotide synthesis

Purine nucleotides are synthesised by two pathways:

- the *de novo* pathway, which uses simple intermediates, is found in most tissues of the body (Fig. 108)
- the salvage pathway, which allows free purine bases produced by the degradation of nucleic acids or purine nucleotides to be reclaimed.

The de novo pathway starts with PRPP

This pathway is complex; the essential features are as follows:

1. The starting point for the de novo synthesis of a purine nucleotide is an activated ribose phosphate (phosphoribosylpyrophosphate; PRPP), which is synthesised by transfer of a pyrophosphate group from ATP to the carbon-1 of ribose 5-phosphate catalysed by *PRPP synthetase*.
2. The committed step in purine biosynthesis is the formation of 5-phosphoribosylamine from PRPP and glutamine catalysed by *PRPP–glutamine amidotransferase*. The reaction is driven forward by the hydrolysis of pyrophosphate.
3. Additional carbon and nitrogen atoms are added until the parent purine nucleotide is formed. Nitrogens are provided by the amide groups of glutamine, aspartate and glycine. Carbons are derived from glycine and bicarbonate, as well as from two tetrahydrofolate (FH_4) derivatives (Fig. 108).
4. Altogether, ten reactions lead to the synthesis of IMP, which is not a component of the nucleotide pool or a constituent of the nucleic acids. The purine base of inosinate is called hypoxanthine.

5. IMP is the precursor of AMP and GMP. AMP is synthesised by the substitution of an amino group for the carbonyl group at carbon-6; this is accomplished by the addition of aspartate followed by elimination of fumarate (as in the urea cycle).

GTP is required in the synthesis of AMP. Guanylate (GMP) is synthesised by the NAD$^+$-dependent oxidation of IMP to xanthylate (XMP), followed by the transfer of an amino group from the amide of glutamine. ATP is required for GMP synthesis.

Table 16 Purine and pyrimidine nucleotide nomenclature

Base	Abbreviation	Type	Nucleoside	Nucleotide[a]
Adenine	A	Purine	Adenosine	Adenylate
Guanine	G	Purine	Guanosine	Guanylate
Hypoxanthine	H	Purine	Inosine	Inosinate
Cytosine	C	Pyrimidine	Cytidine	Cytidylate
Thymine	T	Pyrimidine	Thymidine	Thymidylate
Uracil	U	Pyrimidine	Uridine	Uridylate

[a]Nucleotides are named by adding the position and number of phosphate groups to the name of the nucleoside, e.g. adenosine 5'-triphosphate (ATP). Ribonucleotides are assumed unless the prefix d- or deoxy is used.

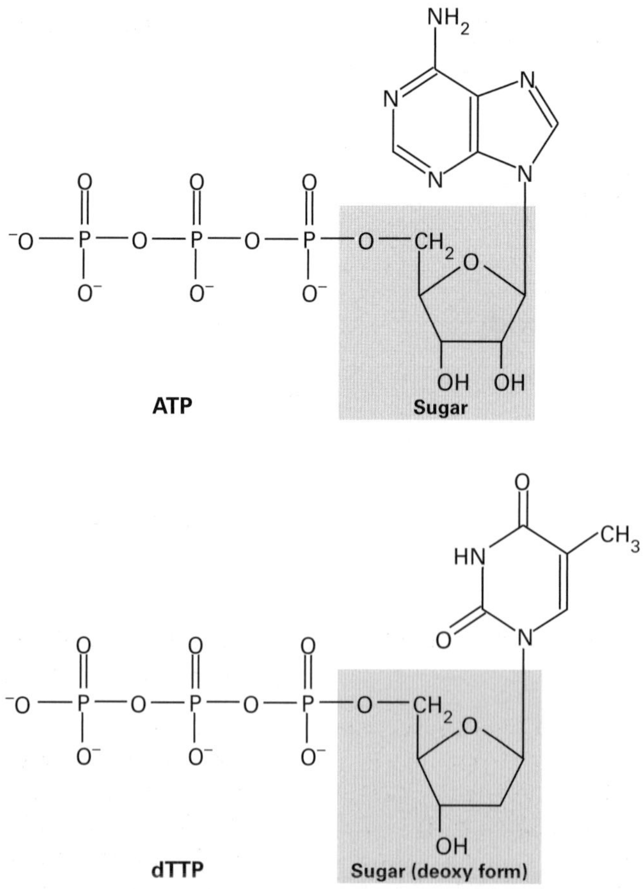

ATP   **Sugar**

dTTP   **Sugar (deoxy form)**

Fig. 107 The structures of a purine ribonucleotide (ATP) and a pyrimidine deoxyribonucleotide (dTTP). The corresponding nucleosides would have only base and sugar.

Table 17 The roles of purine and pyrimidine nucleotides and nucleosides

Nucleic acid biosynthesis	NTP and dNTP
Energy metabolism	ATP, GTP
Allosteric modifiers	ATP, ADP, AMP, NADH
Cell signalling	Cyclic AMP, cyclic GMP, GTP
Coenzymes	$NAD^+/NADH^+$, $NADP^+/NADPH$, FAD, *S*-Adenosylmethionine, adenosyl-vitamin B_{12}, coenzyme A
Carbohydrate, glycoprotein and glycolipid biosynthesis	UDP-glucose, UDP-NAGA, UDP-galactose, GDP-mannose
Ganglioside biosynthesis	CMP-NANA
Phospholipid biosynthesis	CDP-choline, CDP-ethanolamine, CDP-diacylglycerol
Bile pigment metabolism and xenobiotic metabolism	UDP-glucuronate
Transmethylation reactions	*S*-Adenosylmethionine

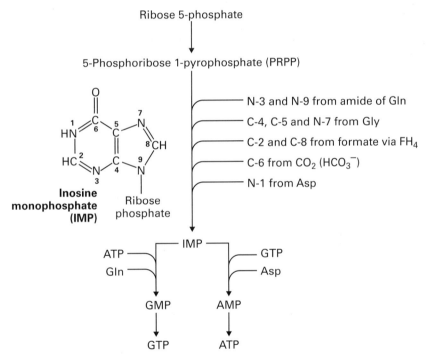

Fig. 108 The de novo pathway of purine nucleotide biosynthesis.

In the salvage pathway PRPP is added to purine bases

Free purine bases formed by degradation of nucleic acids are recycled by transfer of a 5′-phosphoribosyl group from PRPP to the base. This is more efficient and economical than de novo synthesis. The salvage pathway is outlined in Figure 109. The relevance of the salvage pathway is indicated in the inherited disorder Lesch–Nyhan syndrome, in which hypoxanthine–guanine phosphoribosyltransferase (HGPRTase) is absent.

'Product inhibition' is a feature of the control of purine nucleotide biosynthesis

The initial steps catalysed by PRPP synthetase and PRPP amidotransferase are inhibited by the purine nucleotide products AMP, GMP and IMP acting synergistically (Fig. 110). In contrast, PRPP has a positive effect, causing the PRPP amidotransferase (for which it is substrate) to shift to the active form. There is also regulation at the branch point at IMP, with AMP inhibiting the conversion of IMP into adenylosuccinate, which is its

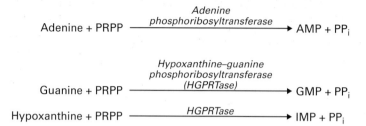

$$\text{Adenine + PRPP} \xrightarrow{\substack{\textit{Adenine} \\ \textit{phosphoribosyltransferase}}} \text{AMP + PP}_i$$

$$\text{Guanine + PRPP} \xrightarrow{\substack{\textit{Hypoxanthine–guanine} \\ \textit{phosphoribosyltransferase} \\ \textit{(HGPRTase)}}} \text{GMP + PP}_i$$

$$\text{Hypoxanthine + PRPP} \xrightarrow{\textit{HGPRTase}} \text{IMP + PP}_i$$

Fig. 109 The salvage pathway of purine nucleotide synthesis.

Clinical note:
Lesch–Nyhan syndrome

A severe or complete deficiency of HGPRTase activity results in Lesch–Nyhan syndrome, which is characterised by mental retardation and, in the most severe cases, self-mutilation. Lack of HGPRTase precludes the salvage of hypoxanthine and guanine, leading to decreased levels of IMP or GMP and increased levels of PRPP. Both these factors increase the de novo pathway of purine biosynthesis as the pathway is no longer subject to proper regulation (Fig. 110). The disease is characterised by excessive uric acid production and hyperuricaemia.

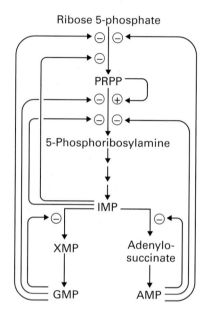

Fig. 110 The control of purine nucleotide synthesis.

precursor, and GMP inhibiting the conversion of IMP into XMP, its precursor (Fig. 110). GTP serves as an energy source for the adenylosuccinate synthase reaction while AMP is a competitive inhibitor of this step. Similarly, ATP is the energy source in the conversion of XMP to GMP while GMP is an inhibitor of XMP formation. These controls serve to balance the synthesis of adenine and guanine nucleotides. For example, an excess of GTP favours the conversion of IMP to adenylosuccinate, which is the immediate precursor of AMP. In the salvage pathways, the products of the phosphoribosyltransferase reactions are feedback inhibitors.

Pyrimidine nucleotide biosynthesis

The de novo pathway for pyrimidine nucleotide biosynthesis contrasts with that for purines in that the sugar and phosphate are added from PRPP *after* the pyrimidine ring has been formed. A salvage pathway also exists for pyrimidine nucleotides.

The de novo pathway

This pathway is complex and involves two multifunctional enzymes (Fig. 111). Key points about this pathway are:

1. Carbamoyl phosphate is required and is produced in a reaction that involves glutamine (not ammonia)

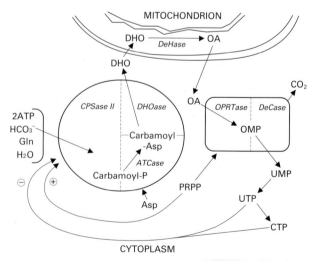

Fig. 111 Pyrimidine nucleotide biosynthesis. (Based on Jones, M.E. (1980) *Annual Review of Biochemistry* 49: 253–279.)

In a clinical condition called orotic aciduria, excessive amounts of orotic acid are produced because of deficiencies in either OPRTase or DeCase, the enzymes in the second multiple enzyme protein. Orotic aciduria can also result from a deficiency of ornithine transcarbamoylase in the urea cycle. Can you reason why?

and the enzyme, *carbamoyl phosphate synthetase II* (CPSII), is in the cytosol.

2. The second step in pyrimidine biosynthesis is the formation of *N*-carbamoylaspartate (Fig. 111) from aspartate and carbamoyl phosphate; this reaction is catalysed by *aspartate transcarbamoylase* (ATCase). *Dihydro-orotase* (DHOase) catalyses the cyclisation of *N*-carbamoylaspartate to dihydro-orotate.

3. In higher eukaryotes or mammals, CPSII, ATCase and DHOase are covalently linked to form a single chain, a 240 kDa multifunctional enzyme called CAD.

4. Dihydro-orotate is oxidised to orotate in an NAD$^+$-dependent reaction in mitochondria, then *orotate phosphoribosyltransferase* (OPRTase) transfers a ribose phosphate group from PRPP to orotate to form the pyrimidine nucleotide orotidylate (OMP). Decarboxylation of OMP catalysed *by orotidine-5′-monophosphate decarboxylase* (DeCase) yields the parent pyrimidine nucleotide, uridylate (UMP).

5. Again, in eukaryotes, OPRTase and DeCase are associated in a single 52 kDa protein. CTP is derived from UTP, a reaction catalysed by CTP synthetase (Fig. 111). The carbonyl oxygen at carbon-4 of UTP is replaced by an amino group donated by the amide group of glutamine.

In the salvage pathway PRPP is added to pyrimidine bases

Pyrimidine bases can be 'salvaged' by conversion to the nucleotides via pyrimidine phosphoribosyltransferase.

Pyrimidine + PRPP→Pyrimidine nucleoside monophosphate + PP$_i$ (pyrophosphate)

Orotate, uracil and thymine are substrates but cytosine is not.

'Product inhibition' is a feature of the control of pyrimidine nucleotide biosynthesis

The main control of pyrimidine nucleotide synthesis in mammals is exerted at the level of CPSII; the enzyme is inhibited by UTP and CTP (Fig. 111). In addition, UMP

and, to a lesser extent, CMP inhibit DeCase. CTP synthetase is inhibited by CTP to prevent all of the UTP from being converted to CTP. Also, since pyrimidine nucleotide synthesis is dependent upon a supply of PRPP and PRPP activates CPSII, the activity of PRPP synthetase is a factor in determining flux through the pathway.

Synthesis of trinucleotides

To convert purine and pyrimidine mononucleotides to trinucleotides (e.g. AMP to ATP and GMP to GTP), two additional kinases are required. These kinases are not specific for the base involved.

11.2 Deoxyribonucleotide and nucleotide coenzyme synthesis

Learning objectives

You should be able to:

- explain the overall structure of ribonucleotide reductase (RR) and the role of thioredoxin

- describe how RR is controlled to achieve balance in dNTPs

- give the details of the reaction for dTMP synthesis and how that reaction is targeted in the treatment of cancer.

During DNA replication (S phase), deoxyribonucleotides are required to support DNA synthesis. The deoxyribonucleotides are formed by reduction of the 2′-hydroxyl of the corresponding ribonucleotide (Fig. 112). Thioredoxin, a small protein (12 kDa), is oxidised at the same time and is regenerated finally by NADPH. The reduction of a specific NDP requires a specific NTP as a positive modulator of RR; the enzyme is also regulated by other NTPs. RR is a multiple subunit enzyme.

Control of deoxyribonucleotide synthesis is vital to survival of an organism

An organism must synthesise the four dNTPs in amounts that will allow for DNA synthesis. One potential consequence of imbalance in dNTP synthesis is mutagenesis. The pathways are controlled by feedback inhibition. From studies of *Escherichia coli* RR, we know that there are two allosteric sites.

- The overall activity of RR is controlled by ATP binding to one of these sites (the activity site).

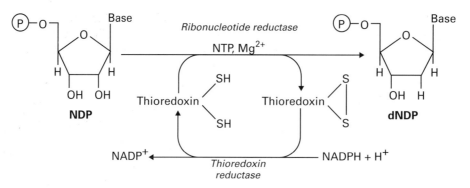

Fig. 112 The synthesis of deoxyribonucleotides catalysed by ribonucleotide reductase.

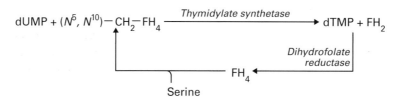

Fig. 113 The synthesis of deoxythymidine (dTMP).

Binding of dATP at the activity site inhibits the enzyme's activity towards all substrates, so abnormally high levels of dATP are toxic!
- The final activity is controlled by the level of modulators at the second site (the specificity site).

The synthesis of deoxythymidylate is a target for anti-cancer drugs

DNA contains thymine (T), the methylated analogue of uracil, rather than uracil (U) (Ch. 12) and deoxythymidy-late is required for DNA synthesis (Ch. 12). A rapidly growing tumour is going to require a high rate of DNA synthesis. *Thymidylate synthase* catalyses the transfer of a one-carbon unit to dUMP and in the process reduces the one-carbon to a methyl group. In addition to serving as a one-carbon donor, N^5,N^{10}-methylene-FH_4 acts as the reducing agent (Fig. 113). For this reason, it is dihydro-folate (FH_2) that is produced in this reaction. FH_2 must be reduced to FH_4 by *dihydrofolate reductase* using NADPH, since it is FH_4 that participates in one-carbon transfers (Ch. 8, p. 118).

Synthesis of nucleotide coenzymes

Many nucleotide coenzymes function in the principal pathways of intermediary metabolism and, clearly, they have to be synthesised in cells. Examples include:

Clinical note:
Anti-cancer drugs

Analogues of FH_4, such as *aminopterin* and *methotrexate*, are potent inhibitors of dihydrofolate reductase and, as such, are most toxic to proliferating cells because they block recycling of FH_2. Methotrexate binds so tightly to dihydrofolate reductase that it is classified as a pseudo-irreversible inhibitor. When tumour cells are treated with methotrexate, the cells die. Although a valuable drug in the treatment of rapidly growing tumours, such as acute leukaemia and choriocarcinoma, it is quite toxic as it also kills rapidly growing non-malignant cells.

5-Fluorouracil (5-FU), another anti-cancer drug, is converted into fluorouridylate (F-dUMP). F-dUMP is a substrate for thymidylate synthase, but catalysis results in a covalent complex formed by F-dUMP, methylene-FH_4 and the sulphydryl of thymidylate synthase. This is another example of suicide inhibition. 5-FU and methotrexate can be used as a cocktail in chemotherapy.

There are several other groups of drugs that have been synthesised or isolated from natural products and are involved in inhibition of nucleotide synthesis or interconversions which are useful as anti-tumour agents. These include 6-mercaptopurine, 8-azaguanine, 6-azauracil, 5-iodouracil and 5-fluoro-orotate.

- NAD$^+$ (nicotinamide adenine dinucleotide), which can be synthesised from dietary nicotinate and also from nicotinate made in the body from tryptophan.
- FAD (flavin adenine dinucleotide), which is synthesised from riboflavin and ATP.
- Coenzyme A, which is synthesised from pantothenate, cysteine and ATP.
- *S*-Adenosylmethionine, which is formed from methionine and ATP by the transfer of an adenine and ribose from ATP.

The biosynthesis of NAD$^+$, FAD and coenzyme A involves the transfer of AMP from ATP to the phosphoryl group of a phosphorylated intermediate, resulting in the formation of pyrophosphate (PP$_i$); cleavage of PP$_i$ to 2P$_i$ has a large negative ΔG which drives the reaction.

11.3 Purine and pyrimidine catabolism

Learning objectives

You should be able to:

- outline the pathway leading to uric acid synthesis
- describe several causes for hyperuricaemia
- explain how allopurinol is successful in the treatment of gout.

Purines are catabolised to uric acid

Hydrolytic reactions of purine nucleotides result in the formation of purine mononucleotides (AMP, GMP, IMP). These are further degraded via a nucleotidase, which removes the phosphate. The nucleoside is then converted to the free base and either ribose 1-phosphate or deoxyribose 1-phosphate by *5′-nucleoside phosphorylase*. There are two potential pathways for AMP. In one, AMP is deaminated by *AMP deaminase* and the product, IMP, is hydrolysed to the nucleoside inosine by the

5′-nucleotidase. In the other, AMP is converted to adenosine by the action of the 5′-nucleotidase then adenosine is deaminated to inosine catalysed by *adenosine deaminase*.

Inosine can be converted to hypoxanthine via purine nucleoside phosphorylase

The purine bases hypoxanthine, adenine, and guanine are oxidised in the liver to uric acid (Fig. 114), which is excreted via the kidneys. Uric acid is not very water-soluble, the mean concentration in adult males being close to the limit of solubility. An increase in uric acid levels for whatever reason can lead to crystallisation out of uric acid crystals in various sites in the body, resulting in gouty arthritis and kidney damage (stones). *Xanthine oxidase* (which contains molybdenum) is the target for drugs (e.g. allopurinol) used to treat patients with gout. Allopurinol is effective because the precursors of uric acid (xanthine and hypoxanthine) are more water-soluble than uric acid is.

Pyrimidine metabolites include β-alanine

Degradation of the pyrimidine nucleotides, primarily UMP, CMP and TMP, involves hydrolysis to their respective bases in reactions comparable to those for purine nucleotides. Degradation of the pyrimidine bases generates ammonia, malonyl-CoA, β-alanine and methylmalonyl-CoA, all very water-soluble. An intermediate in the catabolism of cytosine and uracil, β-alanine, is required for coenzyme A biosynthesis.

Clinical note:
Adenosine deaminase deficiency

Adenosine deaminase deficiency causes severe combined immunodeficiency involving both T and B cells. The adenosine that accumulates is toxic to T and B lymphocytes. Accumulation of dATP is also a consequence of this disorder, leading to inhibition of ribonucleotide reductase; consequently, there is reduced DNA synthesis in T and B cells.

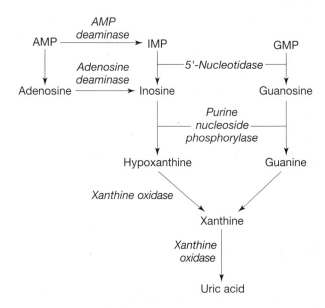

Fig. 114 Purine degradation pathways.

Self-assessment: questions

Single best answer MCQs

1. The de novo biosynthesis of purine nucleotides differs from the de novo biosynthesis of pyrimidine nucleotides in which one of the following features?
   a. Utilises glutamine
   b. Utilises aspartate
   c. Only occurs in the liver
   d. Is inhibited in the presence of high levels of phosphoribosylpyrophosphate (PRPP)
   e. Has PRPP involved (as a substrate) in the initial rate-controlling step

2. In connection with the conversion of ribonucleotides to deoxyribonucleotides by ribonucleotide reductase (RR):
   a. RR has an activity site with ATP being an inhibitor and dATP being an activator
   b. The conversion of ribonucleotides to deoxyribonucleotides is carried out exclusively at the level of the nucleoside diphosphates
   c. The specificity site of RR binds nucleoside triphosphates
   d. Both a and b are correct
   e. Options a, b and c are all correct

3. Your 60-year-old male patient is scheduled for an office visit after describing that he had been awakened from his sleep the night before by an excruciating pain in his big toe. Physical examination is notable for an exquisitely tender and erythematous left first metatarsophalangeal joint (big toe!). Subsequently you ascertain that he has very significant hyperuricaemia and make the diagnosis of gouty arthritis. Potential causes for his condition include which of the following?
   a. Increased sensitivity of PRPP–glutamine amidotransferase to feedback inhibition
   b. Increased sensitivity of PRPP synthetase to feedback inhibition
   c. Increased clearance (excretion) of uric acid by the kidney
   d. Decreased hypoxanthine–guanine phosphoribosyltransferase activity
   e. Decreased intracellular levels of PRPP

4. Which one of the following statements is correct about this pathway in which dUMP is converted to dTMP and the resultant dihydrofolate is reduced to tetrahydrofolate?
   a. The thymidylate synthetase catalysed reaction has a requirement for N^5-methyl-FH_4
   b. Dihydrofolate reductase has a requirement for ATP
   c. Thymidylate synthetase can be inhibited by methotrexate
   d. Dihydrofolate reductase can be inhibited by allopurinol
   e. Chemotherapy of fast-growing tumours involves the use of drug that is metabolised to a suicide inhibitor of thymidylate synthase

5. Select the nucleotide coenzyme in Column A that is correctly matched with its function as described in Column B.

	A	B
a.	*S*-Adenosylmethionine	Methylation of dUMP
b.	FAD	Glycolysis
c.	NAD$^+$	Urea cycle
d.	Coenzyme A	Fatty acid synthase
e.	NADPH	Mixed function oxidases

6. The direct source of the sugar phosphate incorporated in the de novo synthesis of purine nucleotides is:
   a. GMP
   b. Ribulose 5-phosphate
   c. UTP
   d. Glucose 6-phosphate
   e. 5-Phosphoribosyl-1-pyrophosphate (PRPP)

7. In the synthesis of GMP and AMP from IMP:
   a. AMP synthesis involves a deamination
   b. GMP synthesis requires GTP
   c. The NH_2 group in GMP is derived from glutamine and that in AMP is derived from aspartate
   d. AMP synthesis requires ATP
   e. AMP synthesis from IMP occurs via 3′-5′-cyclic AMP

8. Which of the following statements describe pyrimidine biosynthesis in mammals?
   a. The rate of UMP synthesis is regulated by UTP, which inhibits carbamoyl phosphate synthetase II (CPSII)
   b. In the de novo pathway, the first three reactions occur in a multiple enzyme complex (CAD)
   c. CPSII utilises glutamine as the source of an amino group
   d. a and b are both correct
   e. a, b and c are all correct

True/false questions

Are the following statements true or false?

1. The ribose in purine but not in pyrimidine nucleotides is supplied by 5-phosphoribosyl-1-pyrophosphate (PRPP).
2. Tetrahydrofolate donates single-carbon units at several stages in the biosynthesis of purines.
3. F-dUMP is a substrate for thymidylate synthase.
4. Ribonucleotide reductase is closely regulated through feedback inhibition by several different nucleotides.
5. Allopurinol is effective in the treatment of hyperuricaemia because hypoxanthine and xanthine are less water-soluble than uric acid.
6. Many potential anti-cancer drugs are inhibitors of nucleotide biosynthesis.

Short essay questions

1. Discuss the roles of glutamine and aspartate in supplying nitrogens (amino groups) in the biosynthesis of purine and pyrimidine nucleotides in the body.
2. Discuss the importance of the reaction catalysed by thymidylate synthase and its relevance to cancer chemotherapy.

Self-assessment: answers

Single best answer MCQ answers

1. a. **False**. Glutamine is the source of several nitrogens in purine nucleotide biosynthesis and it is also used to form carbamoyl phosphate in the pyrimidine nucleotide pathway.
   b. **False**. Aspartate donates a nitrogen for the purine ring as well as the amino group in AMP. Aspartate supplies three carbons and a nitrogen in the pyrimidine ring.
   c. **False**. Both are vital in the liver.
   d. **False**. PRPP stimulates both.
   e. **True**. PRPP is involved in the initial committed step for purines, but in the case of pyrimidines it is added after the ring is formed.

2. a. **False**. This site is the 'coarse control' for deoxyribonucleotide synthesis.
   b. **True**. NDPs are the substrates for RR.
   c. **True**. This additional allosteric site is the key to balanced production of dNTPs.
   d. **False**. Because c is also correct.
   e. The single best answer!

3. a. **False**. This option would result in less purines being produced.
   b. **False**. This option would also result in less purines being produced.
   c. **False**. Increased excretion would lower uric acid levels in blood.
   d. **True**. Low activity of the salvage pathway raises PRPP levels and these stimulate purine synthesis.
   e. **False**. The result would be reduced purine synthesis.

4. a. **False**. The methyl group comes from $N^{5,10}$-methylene-FH_4.
   b. **False**. FH_2 needs reducing power supplied by NADPH to be reduced to FH_4.
   c. **False**. Dihydrofolate reductase is the target for methotrexate.
   d. **False**. Dihydrofolate reductase is inhibited by methotrexate and related compounds.
   e. **True**. The drug is 5-fluorouracil, which is converted to the actual suicide inhibitor, F-dUMP.

5. a. **False**. $N^{5,10}$-methylene-FH_4 provides the methyl group.
   b. **False**. NAD^+ is what is required.
   c. **False**. There are no oxidative steps in the urea cycle!

d. **False**. Acyl carrier protein is part of fatty acid synthase. Related to but not actually coenzyme A!
   e. **True**. When molecular oxygen (O_2) is used in reactions catalysed by mixed-function oxidases, reducing power is required to handle the second oxygen.

6. a. **False**. GMP is a purine nucleotide.
   b. **False**. Ribulose 5-phosphate isn't activated.
   c. **False**. UTP is a pyrimidine nucleotide important in complex carbohydrate synthesis.
   d. **False**. Glucose 6-phosphate is a precursor of what is used.
   e. **True**. Ribose 5-phosphate produced in the pentose phosphate pathway is activated to PRPP and PRPP is then used in both purine and pyrimidine nucleotide synthesis.

7. a. **False**. AMP synthesis from IMP involves the addition of an amino group.
   b. **False**. ATP is required.
   c. **True**. Both final products require amino groups. Glutamine supplies the one needed for GMP, aspartate supplies the one required for AMP.
   d. **False**. GTP supplies the energy. Note that this helps achieve 'balance' with ATP required for GMP and GTP required for AMP.
   e. **False**. AMP is produced from cyclic AMP by the action of phosphodiesterase.

8. a. **True**. This is a classical example of end-product controlling activity.
   b. **True**. The multiple enzyme is called CAD.
   c. **True**. This distinguishes CPSI (urea cycle) from CPSII (pyrimidines).
   d. Not the best answer.
   e. The single best answer.

True/false answers

1. **False**. PRPP is used in both cases.
2. **True**. There are two steps where this occurs.
3. **True**. It isn't a natural substrate, but when 5-fluorouracil is used in cancer chemotherapy it acts after conversion to F-dUMP. The latter is a suicide inhibitor!
4. **True**. It is vital to have tight control over the relative amounts of deoxyribonucleotides in cells if DNA replication is to occur in a controlled fashion.

5. **False**. By inhibiting xanthine oxidase allopurinol increases production of hypoxanthine and xanthine and they are *more* water-soluble than uric acid.
6. **True**. Examples include 5′-fluorouracil.

Short essay answers

1. It is important to recall that there are two reactions in which amino acids are made by the incorporation of ammonia. One is the glutamate dehydrogenase catalysed reaction in which α-ketoglutarate undergoes reductive amination. The other is the amidation of glutamate to form glutamine. In most other circumstances, it is the amide nitrogen in glutamine or the amino group in aspartate that is used where a nitrogen or an amino group is required in a biosynthetic pathway.

   Glutamine:

   - provides the amino group required for GMP synthesis from IMP
   - provides the amino group for carbamoyl phosphate synthesis in pyrimidine nucleotide biosynthesis
   - provides two of the ring nitrogens during de novo synthesis of the purine nucleotides
   - supplies the amide group required for the synthesis of asparagine from aspartate.

   Aspartate

   - provides one of the nitrogens required during urea synthesis
   - provides the amino group that is required for the formation of AMP from IMP

   - provides one of the ring nitrogens in the de novo synthesis of the pyrimidine nucleotides
   - provides a ring nitrogen in de novo purine nucleotide synthesis.

2. The reaction in question is:

   dUMP + N^5,N^{10}-methylene-FH$_4$→dTMP + FH$_2$ (dihydrofolate)

   By the action of thymidylate synthetase, dUMP is methylated, which means that N^5,N^{10}-methylene-FH$_4$ provides both a methylene group and reducing power. The other product is FH$_2$. Clearly, the continued operation of the system requires that the FH$_2$ be converted to FH$_4$ so that the latter can acquire another one-carbon unit from serine as follows:

   FH$_2$→FH$_4$ (+ serine)→N^5,N^{10}-methylene-FH$_4$

   The formation of FH$_4$ from FH$_2$ involves *dihydrofolate reductase* and requires NADPH.

   Fluorouracil (5-FU) is useful in cancer chemotherapy because it is converted in the body to 5-fluoro-dUMP (F-dUMP), an inhibitor of thymidylate synthetase; indeed, it is a 'suicide' inhibitor of the enzyme.

   Compounds that are related to tetrahydrofolate such as methotrexate can be used in cancer chemotherapy because they inhibit dihydrofolate reductase. They are often used in combination with 5-FU to produce a more efficient inhibition of dTMP synthesis; this will inhibit the growth of rapidly growing tumours since that growth is dependent upon a high rate of DNA synthesis.

12 DNA structure and function

Overview

DNA stores the genetic information for the amino acid sequences of all the proteins in a cell. When the cell divides, precise copies of its DNA are made for each daughter cell. Base pairing within the double helix structure of DNA explains how it can carry out these processes of information storage and exact replication.

Replication of DNA has to overcome the topological difficulty of copying two antiparallel strands at the same time. Another topological problem is condensation of the very long DNA molecules for storage in a cell with much smaller dimensions.

The cell has the ability to repair DNA sequences when they are damaged.

Protein catalysts are responsible for most of the synthetic activities found in living cells, but the synthesis of proteins themselves cannot be carried out entirely by other protein molecules. If it was, then how could the protein molecules responsible for synthesising new proteins themselves be synthesised? Macromolecules other than proteins must be involved. The sequences of its proteins are what makes a species a species and what makes an individual unique. Protein synthesis is under the control of genes.

Nucleic acids are involved in protein synthesis

Proteins are involved in protein synthesis, but another class of macromolecule provides the information about the amino acid sequence of new proteins. *DNA* (deoxyribonucleic acid), the genetic material in all organisms except some viruses, is the archive of protein sequence information that exists in every cell capable of protein synthesis. This archive is known as the *genome*. *RNA* (ribonucleic acid) has several roles in protein synthesis. Messenger RNA (mRNA) is a working copy of the genetic material and carries the information from DNA in the nucleus to the site of protein synthesis outside the nucleus. Further RNA molecules are involved in the cellular machinery that synthesises proteins. This machinery can make any protein, even its own protein components, if given the appropriate mRNA. It also requires amino acid building blocks and a supply of energy in the form of ATP and GTP.

12.1 Genes control protein synthesis

Learning objectives

You should be able to:

- explain why sequence information is needed for protein synthesis

- describe the form in which this sequence information exists in the cell

- define the genome.

12.2 DNA structure and role

Learning objectives

You should be able to

- discuss the relative sizes of the genomes of viruses, bacteria and humans

- describe where DNA is found in the cell

- describe the functions of histones in chromosome structure

175

- define the terms: replication, transcription and translation. Use these terms to outline the central dogma of molecular biology

- describe what is meant by the genetic code

- describe the structures of DNA and RNA, their similarities and their differences

- name the four bases that occur in DNA and identify the purines and the pyrimidines

- explain what is meant by a base pair and name the bases that form them.

DNA content

The size of the genome appears to increase with what we might consider to be the 'complexity' of the organism (Table 18). However, a more extensive list of organisms would show some anomalies. Some organisms have much more DNA in their genome than you might expect. A few amphibians have genomes that are 100 times larger than those of mammals. Similar plants can have genomes of very different size. Most eukaryotic organisms appear to have some DNA that has no identifiable function. Organisms with exceptionally large genomes are assumed to have more of this 'junk' DNA than organisms whose genomes seem to be of an appropriate size for their complexity.

Location of DNA

In eukaryotes, most, but not all, DNA is contained in the nucleus. There is some DNA in mitochondria, which synthesise a small number of the protein molecules that they contain. Human mitochondria contain circular DNA molecules of known sequence. Each molecule contains 16 569 base pairs, which encode for several proteins, two ribosomal RNAs and a set of transfer RNAs (tRNAs). Proteins encoded by mitochondrial DNA include some subunits of the membrane-bound complexes of the electron transport chain (p. 88) and some subunits of the membrane-bound ATP synthase.

Table 18 DNA content of cells

	Genome size (base pairs)	Length (mm)
SV40 virus	5243	0.002
E. coli	4×10^6	1.4
Yeast	1.4×10^7	4.6
Fruit fly	1.7×10^8	56
Human	3.9×10^9	990

Other subunits and the vast majority of mitochondrial membrane and matrix proteins are encoded by nuclear DNA and are imported after being synthesised outside the mitochondria.

Organisation of DNA

DNA is the component of the chromosomes that carries genetic information. Table 18 also shows that the length of DNA in a cell greatly exceeds any linear dimension of the cell containing it. The DNA in each nucleus in human cells has a total length of almost 1 metre. DNA molecules must be coiled and folded. Nuclear DNA is in the form of chromosomes, which condense and become visible during cell division. Human somatic cells contain 46 *chromosomes* in 23 pairs. Each chromosome contains one very long DNA molecule. Chromosomes also contain basic proteins known as *histones*, which associate with the DNA and organise its coiling and folding. This condensation of DNA is the major function of the histones; they are not directly responsible for the control of protein synthesis. They are highly conserved proteins. Histones from animals and plants only differ by a few amino acid residues in their sequences.

Central dogma of molecular biology

Genetic information describing the amino acid sequences of proteins is carried in coded form by base sequences in DNA. Only a small percentage of the total DNA in the human genome actually codes for protein sequences. Other base sequences mark out the parts of the DNA sequence that are used for protein synthesis. Most of the DNA in the human genome is of unknown function. In any organism, each cell with a nucleus contains an identical set of DNA molecules, the genome, and, therefore, has the information to make all the protein molecules found in that organism. In practice, each cell only synthesises small subsets of these possible proteins: proteins it needs for its specialised functions and some proteins that are made in virtually every cell. For example, proteins used by the protein synthesising machinery itself and enzymes required for basic metabolic processes, such as the production of ATP, are common to all cells.

When cells divide, each daughter cell must be provided with the complete DNA archive of sequence information. DNA molecules have a structure that allows them to replicate precisely to produce DNA molecules for each daughter cell that are identical to those found in the mother cell.

The flow of information from DNA to RNA (mRNA) to protein has been represented as the 'Central Dogma of Molecular Biology' (Fig. 115). Of course, the processes

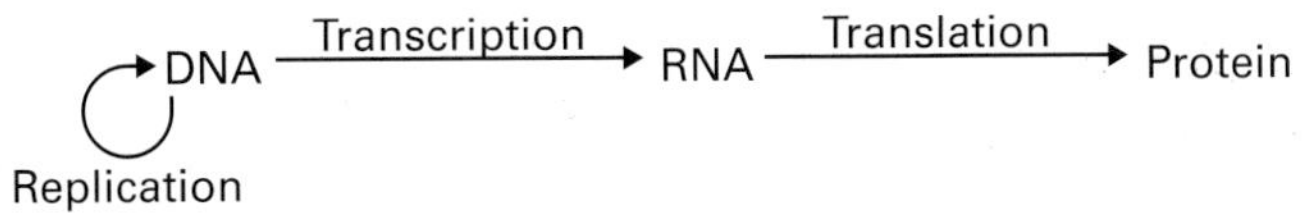

Fig. 115 The 'Central Dogma of Molecular Biology'.

depicted, *replication*, *transcription* and *translation*, also require enzymes and a supply of energy and building blocks for the synthesis of new molecules.

Genetic code

The information for an organism is held in the sequences of bases in the DNA: a 'nucleic acid language'. This can be translated into amino acid sequences in proteins, which can be considered to be in 'protein language'. The process of translation from one language to the other involves the genetic code (p. 202).

Some small viruses with RNA genomes are the only exceptions to the flow of information represented by the Central Dogma (p. 219). The replication of RNA genomes involves either direct replication of RNA or the formation of a DNA version of the genome, which can then direct the formation of new RNA copies. Replication of RNA genomes is a lot more error-prone than replication of DNA; as a result, RNA viruses are very mutable and are limited in the size of the genome that they can maintain.

Structure of nucleic acids

We must study the structures of the nucleic acids if we are to understand how they perform their functions. These structures reveal how the molecules can store information and how copies of this information can be made. DNA molecules can be replicated to make identical copies for passing on to daughter cells during cell division and can also be transcribed to make RNA copies for directing protein synthesis.

Primary structure

DNA and RNA have similar covalent structures consisting of *sugar phosphate backbones* with bases attached. They are linear polymers of building blocks known as nucleotides (Ch. 11). A nucleotide comprises:

- a phosphate group
- pentose sugar (Fig. 116)
  — ribose in RNA
  — 2-deoxyribose in DNA
- a nitrogenous base (Fig. 117)
  — purine derivatives: adenine (A) and guanine (G)
  — pyrimidine derivatives: cytosine (C) and thymine (T) (DNA) or uracil (U) (RNA).

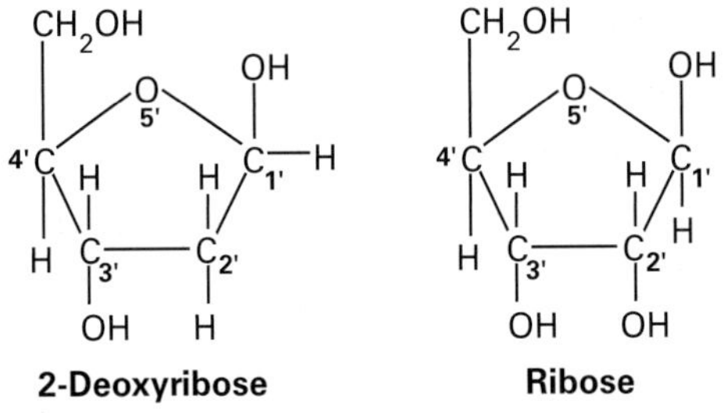

Fig. 116 Pentose sugar in DNA (deoxyribose) and RNA (ribose).

A typical nucleotide, AMP, is shown in Figure 118. A pentose sugar attached to a base but with no phosphate attached is called a *nucleoside*. Adenosine is the nucleoside composed of the base adenine and ribose. The nucleic acid backbone chain is composed of alternating sugar and phosphate groups. Each phosphate group is esterified to the 3'-hydroxyl group on one sugar and to the 5'-hydroxyl group of the next (Fig. 119); this is known as a *phosphodiester linkage*. The chain is unbranched and may contain thousands of sugar and phosphate units, in the case of RNA, or millions, in the case of DNA. Each sugar unit in the chain carries a nitrogenous base attached by an N-glycosidic bond to carbon-1, the anomeric carbon of the sugar. There is no restriction on the sequence of the bases on a single nucleic acid chain. Consequently, the base sequence can be used to encode information. Base sequences that correspond to any possible amino acid sequence for a protein can be carried on DNA.

As befits an archival material, DNA has remarkable chemical stability. This makes it possible to recover bodily material during forensic investigation, extract DNA, and identify base sequences in it that are unique to an individual, so-called *genetic fingerprints*. Intact DNA sequences can also be isolated from archaeological materials many thousands of years old. The 2'-hydroxyl group on the ribose, (absent in 2'-deoxyribose), facilitates the hydrolysis of phosphodiester bonds in RNA by bases. Consequently, RNA is much less stable than DNA.

Polarity of nucleic acids

Nucleic acid chains have direction: both RNA and DNA have ends that can be distinguished. The phosphodiester linkages result in a chain with a nucleotide unit with a 5'-hydroxyl not involved in a linkage at one end

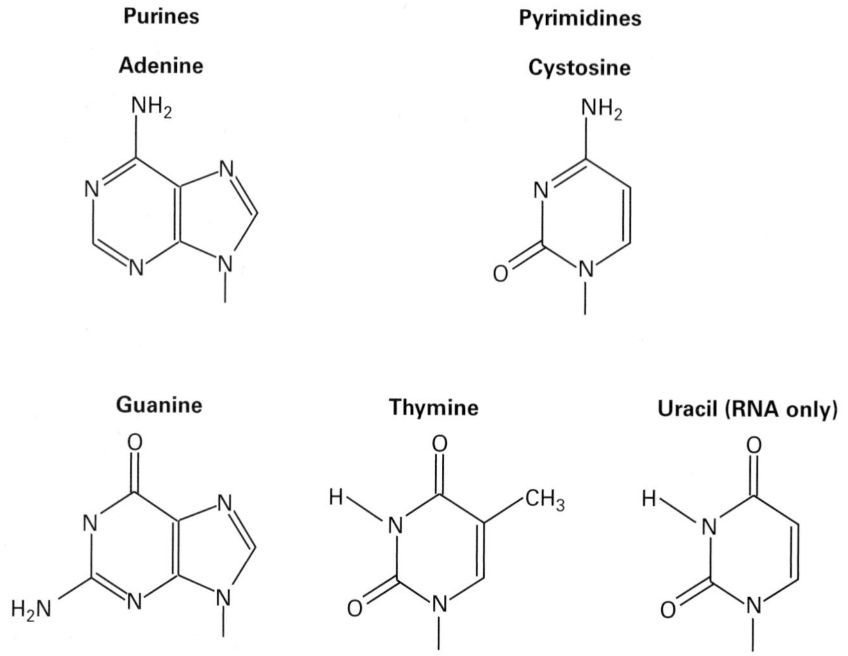

Purines

Pyrimidines

Adenine

Cystosine

Guanine   Thymine   Uracil (RNA only)

Fig. 117 Bases in DNA and RNA.

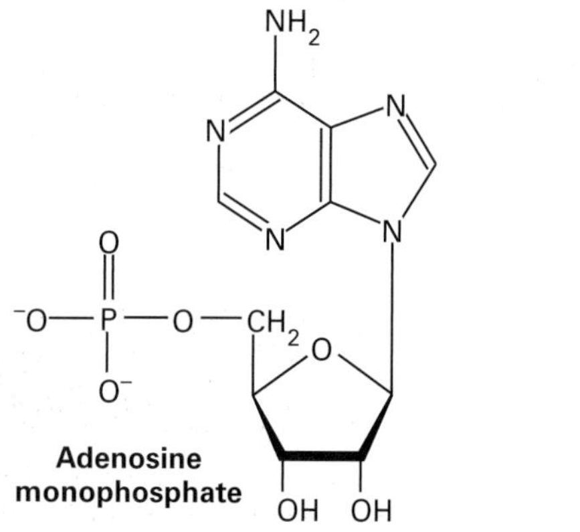

Adenosine
monophosphate   OH   OH

Fig. 118 AMP, a typical nucleotide containing adenine, ribose and a phosphate group.

and a 3′-hydroxyl not involved in a linkage at the other. These ends of the chain are referred to as the 5′ and 3′ ends (Fig. 119). All nucleic acid chains, both DNA and RNA, are synthesised in the 5′ to 3′ direction; that is to say, the chains are elongated by addition of new nucleotide units at the 3′ ends. When we consider the association of two DNA chains to form a DNA double helix, we find they are *antiparallel*: one runs in the 5′ to 3′ direction while the other runs in the 3′ to 5′ direction.

Translation of mRNA occurs in the 5′ to 3′ direction. Since this is the direction for all the processes in which nucleic acids engage, nucleic acid sequences are conventionally written with the 5′ end on the left and the 3′ end on the right. The only exception to this convention

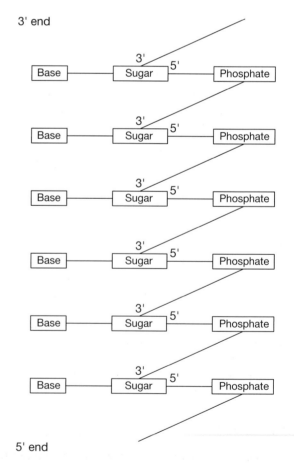

3′ end

5′ end

Fig. 119 Polynucleotide chain structure.

is when a sequence is depicted together with its complementary sequence. Since the chains are antiparallel, the lower one is shown with its 3′ end on the left. Positions in a sequence are often referred to as *upstream* if they are towards the 5′ end, or *downstream* towards the 3′ end.

Higher structural levels

In nucleic acids, as with proteins, higher levels of structure beyond the covalent primary structure must be considered when we try to relate structure to function. In the case of the nucleic acids, this involves the folding and coiling of the chains and, most importantly, the specific association of one chain with another. The association of one chain with another depends on the base sequences of the chains involved. The bases on one chain must be able to make 'base pairs' with the bases on the other (see below). Two base sequences that can make base pairs with one another are said to be *complementary*.

The double helix

The most important structure that involves the association of nucleic acid chains with complementary base sequences is the *double helix* formed by DNA. The description of this structure by Watson and Crick in 1953 triggered the explosion in knowledge of the biochemical basis of genetics that has occurred since then. After studying the results of X-ray crystallography studies and chemical analysis, Watson and Crick proposed that DNA existed as pairs of DNA chains having complementary base sequences. The two chains associated with each other to form a double helix with a distinct character (Fig. 120):

- deoxyribose-phosphate backbones are antiparallel: one chain runs 5′ to 3′ while the other runs 3′ to 5′
- the deoxyribose phosphate backbones wind round each other to form a helix; a complete turn of the helix occurs every 10 base pairs
- base pairs link a base on one chain with a base on the other across the core of the helix
- bases are planar with hydrophobic surfaces (see p. 5); the base pairs stack, one on top of the other like a pile of plates, to fill the core, adding greatly to the stability of the helix
- two helical grooves, one wide and one narrow, allow access to the bases so that they can interact with proteins
- protein binding to specific base sequences is vital for the control of gene expression.

Base pairing

Each base pair must form according to strict base-pairing rules. One base in each pair must be a purine (adenine

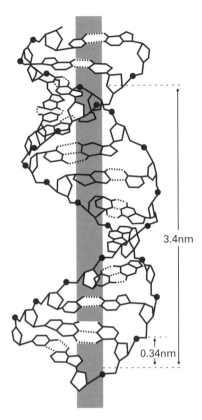

Fig. 120 The DNA double helix. The sugars are represented by pentagons and the phosphates by black circles. (From Bell, Emslie-Smith and Paterson (1976) *Textbook of Physiology and Biochemistry*, 9th edn. Edinburgh: Churchill Livingstone.)

Clinical note:
Many mutagens contain aromatic rings

Some mutagens (and, hence, carcinogens) have planar aromatic ring structures which can insert themselves into the stack of base pairs at the core of the DNA double helix. Examples of such carcinogens are benzanthracene, found in cigarette smoke, and aflatoxins, produced by the action of certain moulds.

or guanine) and the other must be a pyrimidine (cytosine or thymine). Two purines together are too large to fit into the core of the helix and two pyrimidines are too small. Furthermore, hydrogen bond formation dictates that, if one base is adenine, the other in the pair must be thymine, and if one base is guanine, the other must be cytosine. Thus four base pairs are possible: AT, TA, GC and CG (Fig. 121). Notice that the overall sizes and shapes of the base pairs are very similar and that the atoms on the bases linking them to the sugar occupy similar positions in each base pair. An AT base pair and a TA base pair are also similar and are related to each

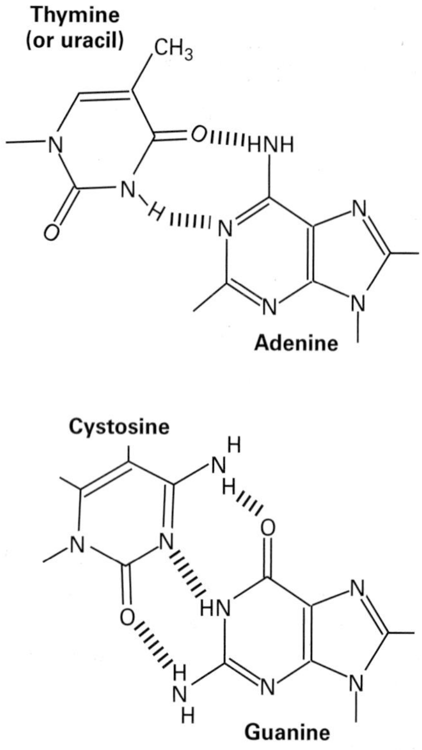

Thymine
(or uracil)

Adenine

Cystosine

Guanine

Fig. 121 Base pair formation.

other by a twofold rotational symmetry; so also for GC and CG base pairs. The double helical structure of DNA can accommodate any sequence of base pairs. One chain in the double helix can have any sequence of bases, but this sequence of bases imposes a complementary, and hence predictable, sequence on the second chain. If one chain were to be taken away or destroyed, an identical chain could be constructed to replace it by constructing a chain with a base sequence complementary to the remaining chain.

12.3 DNA replication

Learning objectives

You should be able to:

- define and explain the following terms: semi-conservative replication, replication bubble, replication fork, leading strand, lagging strand, Okazaki fragments

- name the form in which deoxynucleotide units are required for DNA synthesis

- state the direction of DNA chain growth during DNA synthesis

- distinguish between a primer and a template in DNA synthesis

- describe the functions of DNA polymerase I and DNA ligase in the formation of the lagging strand.

The Watson–Crick structure of DNA lends itself to direct replication. If you separate the chains and obey the base-pairing rules while constructing a new partner chain for each, the result is two double helical molecules that are exact replicas of the original. This mode of replication is described as semi-conservative. Each daughter molecule contains a complete chain from the original. Meselson and Stahl demonstrated by an elegant experiment that DNA did indeed replicate in this way (Fig. 122), but the actual replication process in cells must overcome some practical difficulties. The main difficulty is that the two chains are not separated before being copied; a continuous process of separation and copying passes along the original molecule. Only a very short section of DNA is converted to single-stranded form for copying at one time.

Replication of prokaryotic DNA starts in both directions from a single initiation site on the closed circular DNA molecule and replication proceeds until the replication sites meet on the other side of the circle.

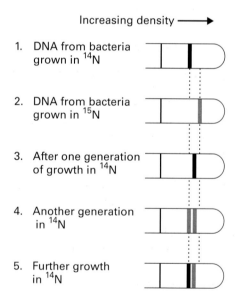

Increasing density ⟶

1. DNA from bacteria grown in ^{14}N

2. DNA from bacteria grown in ^{15}N

3. After one generation of growth in ^{14}N

4. Another generation in ^{14}N

5. Further growth in ^{14}N

Fig. 122 Meselson and Stahl's experiment to show semi-conservative DNA replication. DNA containing ^{14}N can be distinguished from that containing ^{15}N by ultracentrifugation in a caesium chloride density gradient, where they form bands at different positions (tubes 1 and 2). Bacteria grown for several generations in ^{15}N and then grown for one generation in ^{14}N contain a hybrid DNA of intermediate density (tube 3). After another generation in ^{14}N, a ^{14}N band appears in addition to the hybrid band (tube 4); the latter band gets fainter during further generations (tube 5).

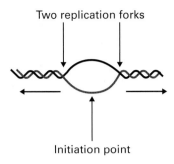

Fig. 123 Replication bubble consisting of two replication forks proceeding in opposite directions.

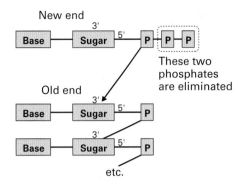

Fig. 124 Addition of a nucleotide unit to a growing chain: 5' to 3' growth.

Replication in eukaryotes, where the DNA molecules are much longer, starts at many initiation sites on each chromosome and proceeds in both directions until the replication process moving in one direction from one site meets the process moving in the other direction from the next site. The two replication processes moving apart from a single initiation site form what is termed a *replication bubble*. Each replication bubble has two regions where the DNA double helix is being unwound and replicated (Fig. 123). These regions are known as *replication forks*. To understand how DNA replication works, we have to consider events at a replication fork. The mechanism of DNA synthesis is very similar in prokaryotes and eukaryotes.

Synthesis of new DNA

DNA polymerases synthesise new DNA from deoxynucleoside 5'-triphosphates. In bacteria at least two forms are involved, *DNA polymerase III*, which synthesises most of the new DNA, and *DNA polymerase I*, which fills in gaps that DNA polymerase III must leave in one of the new chains at each fork. Both enzymes require a supply of deoxynucleotide units in the form of their triphosphates: dATP, dGTP, dCTP and dTTP. During the addition of each unit to the growing chain, two phosphate groups are eliminated as inorganic pyrophosphate, which is quickly hydrolysed by a *pyrophosphatase*. The hydrolysis of two high energy bonds in the triphosphate provides the energy for the addition of one nucleotide unit (Fig. 124).

Addition of new units only occurs at the 3' end of an existing DNA chain. Because they use deoxynucleoside 5'-triphosphates as substrates, DNA polymerases can only catalyse the addition of new nucleotides at the 3' end of an existing DNA molecule. They also require a template: a single-stranded DNA molecule. This controls the base sequence of the new strand, which is complementary to the template. The new strand is formed antiparallel to the template. At a replication fork, DNA

polymerase III and its associated DNA unwinding proteins separate the two chains of the original double helix. The replication process is different for the two chains of the original helix, the so-called *leading* and *lagging* strands.

The leading strand
The leading strand is copied continuously as it runs from 3' to 5', and will be able to act as a continuous template to produce an antiparallel complementary strand (Fig. 125).

The lagging strand
Copying of the other strand, the lagging strand, cannot be continuous, since no DNA polymerase can produce a new strand in the 3' to 5' direction. New DNA for the lagging strand is synthesised in fragments, called *Okazaki fragments* after the biochemist who first described them. These fragments, which are a few hundred base units long, are then joined to form a continuous chain (Fig. 125), a process that requires the cooperation of several enzyme activities.

Formation of Okazaki fragments

Only after the leading strand synthesis has proceeded for several hundred base units can the synthesis of the lagging strand commence to make a complementary chain for the several hundred units length of single-stranded 5' to 3' template now exposed. Synthesis of this chain must be in the direction opposite to the overall direction of movement of the replication fork. That is to say it must start in the fork and grow out from the fork. Each Okazaki fragment has an RNA primer since DNA polymerases absolutely require a 3' end of a nucleic acid chain if they are to attach new units This primer is a short section of RNA made by a form of RNA polymerase known as primase. RNA polymerases

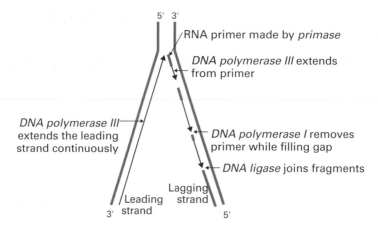

Fig. 125 Replication fork. The leading strand is directly replicated 5′ to 3′. The lagging strand is replicated in Okazaki fragments from RNA primers. The RNA primers are then removed and the gaps filled with DNA.

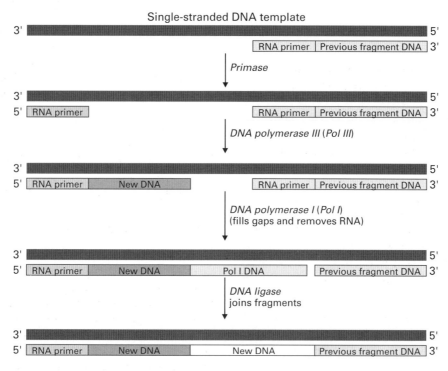

Fig. 126 Mechanism of replication of the lagging strand.

do not need a 3′ end to start synthesis. DNA polymerase can then add a new DNA chain to the RNA primer until it reaches the 5′ end of the previous fragment.

Filling the gaps between fragments

This is done by DNA polymerase I, which removes the RNA primer and replaces it with DNA. DNA ligase then joins the DNA fragments to make a continuous chain (Fig. 126) using the energy of hydrolysis of ATP or NAD^+ to create the phosphodiester bond.

12.4 Fidelity of DNA replication

Learning objectives

You should be able to:

- explain why DNA replication needs to be accurate

- give examples of agents that can damage DNA

- outline the process of DNA repair.

It is evident that to copy the complete genome with very few errors requires tremendous accuracy in the copying process. The $4' \ 10^6$ base pairs in the *E. coli* genome are copied with hardly any error. The accuracy required is, in fact, greater than can be achieved by DNA polymerase in its synthetic reaction alone. It is thought that about 1 in 10^5 of the inserted bases are not complementary to the corresponding base in the template chain. In bacteria, any wrongly inserted nucleotide is removed by a 3'-nuclease activity of DNA polymerase I. After inserting the wrong nucleotide, the enzyme is unable to proceed until the non-complementary nucleotide is removed. Prokaryotic DNA polymerase I, therefore, has a 'proof-reading' function. In both prokaryotes and eukaryotes, enzymes that repair the genome after damage and can also detect and eliminate copying errors.

DNA repair

The DNA of the genome may from time to time sustain damage that needs to be repaired. There are some diseases in which the underlying biochemical lesion has been identified as a reduced activity of one of the enzymes responsible for repair. Subjects suffering from such diseases may be unable to tolerate exposure to direct sunlight, or be particularly prone to some forms of cancer.

Damage to DNA can, in principle, be repaired if one of the DNA chains remains intact in the damaged region. The damaged part of the chain can be excised or cut away and then replaced by newly synthesised DNA that is complementary to the undamaged chain. Damage to DNA can arise from a variety of causes:

- exposure of cells to intense ultraviolet light can induce photochemical reactions between bases on the DNA chains: two thymines if next to each other in a sequence can be linked covalently to form a thymine dimer
- mutagenic chemicals may convert one base into another
- reactive chemical species produced by ionising radiation react with bases and alter them
- the bond between deoxyribose and a base, particularly a purine, is not completely stable and breaks, leaving a sugar group without any base attached.

Proteins that interact with the distorted double helix can detect all these forms of damage. Nucleases then excise the damaged section, DNA polymerase I fills in the gap with new DNA and DNA ligase joins the new DNA to the old.

12.5 DNA in cells

Learning objectives

You should be able to:

- explain why DNA synthesis must be synchronised with the processes of cell division
- explain the role of histones in condensing DNA to form chromosomes in eukaryotic cells
- explain how bacterial DNA is condensed.

DNA synthesis and the cell cycle

Eukaryotic cells that are dividing do not synthesise DNA continuously but only during the S phase of the cell cycle (Fig. 127). Replication of chromosomal DNA must be complete before the start of mitosis, the process by which replicated chromosomes segregate equally toward opposite poles prior to cell division. DNA synthesis does not resume again until after completion of mitosis. S (for synthesis) phase in the cycle is separated from M (for mitosis) phase by gap phases (G_1 and G_2) when neither process is occurring. There is evidence that the controls responsible for the timing of the cell cycle contain 'checkpoints' that halt the cycle while DNA replication or repair is in progress.

DNA in chromosomes

Apart from the enzymes required for replication and repair, many other enzymes and proteins exist which interact with DNA. In eukaryotes, the molecule of DNA that forms a single chromosome may be several centimetres in length. It must be condensed or shortened by coiling and folding if it is to fit in the nucleus. *Histones* are proteins that bind to DNA to promote coiling of DNA and reduction of its length. The first stage of the condensation process is the formation of *nucleosomes*. A length of DNA, about 200 base pairs long, forms a double coil around a 'bobbin' composed of histone proteins (Fig. 128). Eight histone molecules make up the

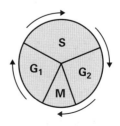

Fig. 127 The cell cycle.

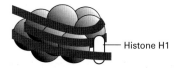

Fig. 128 Nucleosome structure with histones.

core of the nucleosome: two each of H2A, H2B, H3 and H4. A single H1 molecule per nucleosome appears to control when DNA can unwind from the core. Each nucleosome holds DNA of about 200 base pairs in length. Chains of nucleosomes are coiled into a solenoid structure, thus reducing further the length of the DNA. DNA that is being replicated or that is being used as a template for RNA synthesis must be unwound from the nucleosome and from the higher level coiling. This is achieved by local covalent modification of the histones by acetylation, phosphorylation and other processes. Condensed DNA is protected against nuclease action, whereas DNA that is unwound is much more easily attacked.

Mitochondria contain closed circles of DNA similar to those found in bacteria.

Enzymes for uncoiling and untangling DNA

The length and helical double-strand structure of DNA would be expected to cause severe topological problems, tangles and twists, during replication, transcription, condensation and nucleosome formation. Enzymes that can unwind the double helix or that can produce or relieve supercoiling of the structure overcome these problems.

- *Helicases* separate local regions of the helix to produce single strands for replication or transcription. These enzymes use the energy of ATP hydrolysis to separate the strands.

Unwinding of one region produces supercoiling of adjacent regions. This can be overcome by other classes of enzymes, topoisomerases.

- *Type I topoisomerases* relieve supercoiling by temporarily cleaving one strand of the double helix to create a swivel point where one-half of the chain can rotate with respect to the other part.
- *Type II topoisomerases* can introduce negative supercoiling using the energy of ATP hydrolysis to drive the reaction. They operate on two strands of DNA at a time: both chains of one strand are cut temporarily and the second chain is passed through the gap that is formed.

Bacterial DNA

Histones are not found in bacteria. Another method of condensing DNA is used. The DNA is in the form of a closed circle so there is no 5' or 3' end to either chain in the double helix. This circle is negatively supercoiled by type II topoisomerases. Since there are no free ends to rotate, the DNA coils on itself and shortens (Fig. 129). Type I topoisomerases can act as swivel points in the DNA chain and relieve the negative supercoiling. Bacteria must control the extent of supercoiling of their DNA since it influences the accessibility of base sequences for transcription.

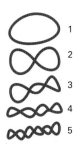

Fig. 129 Supercoiling of circular DNA.

Self-assessment: questions

Single best answer MCQs

1. Identify the single correct statement that describes the relationship between nucleic acids and proteins.
   a. Nucleic acids synthesise proteins
   b. Proteins cannot be directly involved in the synthesis of proteins
   c. Chromosomes are composed of DNA
   d. All cellular DNA is located in the nucleus
   e. Every nucleated cell in the body contains information about the amino acid sequence of every protein that can be synthesised in any cell

2. Identify the statement that applies to the genomes of different species.
   a. Fruit flies have more DNA per cell than bacteria and humans have more than fruit flies, but some frogs and toads have more than humans
   b. DNA is the primary genetic material in animals and RNA is the primary genetic material in plants
   c. Human somatic cells contain 23 chromosomes
   d. Histones are proteins associated with DNA in chromosomes and vary greatly from species to species
   e. Each human chromosome contains one DNA molecule about 1 metre long

3. Select the single correct statement that describes DNA and protein synthesis.
   a. The Central Dogma of Molecular Genetics concerns the flow of sequence information from DNA to RNA to protein
   b. The production of two identical DNA molecules from an original DNA molecule is known as replication; in eukaryotic cells it occurs only in the nucleus
   c. The copying of base sequence information from DNA to RNA is known as translation; it occurs inside the nucleus in eukaryotic cells
   d. The synthesis of a protein with an amino acid sequence specified by the base sequence of an RNA molecule is known as transcription; it occurs outside the nucleus of eukaryotic cells
   e. DNA replication, transcription and translation are sufficient to account for the specificity of protein synthesis in all organisms including viruses

4. Given the significance of bases in nucleic acids, which of the following statements is accurate?
   a. In the DNA double helix, each base pair must contain two purines or two pyrimidines
   b. The bases in DNA and RNA are joined to the sugar phosphate backbone by ester linkages to the phosphate groups
   c. In double-stranded DNA the number of purine bases equals the number of pyrimidine bases
   d. In double-stranded DNA, the number of adenine bases equals the number of guanines and the number of thymines equals the number of cytosines
   e. The two DNA chains in a double helix are parallel

5. Which of the following is a correct description of the chemistry of DNA and RNA?
   a. Uracil is a purine base that occurs in RNA but not in DNA
   b. Thymine is a pyrimidine base that occurs in RNA but not in DNA
   c. Ribose is a pentose sugar that occurs in DNA and RNA
   d. Cytosine is a pyrimidine base that occurs in both RNA and DNA
   e. Adenine and guanine are purine bases that occur in DNA but not in RNA

6. Which one of the following statements accurately describes nucleic acids as polynucleotides?
   a. The two ends of a chain can be distinguished, one is known as the N-terminal end and the other as the C-terminal
   b. A backbone consisting of alternating nitrogenous bases and pentose sugar units
   c. There is no structural restriction on the sequence of bases
   d. Nucleic acid chains are never closed circles
   e. Nucleic acid chains are often branched

7. Which of the following is an accurate description of structural aspects of DNA and RNA?
   a. They differ in the pentose sugar units they contain but have the same nitrogenous bases
   b. RNA is chemically more stable than DNA because it must function outside the nucleus

c. They contain nitrogenous bases attached to the carbon-1' of the pentose sugar units by a carbon–nitrogen bond

d. Nucleotide units are joined by 3',5'-phosphodiester bonds in DNA whereas those in RNA are joined by 2',5' bonds

e. The two strands in the DNA double helix cannot be separated

8. A section of A DNA chain has the sequence A T G G C T A. Which one of the sequences shown is complementary? (The base sequences shown below have their 5' ends on the left and their 3' ends on the right.)

a. A T G G C T A

b. T A G C C A T

c. T A C C G A T

d. A T C G G T A

e. G C T A A C G

9. Which one of the following is NOT required for replication of DNA by DNA polymerase?

a. A template of single-stranded DNA

b. A DNA or RNA primer with a free 3' end

c. 2'-Deoxy-ATP

d. 2'-Deoxy-UTP

e. 2'-Deoxy-CTP

10. In the process of DNA replication:

a. Addition of new nucleotide units can occur at either the 5' or the 3' end of the chain being extended

b. Addition of new nucleotide units cannot occur continuously on the leading strand

c. Addition of new nucleotide units can occur continuously on the lagging strand

d. Each new nucleotide unit added to a growing strand must have a base that can form a complementary base pair with the corresponding base on the template strand

e. DNA polymerase is responsible for the replication of the leading but not the lagging strand

11. Which of the following accurately describes DNA replication?

a. It is conservative; that is to say, each of the original strands from a double helix is

associated with a newly synthesised strand in the daughter molecules

b. It occurs continuously on the two DNA chains in a double helix

c. It involves DNA polymerase III, which requires a DNA primer and a template, which is usually RNA

d. It proceeds in both directions from an initiation site, so a replication bubble is formed

e. Replication of the leading strand in DNA synthesis involves the formation of RNA primers and Okazaki fragments; the fragments are finally sealed together by the actions of DNA polymerase I and DNA ligase

12. Lagging strand replication is a process that:

a. Involves the formation of RNA primers by ribonuclease action

b. Produces fragments that start with an RNA primer; DNA polymerase III adds new nucleotide units to the 5' end of this primer

c. Results in gaps between fragments, which are filled with DNA by reverse transcriptase

d. Produces fragments known as Okazaki fragments, which are eventually joined into a continuous strand by DNA ligase

e. Involves DNA polymerase III, which is also involved in DNA repair

13. Which statement is correct concerning DNA in chromosomes?

a. It is replicated continuously in dividing cells

b. The final stage of condensation of nuclear DNA in eukaryotes involves the formation of nucleosomes

c. Nucleosomes each consist of about 200 base pairs length of double helix wound inside a coat composed of histone proteins

d. In prokaryotes, DNA exists as closed circles and is condensed by supercoiling

e. It is supercoiled; supercoiling can be increased but not decreased by enzymes

Short essay question

Describe the features of DNA that fit it for its function as the primary genetic material in most organisms.

Self-assessment: answers

Single best answer MCQ answers

1. a. **False**. Proteins are also involved.
   b. **False**. Many proteins are involved in nucleic acid synthesis as enzymes and constituents of the ribosome,.
   c. **False**. Chromosomes are about 50% protein, mostly histone.
   d. **False**. Some DNA is found in organelles, particularly mitochondria.
   e. **True**. Every diploid nucleated cell has a complete set of chromosomes.

2. a. **True**. As a general rule, the more complex the organism, the more DNA it has in its genome, but some frogs and toads have much more DNA than would be expected.
   b. **False**. Both animals and plants have DNA as the primary genetic material.
   c. **False**. There are 23 pairs of chromosomes in human somatic cells.
   d. **False**. Histones are remarkably similar from species to species.
   e. **False**. Each chromosome contains one molecule. The total length is near 1 metre.

3. a. **True**. It applies in all organisms except some viruses.
   b. **False**. Mitochondrial DNA is an exception.
   c. **False**. This is transcription.
   d. **True**. This is translation.
   e. **False**. RNA viruses need RNA replication to replicate their genome.

4. a. **False**. Each base pair contains a purine and a pyrimidine.
   b. **False**. They are joined to carbon-1 of the sugars by glycosidic bonds.
   c. **True**. This is a consequence of specific base pairing.
   d. **False**. Adenine pairs with thymine so they are present in equal numbers. Similarly guanine and cytosine.
   e. **False**. They are antiparallel. One runs in the 5′ to 3′ direction, the other 3′ to 5′.

5. a. **False**. Uracil is a pyrimidine base.
   b. **False**. Thymine only occurs in DNA.
   c. **False**. 2′-Deoxyribose is found in DNA.
   d. **True**.
   e. **False**. These two purines occur in both DNA and RNA.

6. a. **False**. The ends are known as 3′ or 5′ since the nucleotide units at the ends of chain have either a free 3′ or a free 5′ not involved in a phosphodiester link.
   b. **False**. The backbone is alternating pentose sugar units and phosphate in both RNA and DNA.
   c. **True**. This allows nucleic acids to act as information carriers.
   d. **False**. Bacterial DNA usually occurs as closed circular molecules, as does mitochondrial DNA.
   e. **False**. Nucleic acids are never branched.

7. a. **False**. They also differ in the bases they contain. DNA contains thymine whereas RNA has uracil.
   b. **False**. RNA is much more easily hydrolysed, especially in alkali.
   c. **True**. This applies to all nucleotides and polynucleotides.
   d. **False**. Both have 3′,5′-phosphodiester bonds.
   e. **False**. Heating separates the chains. This process is sometimes referred to as *melting* of DNA.

8. b. is the correct answer. Base-paired chains are always antiparallel. 5′-T A G C C A T-3′ becomes 3′-T A C C G A T-5′ when written with its 3′ end on the left and is complementary to 5′-A T G G C T A-3′.

9. a. **False**. The template is needed to direct the sequence of the new strand.
   b. **False**. DNA polymerases need primers and cannot start a chain without one.
   c. **False**. 2′-Deoxy-ATP provides nucleotide residues for the new chain.
   d. **True**. Uracil does not occur in DNA. 2′-Deoxy-TTP is required.
   e. **True**. 2′-Deoxy-CTP provides nucleotide residues for the new chain.

10. a. **False**. Addition occurs only at the 3' end.
    b. **False**. The leading strand grows continuously at its 3' end.
    c. **False**. The lagging strand is replicated in fragments, not continuously.
    d. **True**. This is how the template directs the base sequence of the new strand (some mismatching can occur, which requires subsequent repair).
    e. **False**. It is a very complex enzyme and is responsible for the elongation of both strands.

11. a. **False**. This association of new strands with old is described as semi-conservative.
    b. **False**. The leading strand is replicated continuously but the lagging strand is replicated in fragments.
    c. **False**. The template is DNA and the primer is usually RNA.
    d. **True**. The replication bubble consists of two replication forks.
    e. **False**. The mechanism describes DNA formation on the lagging strand.

12. a. **False**. The enzyme involved is not ribonuclease but an RNA polymerase known as primase.
    b. **False**. New nucleotide units are always added at the 3' end in all nucleic acid synthesis.
    c. **False**. The gaps are filled by DNA polymerase I.
    d. **True**. DNA ligase joins the 3' end of one fragment to the 5' end of the next.
    e. **False**. Damaged strands are repaired by DNA polymerase I and DNA ligase.

13. a. **False**. Nuclear DNA is replicated only during S phase of the cell cycle.
    b. **False**. Nucleosome formation is the first stage of condensation.
    c. **False**. Nucleosomes have a histone core with DNA wound around it.
    d. **True**. Bacterial genomes and plasmids are circular DNA molecules.
    e. **False**. Enzymes exist to increase and decrease supercoiling.

Short essay answer

Points that should be mentioned include its double helical structure, which allows for straightforward replication, its ability to carry information in its sequence of bases and its chemical stability.

13 RNA structure and function

Overview

RNA has several functions in the cell. Ribosomal RNA has structural and catalytic functions in ribosomes, the particles responsible for protein synthesis. Messenger RNA carries sequence information from DNA in the cell nucleus to the sites of protein synthesis. Transfer RNA molecules are adaptors that match each amino acid with the triplet sequence of bases indicating its position in the protein chain. Other RNA molecules have catalytic roles during the synthesis of messenger RNA.

Transcription, the copying of DNA base sequences into RNA, is one of the main points at which protein synthesis is controlled.

13.1 Types of RNA

Learning objectives

You should be able to:

- name three forms of RNA involved in protein synthesis and name the function of each
- describe how RNA differs from DNA in structure, base content, size and higher order structure
- describe the constituents of a ribosome
- sketch the secondary structure of tRNA to show the position of the anticodon and the amino acid attachment site.

Although DNA carries the information that is needed for the synthesis of proteins, it is not directly involved in protein synthesis. There are three types of RNA needed for protein synthesis:

- messenger RNA (mRNA): carries the sequence information from DNA in the nucleus to the protein synthetic machinery in the cytoplasm
- ribosomal RNA: forms about 50% of the weight of ribosomes, on which protein synthesis occurs
- transfer RNA (tRNA): acts as an adaptor matching a specific amino acid to the codon on the mRNA.

RNA structures

RNA has a covalent structure very similar to that of DNA. It has ribose in place of deoxyribose and the pyrimidine base uracil in place of thymine. The extra hydroxyl group on the 2′ position of the sugar facilitates the cleavage of the phosphodiester bond to the hydroxyl group on the 3′-hydroxyl, so RNA is more easily hydrolysed than DNA. Uracil is very similar to thymine, lacking only the methyl substituent at the 5 position on the ring. Like thymine, it can form a base pair with adenine.

mRNA does not have a higher-order structure like the double helix formed by DNA. Ribosomal RNA and tRNA have structures containing base pairing, not between separate chains as in DNA but between different parts of the same chain. An RNA chain can be folded back on itself to form a stem loop structure. The stem is a double helix stabilised by complementary base pairs and the loop is formed from the chain between the stem sequences (Fig. 130). Table 19 summarises the properties and functions of the various RNAs.

Transfer RNAs

There are 30–40 distinct tRNA molecules, each responsible for bringing a single amino acid to the growing polypeptide chain. Each of these tRNA molecules contains a sequence of approximately 80 nucleotide units and has the same basic shape. Base pairing by parts of these sequences leads to folded forms in a 'clover leaf' structure, containing three major stem loops (Fig. 130).

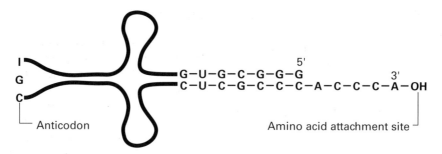

Fig. 130 Secondary structure of tRNA.

Table 19 Principal forms of eukaryotic RNA

Form of RNA	Size (bases)	Role
mRNA	Varies with size of protein to be synthesised	Carries protein sequence information from nucleus to ribosomes. Some mRNA species are very short-lived, others more stable. mRNA is processed in the nucleus from initial transcripts
Ribosomal RNA		
16S	1542	Together with about 20 proteins, makes up the structure of the small ribosomal subunit
23S	About 3000	23S and 5S rRNA with about 30 proteins, make up the structure of the small ribosomal subunit
5S	About 120	Small ribosomal subunit
tRNA	About 80	There are between 30 and 40 different species to act as adaptors, matching amino acids to codons
Small nuclear RNAs (snRNAs)	Up to 200	Associated with proteins to form complexes involved in splicing during mRNA processing
Small cytoplasmic RNA (scRNA)	About 300	Associates with proteins to form a signal recognition particle that is involved in intracellular transport of newly synthesised proteins
RNA primers	About 5	Primers for Okazaki fragments during replication of the lagging strand in DNA replication (Ch. 22); these primers are then replaced by DNA

Base pairing occurs between different parts of the same chain, which folds back on itself; the remaining unpaired bases are exposed in loops where the chain turns. There are three bases at the end of one loop that are not base paired and form the *anticodon*, which interacts with three bases forming a codon on mRNA. Amino acids are attached to the 3′ end of the tRNA that carries their specific anticodon by aminoacyl-tRNA synthetases (p. 203).

Ribosomal RNA

The molecules of ribosomal RNA also contain sequences that bring about folding to form a structure containing many stem loops. Ribosomal RNA adopts a specific three-dimensional configuration that is required for

its function. The role of ribosomes is discussed in Chapter 14.

Messenger RNA

mRNA has a base sequence that directs the synthesis of a protein with a particular amino acid sequence so it cannot adopt a specific three-dimensional shape by base pairing. Nevertheless, stem loops may form in sections of the mRNA sequence that are not used for coding.

Other RNAs

Other forms of RNA exist, especially in eukaryotic cells. RNA molecules having specific catalytic action participate in the processing and maturation of eukaryotic

RNA before it leaves the nucleus. Further RNA molecules direct newly synthesised proteins to their destinations in the cell. These forms of RNA have specific three-dimensional structures that depend on base pairing.

13.2 Transcription: synthesis of RNA

Learning objectives

You should be able to:

- list the precursors of RNA used in its synthesis
- describe the processes occurring during the three phases of transcription.

RNA is synthesised by *RNA polymerase* from the precursor nucleoside triphosphates ATP, GTP, UTP and CTP. RNA polymerase, like DNA polymerase, requires a template to direct the sequence of the RNA product. The template in this case is DNA and the enzyme synthesises an RNA molecule with a sequence that is complementary to one chain of the DNA molecule. Each adenine in the DNA sequence is copied as uracil, each thymine as adenine, each guanine as cytosine and each cytosine as guanine. As in DNA synthesis, pyrophosphate is eliminated during the polymerisation, and the subsequent hydrolysis of this drives the reaction in the direction of synthesis. The growing RNA chain has each new nucleotide unit added at its 3′ end. As in DNA synthesis, the template and the new chain are antiparallel, so the DNA chain is copied in its 3′ to 5′ direction. For any one region of the double helix, only one chain acts as a template. In other regions the other chain is used, i.e. all the coding sequences are not on just one of the two chains. In eukaryotes, different molecular species of RNA polymerase catalyse the synthesis of mRNA, ribosomal RNA and tRNA (Table 20).

The process of RNA synthesis can be considered in three phases:

- initiation
- elongation
- termination.

Table 20 RNA polymerases in eukaryotic cells

Form	RNA species for which transcript is produced
I	23S and 16S ribosomal RNA
II	mRNA
III	tRNAs and 5S ribosomal RNA

Initiation

Initiation has been much studied because it is during this phase that the starting points on the DNA sequence are identified. These starting points are known as *promoters*. It is the efficiency of initiation at each promoter that determines how much of each particular mRNA is made and hence how much of the corresponding protein. Some promoters are subject to control and can be switched on and off. Control of promoter action is the most important mechanism by which the cell controls the proteins that it synthesises and the amount of each.

Formation of a transcription complex

RNA polymerase binds at promoter sequences. RNA polymerase is responsible for all RNA synthesis in prokaryotes and is simpler than the eukaryotic enzymes. It contains five subunits: two alpha subunits, two similar beta subunits (β and β′) and the sigma subunit. The sigma subunit is involved in promoter recognition and in the formation of a transcription complex before the synthesis of each RNA molecule. It is not required for elongation and dissociates once transcription has started. Promoters are recognised by their sequences. By convention, the base in DNA that is complementary to the first base in the RNA molecule is designated +1. The bases of the template are then numbered in sequence: +2, +3 and so on. Bases further down the chain in this direction are said to be *downstream*. The base on the *upstream* side of +1 is designated −1.

The recognition sequences for the promoter are situated around −10 and −35. Promoter sequences are similar but not identical; they are said to resemble a consensus sequence. Around −10, the sequence often includes the bases TATA. When DNA is acting as a template for RNA synthesis, the DNA chains must be temporarily unwound and separated. This involves breaking the base pairs, and it may be significant that the section of chain where separation starts has predominantly AT base pairs. Adenine forms only two hydrogen bonds with thymine, whereas a guanine–cytosine base pair is stabilised by three hydrogen bonds. The TATA sequence is therefore more easily separated than a sequence made up of GC base pairs. A schematic drawing to represent initiation and elongation during transcription is shown as Figure 131.

Elongation

Once the initiation complex is formed and nucleotide units are bound to start transcription, the sigma unit is no longer required and dissociates. Core enzyme of RNA polymerase then catalyses elongation of the RNA chain as it moves along the DNA.

1. Initiation: *RNA polymerase* binds at promoter

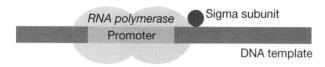

2. DNA chain separation

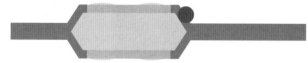

3. Transcription starts

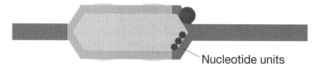

4. Elongation

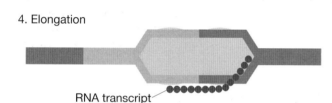

Fig. 131 Initiation and elongation stages of transcription.

Termination

RNA polymerase continues elongating the RNA transcript until it encounters a termination sequence. Some of these sequences require a termination protein called the *rho factor*, which binds to DNA and separates the enzyme from its template.

13.3 Control of transcription

Learning objectives

You should be able to:

- explain the terms: constitutive, inducible and repressible as applied to cell proteins
- describe the functions of the *lac* and *trp* operons in *Escherichia coli*
- give examples of factors which may influence the rate of synthesis of proteins in bacterial and eukaryotic cells

- explain how control of transcription differs between prokaryotes and eukaryotes.

Protein synthesis is largely controlled by transcription. Specific DNA binding proteins control initiation at many promoters. Cells have the ability to switch the synthesis of specific proteins on and off. In each cell proteins can be classified as:

- constitutive, synthesised whatever the circumstances
- repressible, normally synthesised but synthesis can be turned off
- inducible, not normally synthesised but synthesis can be turned on.

Control, which is a combination of *induction* and *repression*, is observed in some cases, such as that of the lactose-catabolising proteins of *E. coli* described below. Repression is often seen in anabolic pathways where a surplus of the end-product of the pathway represses synthesis of all the enzymes in the path. *Repressible proteins* in bacteria include the enzymes responsible for the synthesis of some amino acids or other cellular building blocks. If these amino acids or building blocks are abundant in the growth medium, then bacteria can save energy and material by repressing the synthesis of these enzymes.

Inducible proteins often carry out functions that the cell does not always need, such as the catabolism of some rarely encountered nutrient. *E. coli* can grow on glucose and a variety of other sugars including lactose. The enzymes for glucose catabolism are *constitutive*, but those for lactose catabolism are *inducible*: they are only synthesised if lactose is present and if glucose is absent. The mechanism by which this control is exerted on the synthesis of lactose-catabolising proteins in *E. coli* is well understood (see below).

Control of transcription in prokaryotes

Control of protein synthesis in bacteria has been much studied and some important control mechanisms have been described.

Control of the lac operon in E. coli

Lactose is a disaccharide containing a galactose unit joined to a glucose by a glycosidic bond joining carbon-1, the anomeric carbon of galactose, to carbon-4 of glucose. It is a β-galactoside and must be hydrolysed before it can be catabolised. *β-Galactosidase* is one of the enzymes required for lactose utilisation in *E. coli*. A *lactose transporter protein* is also required for entry of lactose into

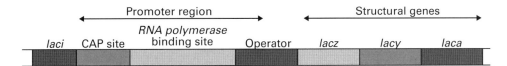

Fig. 132 Map of the *lac* operon of *E. coli* (not to scale).

the bacterium. These two proteins and a third protein, a *transacetylase*, whose function is not clear, are only synthesised when *E. coli* is grown in the presence of lactose or some synthetic analogues of lactose. Synthesis of these proteins is inhibited if glucose is present. *E. coli* can use glucose for energy and as a carbon source, so lactose utilisation is not required if glucose is present. If *E. coli* cells growing in a glucose-containing medium are transferred to a medium containing lactose but no glucose, growth ceases and only resumes after a 'lag' phase lasting about 20 minutes. The proteins required for lactose catabolism are synthesised from amino acids during this interval. They are not produced by the activation of previously synthesised inactive precursors.

Bacterial genes for proteins with related functions often map side by side on the bacterial genome and form a group of genes that are controlled as a unit. Such a group of genes is called an *operon*. The structural genes of the operon are transcribed to give a single mRNA molecule that carries within its length sequences corresponding to the sequences of the polypeptide chains. The three proteins required for lactose catabolism are coded for by the three structural genes of the *lac* operon, *lacz*, *lacy* and *laca*, which code for β-galactosidase, the galactoside transporter protein and the transacetylase, respectively. A map of the genes of the *lac* operon is given in Figure 132.

Downstream from the promoter of the *lac* operon there is a base sequence, the *operator*, which controls initiation at the promoter. This base sequence is recognised by an allosteric control protein, the *lac repressor protein* coded for by the gene *laci*. When this protein binds to the operator, initiation of RNA synthesis at the promoter is completely blocked. The second ligand of the repressor protein is *allolactose*, made from lactose by β-galactosidase, which is always present in the bacterium but at a very low level of activity if it has not been induced. When the repressor binds allolactose it is no longer able to bind to the operator and initiation at the promoter can occur (Fig. 133). Lactose thus induces the proteins required for its own catabolism.

Role of glucose

Glucose can decrease transcription of the *lac* operon. The *lac* promoter does not bind RNA polymerase with high affinity so that even with lactose present very little

transcription occurs. The efficiency of the promoter is greatly increased if another protein binds to its control sequence, which is beside and upstream of the promoter. This protein is the *catabolite gene activator protein* or *CAP*, and the control sequence to which it binds is known as the *CAP site*. When CAP binds to its site it can make contacts with RNA polymerase that greatly favour the initiation of transcription. CAP is also an allosteric protein and can only bind to its site if it has first bound a molecule of the signal molecule, cyclic AMP. Cells that are catabolising glucose contain very low concentrations of cyclic AMP (or cAMP), so induction of the lactose-catabolising proteins does not occur if glucose is available. This control by glucose of operons involved in the synthesis of enzymes required for the catabolism of lactose and other sugars is known as *catabolite repression* (Fig. 134).

Control of the trp operon in E. coli

E. coli can synthesise the tryptophan it needs for protein synthesis if this amino acid is not available in the growth medium. The enzymes required are coded for by genes carried on the *trp* operon, which is controlled as a single unit. *E. coli* either synthesises all the enzymes coded for by the genes on the *trp* operon or none of them. An allosteric repressor protein exerts control by binding to an operator sequence between the promoter and the structural genes. In this case, the repressor protein on its own cannot bind to the operator to block transcription. Only when it has bound its other ligand (tryptophan, of course) can it bind to the operator. Tryptophan acts as a co-repressor (Fig. 135). The presence of tryptophan in the growth medium, therefore, switches off the synthesis of the enzymes required for tryptophan synthesis.

Control of termination

Termination of transcription can also control protein synthesis. In some bacteriophages, proteins that are anti-termination factors control the production of different proteins at different stages of the phage infection cycle. In the presence of these factors, RNA polymerase no longer responds to the termination signal and reads through it to transcribe a further section of the phage genome.

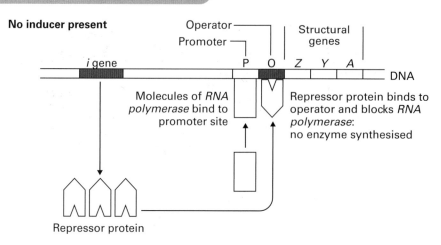

No inducer present

Operator
Promoter
Structural genes

i gene P O Z Y A DNA

Molecules of *RNA polymerase* bind to promoter site

Repressor protein binds to operator and blocks *RNA polymerase*: no enzyme synthesised

Repressor protein

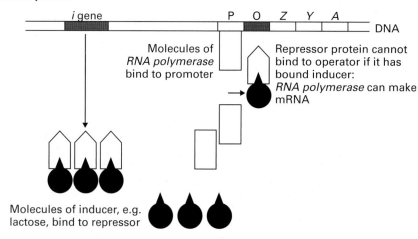

Inducer present

i gene P O Z Y A DNA

Molecules of *RNA polymerase* bind to promoter

Repressor protein cannot bind to operator if it has bound inducer: *RNA polymerase* can make mRNA

Molecules of inducer, e.g. lactose, bind to repressor

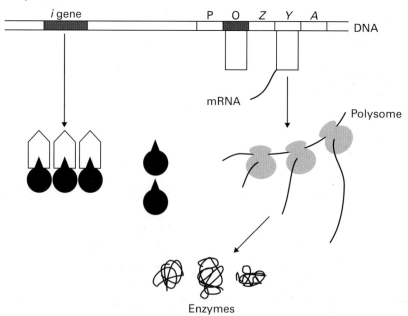

Induction process

i gene P O Z Y A DNA

mRNA

Polysome

Enzymes

Fig. 133 Repressor function in the *lac* operon. An example of an inducible operon. (Molecules of inducer, repressor, etc. are not shown to scale.)

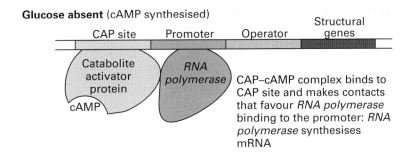

Glucose absent (cAMP synthesised)

CAP–cAMP complex binds to CAP site and makes contacts that favour *RNA polymerase* binding to the promoter: *RNA polymerase* synthesises mRNA

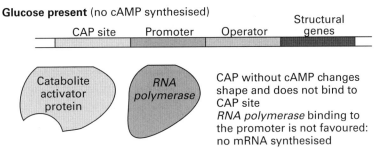

Glucose present (no cAMP synthesised)

CAP without cAMP changes shape and does not bind to CAP site

RNA polymerase binding to the promoter is not favoured: no mRNA synthesised

Fig. 134 Catabolite repression.

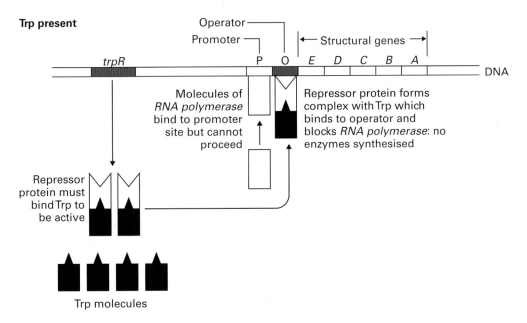

Trp present

Molecules of *RNA polymerase* bind to promoter site but cannot proceed

Repressor protein forms complex with Trp which binds to operator and blocks *RNA polymerase*: no enzymes synthesised

Repressor protein must bind Trp to be active

Trp molecules

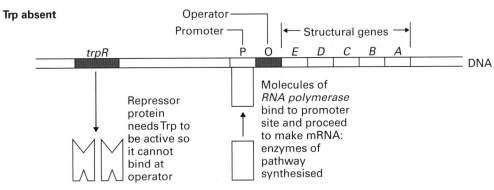

Trp absent

Repressor protein needs Trp to be active so it cannot bind at operator

Molecules of *RNA polymerase* bind to promoter site and proceed to make mRNA: enzymes of pathway synthesised

Fig. 135 Co-repressor function in the *trp* operon. An example of a repressible operon. (Molecules of Trp, repressor, etc. are not shown to scale.)

Control of transcription in eukaryotes

As might be expected, the processes controlling transcription in eukaryotes are much more complex than those found in bacteria. Proteins have to be synthesised that are appropriate to each cell type and its state of differentiation and growth. Protein synthesis must also respond to nutritional state and to stimulation by many hormones.

Operons do not occur in eukaryotes. Each gene has its own promoter and control sequences. Identification of these control sequences is a very active area of research at the present time. They have been found not only upstream and downstream of the genes being controlled but within the genes themselves. Some control sequences are remote, being thousands of bases away from the genes they control. Eukaryotic genes are subject to control by several *DNA binding proteins*, each specific for its particular control sequence. Some of these proteins recognise sequences that identify genes coding for proteins required in a particular cell type; others are allosteric and will only bind to their control sequences if they have also bound a specific steroid or thyroid hormone. The action of each promoter appears to depend on an exact combination of control proteins that have bound to their specific sequences. These control proteins not only bind to control sequences on the DNA but often bind to each other. Only such a combinatorial mechanism could possibly account for the specific expression of the large number of genes found in the eukaryotic genome.

Many of the proteins that control transcription have been isolated and have had their structures determined. The structures often show shared structural motifs for interacting with specific DNA sequences (e.g. *zinc fingers*) or for interacting with each other (e.g. *leucine zippers*) (Fig. 136). For transcription to occur at any potential promoter, the correct combination of DNA binding proteins must be built up, with each protein binding to its specific DNA sequence and able to interact with the other DNA-bound proteins in the complex.

Zinc fingers

These have a zinc ion bound by two cysteine and two histidine side chains; this stabilises a finger-shaped structure that can make contact with the bases within the major groove of DNA. Other amino acid side chains vary to give interaction with specific base sequences.

Leucine zippers.

Protein subunits with a leucine zipper have leucine residues at every seventh position in an alpha helix. Such subunits can be brought together by these to form homo- or heterodimers. Other parts of the subunits bind to specific sequences within DNA.

13.4 RNA processing

Learning objectives

You should be able to:

- explain what is meant by RNA processing

- describe the following terms: RNA splicing, exon, intron, capping and tailing.

After being produced by RNA polymerase, most RNA molecules are extensively modified before reaching their functional state.

Transfer RNA

tRNA contains several modified bases as well as the usual ones. tRNA sequences are transcribed in long sequences which are then cleaved to give precursor tRNA molecules. These have some bases methylated and others rearranged so that they are attached to the ribose by carbon–carbon bonds. Every functional tRNA molecule has the sequence CCA at its 3' end. In eukaryotic cells, this sequence is added enzymatically to a precursor molecule after it has left the nucleus.

Ribosomal RNA

Ribosomal RNA is also transcribed as a long precursor sequence which is then cleaved to give the three RNA molecules that are components of the ribosomal subunits. Ribosomal RNA is transcribed from DNA sequences in the nucleolus of the eukaryotic cell, which

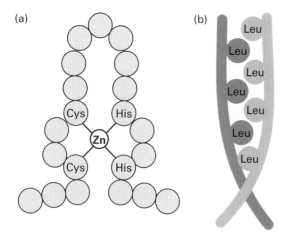

Fig. 136 Structural motifs in DNA binding proteins: (a) zinc finger; (b) leucine zipper.

contains multiple copies of the ribosomal RNA genes. These multiple copies are necessary to allow the high rate of transcription that is needed to form all the ribosomal RNA needed for ribosome formation.

Messenger RNA

mRNA in eukaryotes is subject to several different modifications before becoming functional.

RNA capping and tailing

The ends of mRNA molecules are modified, probably to protect them from rapid degradation by exonuclease action. The 5' end has a methylated guanine-containing nucleotide unit (cap) attached by a 5' to 5' phosphodiester bond, i.e. it has the reverse of the usual orientation. The cap on mRNA is required for recognition by the ribosome. The 3' end of the RNA transcript has a few hundred adenine-containing nucleotide units added enzymatically, a process known as *tailing*. Possession of this polyA tail by most eukaryotic mRNA molecules is exploited for their purification. Their tails will hybridise with a nucleic acid containing only thymine (polyT), so they will stick to an affinity chromatography column on which polyT has been immobilised.

RNA splicing

Eukaryotic structural genes are not stored as continuous base sequences in DNA. Sequences called exons that code for protein sequence are separated by intervening sequences or introns. Both exons and introns are transcribed into a primary RNA transcript. The introns, which are often hundreds of nucleotide units long, must then be precisely *spliced* out of the RNA before it can be used as messenger. Sites where splicing is to occur are marked by specific base sequences. These are recognised by catalytic RNA–protein complexes known as *spliceosomes*. The intron is removed and the exons that were formerly at each end of the intron are joined to form a continuous chain (Fig. 137). Some mRNA molecules are formed from many exons joined in this way. The gene for human haemoglobin beta chains contains three exons separated by two introns.

Splicing of the original transcript may not be carried out in the same way in different cell types. By using alternative splice sites, different cell-specific mRNAs, and hence proteins, can be synthesised from identical original transcripts.

Clinical note:
Some genetic defects are caused by splicing errors

Splicing must be carried out with great precision. It can be affected by alterations in base sequence, i.e. by mutations. Some *thalassaemias* (inherited disorders of haemoglobin synthesis) are caused by mutations that alter the base sequence at splice sites.

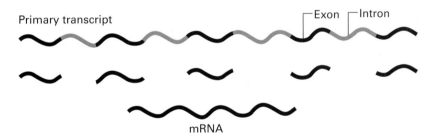

Fig. 137 Splicing of RNA.

Self-assessment: questions

Single best answer MCQs

1. Identify a statement that accurately describes the properties of RNA.
   a. RNA occurs in the cytosol of eukaryotic cells but not in the nucleus
   b. RNA does not form structures in which base pairing is important
   c. Uracil, which is found in RNA, is similar to thymine but has an additional methyl group
   d. mRNA molecules occur in a large range of sizes but tRNA molecules are all very similar in size
   e. Ribosomes are made of ribosomal RNA and ribosomal proteins; eukaryotic ribosomes are made up of two subunits, the smaller, 40S, containing 40 nucleotide units and the larger, 60S, containing 60 nucleotide units

2. Identify the correct list of materials needed for RNA synthesis.
   a. ATP, UTP, CTP, GTP, a DNA primer and a DNA template
   b. ATP, CTP, GTP, a DNA primer and a DNA template
   c. ATP, UTP, GTP, a DNA primer and a DNA template
   d. ATP, UTP, CTP, GTP and a DNA template
   e. ATP, UTP, CTP, GTP and a DNA primer

3. The process of RNA synthesis:
   a. Occurs in the 3′ to 5′ direction
   b. Eliminates pyrophosphate during the addition of every nucleotide unit
   c. Uses a template that is read in the 5′ to 3′ direction
   d. For structural genes that map close together on the eukaryotic chromosome may produce a single molecule of mRNA, a polycistronic messenger that codes for several polypeptide chains
   e. Is initiated at special DNA sequences known as start codons

4. Understanding RNA synthesis and its control is essential for students of molecular medicine. Which one of the following statements on that topic is correct?
   a. Promoter sequences are rich in GC base pairs at the point where the DNA chains are unwound
   b. Initiation of transcription is an important control point for the control of protein synthesis

   c. Eukaryotes have a single RNA polymerase whereas prokaryotes have separate enzymes for the synthesis of different classes of RNA
   d. Termination is by stop codons
   e. In prokaryotes all the DNA sequences used as template are on one strand of the double helix; the other strand does not code for protein synthesis but functions during DNA replication

5. In connection with protein synthesis in bacteria:
   a. Proteins required for glucose catabolism are examples of inducible proteins
   b. Proteins required for lactose catabolism are examples of constitutive proteins
   c. Proteins required for tryptophan synthesis are examples of repressible proteins
   d. Synthesis of the proteins required for lactose catabolism only occurs when glucose is available
   e. Synthesis of the proteins required for lactose catabolism does not occur in a bacterial cell containing a higher than normal concentration of cyclic AMP

6. Select the one correct statement about promoters and operators.
   a. Transcription starts at a sequence on DNA that can bind RNA polymerase and which is known as an operator
   b. Promoters are usually upstream of the operators that they control
   c. Repressors are specific DNA sequences that bind the proteins that block transcription
   d. The *lac* repressor must bind allolactose, its co-repressor, before it can block transcription of the *lac* operon
   e. The *trp* repressor must bind tryptophan, its co-repressor, before it can block transcription of the *trp* operon

7. Transcription in eukaryotes involves:
   a. Structural genes that are arranged in operons with a single promoter for several genes
   b. Control sequences to which regulatory proteins bind and which are clustered around the promoter
   c. Zinc fingers and leucine zippers, which are structural motifs found in regulatory proteins in eukaryotes
   d. Histone proteins for the specific control of protein synthesis

e. Hormones such as steroids that bind directly to specific DNA sequences

8. RNA processing in eukaryotes is a process in which:
   a. The first transcript of ribosomal RNA is subject to specific cleavage before becoming functional
   b. Several modified bases as well as adenine, cytosine, guanine and uracil are incorporated into tRNA during transcription
   c. mRNA has a methylated guanine nucleotide added to its 3′ end
   d. mRNA has a long tail of polyA added to its 5′ end
   e. RNA splicing is the joining of intron sequences with the exclusion of exons

Short essay question

Write an essay about the central role of transcription in controlling the activities of prokaryotic and eukaryotic cells.

Self-assessment: answers

Single best answer MCQ answers

1. a. **False**. RNA is synthesised in the nucleus and moves out after processing.
    b. **False**. Base pairing occurs in many RNA structures, e.g. tRNA, ribosomes.
    c. **False**. It is thymine that has the additional methyl group.
    d. **True**. tRNA molecules all contain about 80 nucleotide units. mRNA varies in size depending on the length of the polypeptide for which it codes.
    e. **False**. 40S and 60S refer to the sedimentation constants of the subunits, not the numbers of nucleotide units which are much greater.

2. d. This is the correct list. No primer is needed for RNA synthesis.

3. a. **False**. All nucleic acid chain synthesis occurs in the 5′ to 3′ direction.
    b. **True**. The nucleoside triphosphate eliminates two phosphate groups as pyrophosphate during the addition of each nucleotide unit to the chain.
    c. **False**. The template is used in the 3′ to 5′ direction. Template and newly synthesised strand are antiparallel in all nucleic acid synthesis.
    d. **False**. This only occurs in prokaryotes.
    e. **False**. The special sequences are known as promoters.

4. a. **False**. Chain separation must occur at promoters that are rich in AT base pairs. These are more easily broken than are GCs.
    b. **True**. Control of transcription allows the cell to control the synthesis of each specific protein.
    c. **False**. It is eukaryotes that have separate RNA polymerases for mRNA, tRNA and ribosomal RNA.
    d. **False**. Stop codons are signals in mRNA for the termination of translation.
    e. **False**. Coding sequences occur on both strands.

5. a. **False**. Glucose catabolism is central and proteins required for it are constitutive.
    b. **False**. The *lac* operon was the first inducible operon to be studied.
    c. **True**. Enzymes for the synthesis of tryptophan and several other amino acids are repressible.
    d. **False**. Induction of the *lac* operon does not occur if glucose is present. This phenomenon is known as catabolite repression.

e. **False**. Induction of the *lac* operon requires a raised concentration of cyclic AMP.

6. a. **False**. The sequence where transcription starts is known as a promoter.
    b. **False**. Operators are usually downstream of the promoters they control.
    c. **False**. Repressors are proteins that bind to DNA sequences known as operators.
    d. **False**. The *lac* repressor can bind allolactose or the *lac* operator but not both at once. Allolactose is thus an inducer of the *lac* operon.
    e. **True**. As in the control of the *trp* operon.

7. a. **False**. This organisation of genes is only found in prokaryotes.
    b. **False**. Control sequences in eukaryotes are often remote from the promoter.
    c. **True**. These motifs allow these proteins to bind to DNA and to each other.
    d. **False**. Histones are the same in every cell of an organism and vary only slightly from species to species.
    e. **False**. Steroid hormones must first be recognised and bound by regulatory proteins.

8. a. **True**. Both ribosomal RNA and tRNA are cleaved from longer precursors.
    b. **False**. These bases are modified after transcription.
    c. **False**. Addition of this nucleotide to the 5′ end unit is known as 'capping'.
    d. **False**. 'Tailing' occurs at the 3′ end.
    e. **False**. It is the introns that are eliminated. The exon sequences are joined together to form the mature mRNA which is then expressed.

Short essay answer

Several points should be mentioned. Controlling transcription is the most important way in which cells control the proteins that they make. It obviously saves material and energy if cells only make mRNA for the proteins that they actually need. Transcription ensures appropriate amplification of the genetic information before it is used. One or two structural genes can be transcribed to give thousands of mRNA molecules, which can in turn be translated to give millions of protein molecules.

14 The synthesis of proteins

Overview

Messenger RNA supplies sequence information for protein synthesis using a base triplet, a group of three bases, to represent each amino acid. There are four different bases in DNA (and RNA), so there are 4×4×4 or 64 possible triplets to be allocated by the genetic code; 61 of these specify amino acids and the remaining three indicate chain termination. Each of the 20 amino acids is represented by between one and six triplets. When more than one triplet represents an amino acid, these triplets are very similar. Similar amino acids often have related triplets.

Amino acids are activated by being attached to their specific transfer RNA. Transfer RNA molecules, each loaded with its amino acid, are matched with successive triplets in messenger RNA and add their amino acid to the growing peptide chain.

Peptide chains, once synthesised, are often subject to chemical modification before becoming functional. This modification is often associated with transport of the protein to where it is needed in the cell or to its assembly into larger structures.

14.1 The genetic code

Learning objectives

You should be able to:

- explain what is meant by the genetic code and describe its general features

- explain the following terms as applied to the genetic code: universal, degenerate, unpunctuated, non-overlapping.

Many activities of the cell, particularly growth, cell division, adaptation and repair, involve the synthesis of new protein molecules. Even in the adult human when growth has ceased, turnover of tissue protein involves the synthesis of hundreds of grams of protein every day (Ch. 8).

Different cells synthesise different proteins. The mechanism of protein synthesis must account for the large number of proteins that are found in a typical cell and for the specificity of these proteins. It also has to explain how different proteins are synthesised in different cells of the same organism. Muscle cells make some proteins found only in muscle, and liver cells make proteins found only in liver, yet other proteins such as some enzymes catalysing glycolysis are common to many different cell types. In protein synthesis, the amino acids that make up the polypeptide chains must be joined in the required order by peptide bonds. The information concerning the order of the amino acids is supplied by messenger RNA (mRNA), which is translated at the ribosomes (Ch. 13). mRNA is translated in the same direction as it is synthesised, in the 5′ to 3′ direction. Translation starts near but not at the 5′ end. Prokaryotic mRNA, which may code for more than one polypeptide chain, will contain further starting points along its length. The identification of the precise starting points for translation is an important feature of the initiation of polypeptide synthesis.

The correspondence between the base sequence in RNA and the amino acid sequence of the protein is known as the genetic code. The sequence of bases on the DNA and mRNA is divided into groups of three bases, each of which is treated as an instruction to insert a specific amino acid into the growing chain (or sometimes to terminate the chain). The group of three bases is known as a *codon* and the matching set of three bases on the tRNA that brings the amino acids into line for protein synthesis is called the *anticodon*. Since there are four bases there are 4×4×4 or 64 possible codons. Of these, 61 specify an amino acid while the remaining three are *chain termination signals*. The genetic code is set out in Table 21. The same code applies in prokaryotes and

Table 21 The genetic code

First position	Second position				Third position
	U	**C**	**A**	**G**	
U	Phe	Ser	Tyr	Cys	U
	Phe	Ser	Tyr	Cys	C
	Leu	Ser	Stop	Stop	A
	Leu	Ser	Stop	Trp	G
C	Leu	Pro	His	Arg	U
	Leu	Pro	His	Arg	C
	Leu	Pro	Gln	Arg	A
	Leu	Pro	Gln	Arg	G
A	Ile	Thr	Asn	Ser	U
	Ile	Thr	Asn	Ser	C
	Ile	Thr	Lys	Arg	A
	Met	Thr	Lys	Arg	G
G	Val	Ala	Asp	Gly	U
	Val	Ala	Asp	Gly	C
	Val	Ala	Glu	Gly	A
	Val	Ala	Glu	Gly	G

eukaryotes; that is to say, the code is universal. Only a very few minor exceptions to the universality of the code have been identified. The nucleic acid sequence and the amino acid sequence it codes are said to be *collinear*; that is, the base triplets are in the same order as the amino acids in the corresponding protein chain.

Some amino acids are represented by just one codon, others by two or four and some even by six: the code is said to be *degenerate*. While it is possible to translate a nucleic acid base sequence into an amino acid sequence, the reverse process is not possible. Given the amino acid sequence of a polypeptide, the base sequence of the mRNA involved in its synthesis cannot be predicted. As many amino acids are represented by more than one codon, there is no way of telling which one of these codons was used in any instance.

Do not attempt to memorise the genetic code table, but notice that:

- Where multiple codons represent one amino acid, these codons are often similar. For example, UUU and UUC both represent phenylalanine and UAU and UAC both represent tyrosine. In this and in other cases where there are just two codons representing an amino acid, the codons are identical in the first two positions, and the third positions contain either the purines A and G or the pyrimidines C and U.
- In the cases of amino acids that are represented by four codons, these codons always have the same first and second bases, the identity of the third base being immaterial. Thus GGX always represents glycine whether X is A or G or C or U.

- Chemically similar amino acids are often represented by similar codons, as in the case of phenylalanine and tyrosine (above) or in the case of aspartate (GAU or GAC) and glutamate (GAA or GAG).

The effect of mutations

The code is unpunctuated; that is to say, there is no feature in the structure of mRNA that shows where one codon ends and the next one begins. Translation, once started, proceeds three bases at a time along the messenger in the 5' to 3' direction. A change that affects the sequence can alter the protein product.

Frameshift mutations
If an extra base were to be inserted in the sequence, the whole message would be corrupted and the sequence of the protein that was synthesised would be completely changed subsequent to the site of the insertion. The same would happen if one base were to be deleted. Such changes are known as frameshift mutations.

Point mutations
The replacement of one base by another is much less damaging. If the replacement occurs in the third position of a codon, either the original amino acid or one similar to it will be used. Changes in the first or second positions will almost always result in a change of amino acid but, since only one codon has been altered, only one amino acid will be changed in the sequence. This may not alter the activity of the protein or it may result in poor or no activity; for example, a single base change resulting in valine instead of glutamate in haemoglobin causes sickle cell disease (p. 65). If the change creates a stop codon, incomplete proteins will form.

Range of potential sequences

The code is also non-overlapping. The meaning of each codon depends only on its own base sequence and not on any other sequence in the mRNA. This makes it possible to synthesise a polypeptide containing any sequence of the 20 amino acids. The nature of the code imposes no restriction on the protein sequences that can be produced.

14.2 Synthesis of protein chains

Learning objectives

You should be able to:

- explain what is meant by 'wobble' in the context of the genetic code

- describe the importance of aminoacyl-tRNA synthetases and the reactions that they catalyse

- describe the role of ATP in the synthesis of aminoacyl-tRNA

- describe the role of the ribosome in protein synthesis

- name and describe the phases of synthesis of a peptide chain

- describe the role of GTP hydrolysis in protein synthesis.

tRNA molecules act as adaptors

Selection of the amino acid specified by each codon is achieved by having tRNA molecules (p. 189) that attach and activate the amino acids and bring them to the required position in the growing polypeptide chain. The anticodon on the tRNA is complementary (under somewhat less strict base-pairing rules than apply during DNA replication and transcription) to codons on the messenger. Between them, the tRNA molecules can form base pairs with all the 61 codons, which specify amino acids. Some of the tRNA molecules can pair with more than one codon, but, when they do this, all the codons they pair with must specify the same amino acid. The codon and anticodon are antiparallel when they associate by base pairing: the third position of the codon is the base at the 3' end of the codon, while the third position of the anticodon is at its 5' end.

Wobble

Base pairing is strict between the first and second bases of the codon and the first and second bases of the anticodon. Base pairing is less strict in the third position, a phenomenon named *wobble* by Crick (Table 22). For example, an inosine base in the third position of the anticodon can base pair with A, U and C in the third position of the codon. Wobble allows all 61 codons specifying amino acids to be recognised by fewer than 40 species of tRNA molecule.

Table 22 'Wobble' pairing

Third position in codon	
Anticodon Base	Codon bases matched
C	G
A	U
G	C or U
U	G or A
Inosine	U, C or A

Attachment of amino acids to tRNA

The tRNA molecules are charged with their specific amino acids by a set of enzymes, the *aminoacyl-tRNA synthetases*. Each amino acid has one of these enzymes, which specifically attaches it to its tRNA. These enzymes, which require ATP as well as the amino acid and the tRNA molecule, attach the amino acid to its tRNA by an ester linkage between the carboxyl group of the amino acid and an hydroxyl group on the ribose of the adenosine at the 3' end of the tRNA molecule. The reaction proceeds in two stages. ATP is used to adenylate the amino acid on its carboxyl group and pyrophosphate (PP_i) is eliminated. During the second stage the amino acid is transferred to the tRNA molecule. The reaction is irreversible since the pyrophosphate is hydrolysed to two molecules of inorganic phosphate by pyrophosphatase.

$$\text{Amino acid} + \text{ATP} \rightarrow \text{Aminoacyl-AMP} + PP_i$$
$$\text{Aminoacyl-AMP} + \text{tRNA} \rightarrow \text{Aminoacyl-tRNA} + \text{AMP}$$
$$PP_i + H_2O \rightarrow 2P_i$$

Each of these aminoacyl-tRNA synthetases shows very high specificity and will only join its amino acid to its corresponding tRNA. Some of these enzymes must distinguish between very similar amino acids; for example, pairs such as valine and leucine or glycine and alanine differ only by a single methylene group. Some of the synthetases have associated hydrolase activities, which proof-read and correct the mistake if the 'wrong' amino acid is joined to a tRNA. The proof-reading is by a double sieve mechanism. Leucine should never be mistaken for valine since it is larger and will not fit an active centre that was specific for valine, but valine can be mistaken for leucine since it fits an active centre created to fit the larger leucine. The hydrolase associated with leucyl-tRNA synthetase is specific for valyl-tRNA^{Leu}, which can fit its active centre and be hydrolysed. When the synthetase makes the correct leucyl-tRNA^{Leu} it is too large to fit the active centre of the hydrolase and will not be cleaved.

Role of ribosomes

The constituents required for protein synthesis are brought together by ribosomes, ribonucleoprotein structures found in the cytoplasm. These subcellular particles, which can be seen in the electron microscope, are particularly numerous in tissues such as liver and pancreas where protein synthesis is most active. They can be isolated from disrupted bacteria or from homogenised cells by high speed centrifugation. Ribosomes prepared in this way are often found in the form of *polysomes*, several ribosomes associated with a single mRNA molecule. These ribosomes are

Table 23 Prokaryotic and eukaryotic ribosomal subunits

	Sedimentation constant (Svedberg units(S))	
	Prokaryotic	Eukaryotic
Ribosome	70	80
Large subunit	50	60
Small subunit	30	40

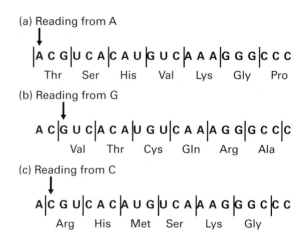

(a) Reading from A

A C G | U C A | C A U | G U C | A A A | G G G | C C C
Thr   Ser   His   Val   Lys   Gly   Pro

(b) Reading from G

A C | G U C | A C A | U G U | C A A | A G G | G C C | C
Val   Thr   Cys   Gln   Arg   Ala

(c) Reading from C

A | C G U | C A C | A U G | U C A | A A G | G G C | C C
Arg   His   Met   Ser   Lys   Gly

Fig. 138 Reading frame for translation. Moving the start position alters the triplet sequence and gives three different polypeptide sequences.

simultaneously translating the single messenger but with the resulting polypeptide chains at different stages of completion. Each individual ribosome can engage in the synthesis of only one polypeptide chain at a time. Ribosomes are not specific for the polypeptide sequences that they synthesise. The sequences they produce depend on the mRNA message.

Biochemists separate ribosomes from other cellular materials using ultracentrifugation, so ribosomes and their subunits are identified by their *sedimentation constants*, measures of the rates at which they sediment in the ultracentrifuge (Table 23). The sedimentation constant of a particle depends on its size, shape and density. Sedimentation constants are quoted in Svedberg (S) units. Prokaryotic ribosomes are smaller than those from eukaryotes.

Ribosomes are composed of three RNA molecules and about 50 proteins, forming two subunits with distinct functions. The small and large ribosomal subunits only come together during protein synthesis. They join the assembly responsible for translation one after the other, first the small subunit, then the large.

Phases of chain synthesis

Synthesis of a polypeptide chain can be considered in three phases, initiation, elongation and termination.

Chain initiation

Initiation of a new chain is a critical stage in protein synthesis because it is at this stage that the 'reading frame' is set for translation. Bases on mRNA are recognised in groups of three, but there is no structural feature on the RNA to act as punctuation to indicate which of the three possible reading frames is to be used. Use of either of the two incorrect reading frames would produce a polypeptide that was completely unrelated in sequence to the required polypeptide (Fig. 138). Mechanisms for initiation and setting of the correct reading frame differ slightly between prokaryotes and eukaryotes.

Initiation in prokaryotes

In prokaryotes, the small ribosomal subunit binds to a ribosome-binding sequence by base pairing with a complementary sequence in the ribosomal RNA. The ribosome-binding sequence, also known as a *Shine–Dalgarno sequence*, is located within the untranslated region upstream from each translated region of the mRNA. These sequences are rich in A and G but are not identical. Different mRNAs bind the ribosomal subunit with different affinities, this being yet another way in which the amount of protein produced can be controlled. Once bound to mRNA, the ribosomal subunit moves downstream until it encounters a start codon: AUG (Fig. 139.

AUG codes for the amino acid methionine, which is found at the N-terminus of prokaryotic proteins when they are first synthesised, although it may be cleaved off later. A special form of tRNA^{Met} is used for initiation. This is first charged with methionine, which is thus activated in its carboxyl group. The amino group of the amino acid is then modified by the addition of a *methanoyl* (formyl) group.

Initiation in eukaryotes

In eukaryotes, each mRNA molecule codes for a single polypeptide chain and there is no sequence corresponding to the Shine–Dalgarno ribosome binding sequence. Recognition appears to depend on the presence of the cap, the modified G nucleotide found at the 5' end of every eukaryotic mRNA. Once bound, the small ribosomal subunit moves along the mRNA until an AUG start codon is encountered. A species of tRNA that carries methionine is required for initiation. The N-terminal methionine is not formylated in eukaryotes. Another tRNA is used for inserting methionine residues where they are needed in other positions in the polypeptide sequence.

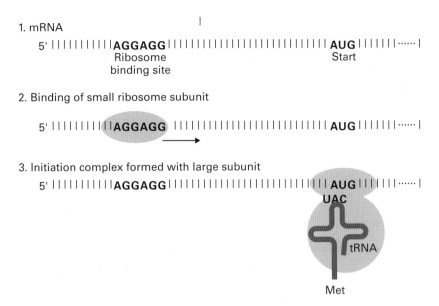

1. mRNA

5' | | | | | | | | | | | **AGGAGG** | | | | | | | | | | | | | | | | | | | | | | | | | | | | | | | **AUG** | | | | | | ······ |
Ribosome   Start
binding site

2. Binding of small ribosome subunit

5' | | | | | | | | | | | **AGGAGG** | | | | | | | | | | | | | | | | | | | | | | | | | | | | | **AUG** | | | | | | ······ |

3. Initiation complex formed with large subunit

5' | | | | | | | | | | | **AGGAGG** | | | | | | | | | | | | | | | | | | | | | | | | | | | | | | | **AUG** | | | | | | ······ |
UAC
tRNA
Met

Fig. 139 Initiation of translation in prokaryotes.

Clinical note:
Many antibiotics inhibit protein synthesis in bacteria

Several antibiotics in clinical use are inhibitors of protein synthesis, particularly in bacteria.
Chloramphenicol inhibits peptide bond formation in parokaryotes. *Tetracycline* inhibits binding of aminoacyl-tRNAs to ribosomes in both eukaryotes and prokaryotes but cannot cross eukaryotic membranes. *Erythromycin* blocks translocation of the peptidyl-tRNA during elongation.

Initiation complex formation

Having located the start codon, AUG, the small ribosomal subunit binds the large subunit and formylmethionyl-tRNA^{Met} (or methionyl-tRNA^{Met} in eukaryotes,) and creates an initiation complex. Assembly of the initiation complex also involves three protein initiation factors. The reading frame for translation is set and the elongation phase of translation can begin.

Chain elongation

The ribosome has two sites where it can bind tRNA: a *P* or *peptidyl site* and an *A* or *aminoacyl site*. In the initiation complex, methionyl-tRNA^{Met} occupies the P site. Later it will be occupied by a tRNA carrying the growing polypeptide chain. There are three stages during each round of the elongation process (Fig. 140).

In the first stage, a tRNA molecule charged with its amino acid binds to the A site. Which tRNA and thus which amino acid binds at the A site depends on the next three bases on the mRNA. The binding of each charged tRNA molecule to the ribosome is an energy-requiring process and involves a catalytic protein or elongation factor. One molecule of GTP is hydrolysed to GDP and phosphate for every aminoacyl-tRNA that is bound.

In the second stage, with a tRNA molecule bound at both sites, a new peptide bond can be formed. The amino acid, or peptide, bound by its carboxyl group to the tRNA in the P site is transferred to the amino group of the amino acid bound to the tRNA in the A site. Synthesis of this new peptide bond is driven by the (ATP) energy used earlier to activate the amino acid by joining it to its tRNA.

In the third stage, the growing peptide chain attached to tRNA in the A site is translocated. The tRNA in the P site, now without any attached amino acid or peptide, is ejected and moves away to pick up another molecule of its amino acid. The tRNA in the A site, which carries the growing polypeptide chain, moves into the P site as the ribosome moves along the mRNA molecule. The A site is now vacant so another round of elongation can begin. Translocation is another energy-requiring process and, like tRNA binding, it involves a catalytic protein, another elongation factor and the hydrolysis of GTP to GDP and phosphate.

Energy requirements of peptide bond synthesis

Each round of elongation requires the equivalent of four molecules of ATP to be hydrolysed to ADP and phosphate. Two of these four are used to drive the activation of the amino acid by joining it to its tRNA. One molecule of ATP is used directly and one indirectly to convert the AMP formed into ADP. The two GDP molecules produced by the use of one GTP to drive tRNA binding and another to drive translocation are each reconverted to GTP by phosphate transfer from ATP.

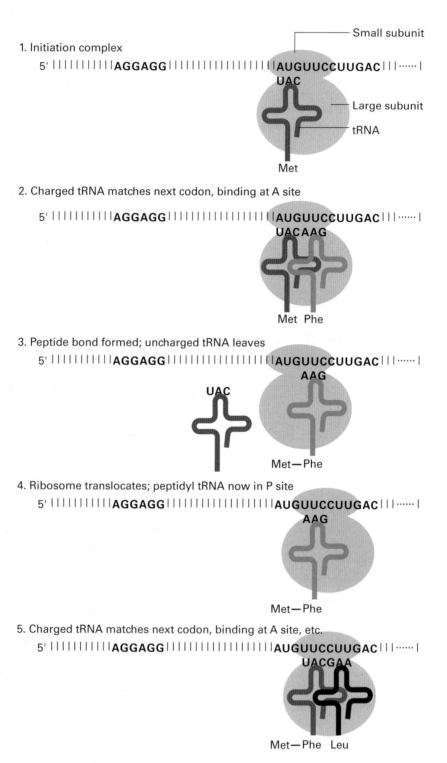

1. Initiation complex

5' | | | | | | | | | | **AGGAGG** | | | | | | | | | | | | | | | **AUGUUCCUUGAC** | | | ······ |
UAC

Small subunit

Large subunit

tRNA

Met

2. Charged tRNA matches next codon, binding at A site

5' | | | | | | | | | | **AGGAGG** | | | | | | | | | | | | | | | | | | **AUGUUCCUUGAC** | | | ······ |
UACAAG

Met Phe

3. Peptide bond formed; uncharged tRNA leaves

5' | | | | | | | | | | **AGGAGG** | | | | | | | | | | | | | | | | | | **AUGUUCCUUGAC** | | | ······ |
AAG

UAC

Met—Phe

4. Ribosome translocates; peptidyl tRNA now in P site

5' | | | | | | | | | | **AGGAGG** | | | | | | | | | | | | | | | | | | | **AUGUUCCUUGAC** | | | ······ |
AAG

Met—Phe

5. Charged tRNA matches next codon, binding at A site, etc.

5' | | | | | | | | | | **AGGAGG** | | | | | | | | | | | | | | | | | | | **AUGUUCCUUGAC** | | | ······ |
UACGAA

Met—Phe Leu

Fig. 140 The elongation phase of protein synthesis.

Chain termination

Elongation steps continue until the ribosome encounters a codon for which there is no corresponding tRNA. There are three such codons: *UAA*, *UAG* and *UGA*. These codons trigger release factors, enzymes that cleave the completed polypeptide from the tRNA that carried the C-terminal amino acid. The final tRNA can then dissociate and the ribosomal subunits separate, ready to start the translation of another molecule of mRNA.

As one ribosome moves along an mRNA molecule, enough of the 5′ end of the mRNA will become available for another ribosome to attach and start translation of the same messenger. As a result, several ribosomes may be simultaneously translating one mRNA molecule, each with a polypeptide at a different stage of completion. Ribosomes isolated from reticulocytes, red cell precursor cells in which mRNA coding for haemoglobin polypeptide chains is being translated, are found in clusters of four or five, held together by mRNA. In prokaryotes, an mRNA molecule does not even have to be completely transcribed before its translation can begin.

14.3 Post-translational modification and transport of proteins

Learning objectives

You should be able to:

- define the term, post-translational modification and explain the importance of this process

- give examples of how newly synthesised proteins are transported to destination, both inside and outside the cell

- describe how a newly synthesised protein can be transported across a membrane

- describe the importance of the post-translational modification of collagen.

Once synthesised, polypeptide chains are often substantially modified before becoming functional proteins. Typically, amino acid side chains may be modified and specific peptide bonds cleaved. This post-translational modification is often associated with the transport of the newly synthesised protein to its destination inside or outside the cell.

Signal sequences

Polypeptide chains that are to be transported to different destinations within the cell often contain sequences

Clinical note:
Genetic disease can be due to errors during protein transport

Inherited defects may affect the transport of newly synthesised proteins so that normal protein function is lost because the protein ends up in the wrong place. In the rare fatal condition, I-cell disease, a molecular signal which directs lysosomal enzymes to lysosomes is not generated and the enzymes follow the default transport route, which is secretion from the cell.

known as signal sequences that act as address labels during the transport process. The signal sequence that marks a protein for transport to the Golgi apparatus via the *endoplasmic reticulum* is typical. This sequence is at the N-terminal end of the polypeptide chain and is, therefore, synthesised before the remainder of the chain. It is often cleaved off after the protein reaches its destination. Its sequence varies somewhat, but it is generally about 20 residues long and contains a highly hydrophobic stretch of about 12 residues and also one positively charged residue.

Once the signal sequence has been synthesised, it is taken up by the transport system, which carries it across the endoplasmic reticulum membrane and the synthesis of the rest of the chain is coupled to its movement through the membrane (Fig. 141). This prevents the polypeptide chain from folding before it passes through. Folding occurs after the chain has crossed the membrane.

The newly synthesised signal sequence, attached to its ribosome, is recognised by a *signal recognition particle* (SRP), a ribonucleoprotein particle, which binds to it. This binding arrests further translation temporarily. The complex binds to an SRP receptor on the endoplasmic reticulum and the signal peptide is taken up by the translocation machinery and fed through a pore in the membrane. At this point the SRP is no longer required. It can dissociate from the complex and the ribosome can resume translation. Elongation of the polypeptide and its passage through the endoplasmic reticulum membrane can now proceed concurrently.

Different signal sequences mark proteins for entry to mitochondria. Most mitochondrial proteins are synthesised in the cytosol and carry N-terminal sequences that are recognised by transport mechanisms in the mitochondrial membrane. Folding is delayed by *chaperonins* since folded proteins are not readily transported across intracellular membranes. Chaperonins are cytosolic proteins, one function of which is to bind unfolded peptide chains and deliver them to the transport mechanism. Once in the mitochondrial matrix the chains fold to their functional forms.

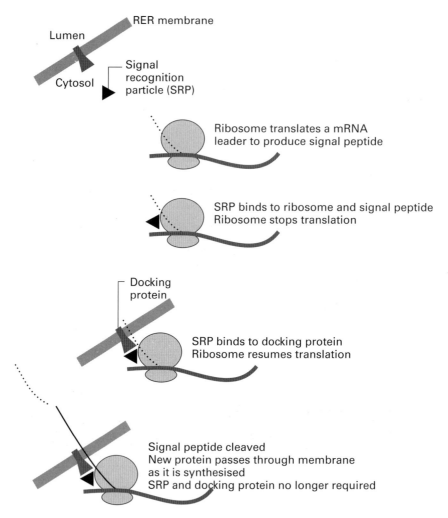

RER membrane

Lumen

Signal recognition particle (SRP)

Cytosol

Ribosome translates a mRNA leader to produce signal peptide

SRP binds to ribosome and signal peptide Ribosome stops translation

Docking protein

SRP binds to docking protein Ribosome resumes translation

Signal peptide cleaved New protein passes through membrane as it is synthesised SRP and docking protein no longer required

Fig. 141 The use of a signal sequence to ensure translocation of newly synthesised protein to the endoplasmic reticulum before sufficient protein is formed to start folding. RER, rough endoplasmic reticulum.

Collagen biosynthesis

The transport and processing steps that occur between synthesis of a polypeptide chain and the formation of a functional protein can be illustrated by considering collagen biosynthesis. Collagen is an extracellular structural protein that has some of its amino acid side chains modified after translation, both by hydroxylation and by the addition of carbohydrate groups. Each collagen triple helix consists of three chains, which are synthesised as precursors and then modified and secreted to form mature collagen fibres. As illustrated in Figure 142, the steps in this process include:

- recognition of a leader sequence in preprocollagen so that the chain is taken up into the endoplasmic reticulum
- cleavage of the leader sequence by an enzyme known as *signal peptidase*

Clinical note:
Role of vitamin C

Many of the symptoms of scurvy (vitamin C deficiency) are explained by the role of this vitamin in collagen synthesis. Poor wound healing, capillary fragility and inadequate maintenance of periodontal structures leading to loosening of the teeth are all the result of deficient collagen synthesis.

- attachment of carbohydrate groups to amino acid side chains
- hydroxylation of some proline and lysine side chains by a process involving ascorbic acid and molecular oxygen
- passage of precursors through the Golgi apparatus, with modification of carbohydrate groups and

(a) Inside the cell

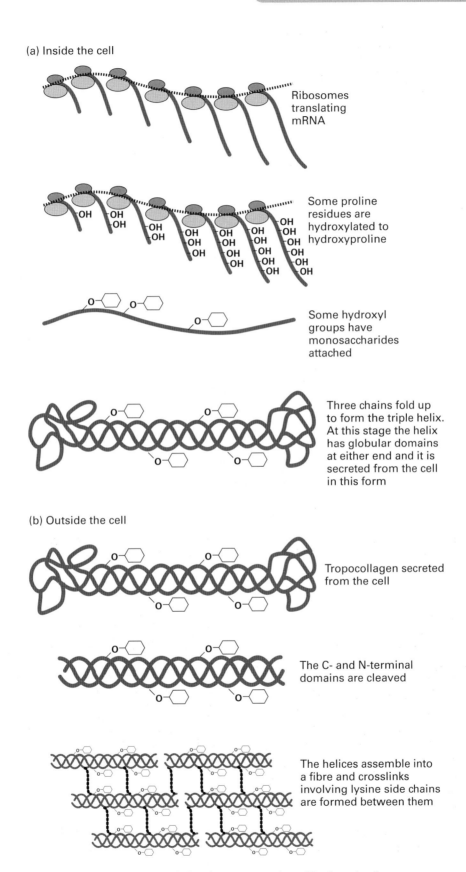

Ribosomes translating mRNA

Some proline residues are hydroxylated to hydroxyproline

Some hydroxyl groups have monosaccharides attached

Three chains fold up to form the triple helix. At this stage the helix has globular domains at either end and it is secreted from the cell in this form

(b) Outside the cell

Tropocollagen secreted from the cell

The C- and N-terminal domains are cleaved

The helices assemble into a fibre and crosslinks involving lysine side chains are formed between them

Fig. 142 Post-translational transport and modification of collagen.

formation of triple helices. Formation of a triple helix involves aggregation of C-terminal extensions and the winding of three chains from their C-terminals towards their N-terminals, forming procollagen
- secretion from cells as procollagen, packaged in membrane-bounded vesicles formed from the Golgi apparatus

- removal of C- and N-terminal extensions on the triple helices by extracellular proteases
- aggregation of triple helical molecules (tropocollagen) to form fibres
- crosslinking between triple helices.

Self-assessment: questions

Single best answer MCQs

Consult a copy of the genetic code (p. 202) for questions 1–5.

1. As you know, during protein synthesis amino acids are represented by codons. Which of the following statements accurately describes this process?
    a. No amino acids are represented by only one codon in the genetic code
    b. No amino acids are represented by three codons in the genetic code
    c. Most amino acids are represented by four codons in the genetic code
    d. No amino acids are represented by more than four codons in the genetic code
    e. Amino acids that have chemically similar side chains often have similar codons

2. When an amino acid is represented by four different codons, these codons are identical in what way?
    a. In the first position only
    b. In the first and second positions
    c. In the first and third positions
    d. In the second and third positions
    e. In the third position only

3. When an amino acid is represented by either of two different codons:
    a. These codons are identical in the first and second positions and can have either purine or either pyrimidine in the third position
    b. These codons are identical in the first and third positions and can have either purine or either pyrimidine in the middle position
    c. These codons are identical in the second and third positions and can have either purine or either pyrimidine in the first position
    d. Only the first base is identical in the two codons
    e. Only the third base is identical in the two codons

4. In order to be competent in the area of molecular medicine you need to know the consequences of mutations in codons. A mutation that changes:
    a. The first base of a codon will always change the amino acid to which the codon corresponds
    b. The second base of a codon will always change the amino acid to which the codon corresponds
    c. The third base of a codon will always change the amino acid to which the codon corresponds
    d. The first base of a codon will never change the amino acid to which the codon corresponds
    e. The third base of a codon will never change the amino acid to which the codon corresponds

5. Which peptide would be produced by translating the following mRNA base sequence? GUG-CAC-CUC-ACC-CCC
    a. Val-His-Leu-Ser-Pro
    b. Val-His-Leu-Thr-Pro
    c. Val-His-Gly-Ser-Pro
    d. Val-Arg-Leu-Thr-Pro
    e. Val-Arg-Gly-Ser-Pro

6. Which one of the following is correct concerning the properties of ribosomes?
    a. They are composed of three proteins and about 50 RNA molecules
    b. They can bind to more than one mRNA molecule at a time and thus form polysomes
    c. Prokaryotic ribosomes are larger than those of eukaryotes
    d. In eukaryotes they are found mostly in the cell nucleus
    e. Are composed of a large and a small subunit which come together when the ribosome is engaged in the synthesis of a polypeptide chain

7. Which of the following statements accurately describes the genetic code?
    a. A codon is a group of three consecutive bases in mRNA that directs the insertion of a specified amino acid during protein synthesis
    b. The code is degenerate because a given codon has only one possible translation
    c. The code is unambiguous because there is often more than one codon corresponding to each amino acid
    d. The genetic code is different for prokaryotes and eukaryotes
    e. mRNA is translated in the 3′ to 5′ direction and polypeptide chain synthesis starts at the N-terminal end

8. Examine the following options and select the one that accurately describes the codons that make up the genetic code.
    a. May contain bases other than A, C, G and U

b. There are structural features in mRNA that show where each codon begins and ends

c. Make up the complete sequence of mRNA

d. There are 64 possible codons; 61 correspond to amino acids

e. Two codons correspond to stop signals, one shows where a new polypeptide chain begins

9. Which of the following is accurate concerning codon recognition by anticodons?

a. Anticodons are three consecutive bases at the end of the tRNA polynucleotide chain

b. Involves complementary base pairs forming between bases in the anticodon and bases in the codon

c. Involves pairing between the base at the 5′ end of the anticodon and the base at the 5′ end of the codon

d. Has base pairing rules that are not so strict for the first base of the codon as for the other two bases

e. Involves 'wobble', the ability of one codon to be recognised by more than one anticodon

10. Properties of tRNA molecules include which one of the following?

a. There are 61 different species of tRNA molecule, one for each codon that corresponds to an amino acid

b. There are 20 different species of tRNA molecule, one for each amino acid that can occur in proteins

c. Some tRNA molecules can carry more than one amino acid

d. Some amino acids can be carried by more than one tRNA molecule

e. Specific tRNA molecules are needed to recognise stop codons

11. Identify the correct statement about amino acid activation in protein synthesis.

a. Amino acids are joined to their cognate tRNA molecules by specific enzymes known as aminoacyl-tRNA synthetases

b. Aminoacyl-tRNA synthetases hydrolyse ATP to ADP and inorganic phosphate at the same time as they join amino acids to their tRNA molecules

c. Amino acids are joined to tRNA by a bond between the amino group on the amino acid and an hydroxyl group on the ribose at the 3′ end of the tRNA

d. If an aminoacyl-tRNA synthetase joins the wrong amino acid to a tRNA molecule, the amino acid must be used for synthesis of a protein which will therefore be defective

e. Aminoacyl-tRNA synthetases almost always match an amino acid to its cognate tRNA, but when mismatches occur it is with a larger amino acid

12. The formation of an initiation complex for polypeptide synthesis in prokaryotes directly requires what?

a. A promoter

b. Formylmethionyl-tRNA^{Met}

c. The 30S ribosomal subunit but not the 50S subunit

d. The 50S ribosomal subunit but not the 30S subunit

e. ATP

13. The elongation phase of protein synthesis is a cyclic process. Which of the following accurately describes that process?

a. For each amino acid added, two molecules of GTP are converted to GMP and inorganic pyrophosphate

b. For each amino acid added, the tRNA molecule to which the growing peptide chain is attached must be translocated from the A (aminoacyl) site on the ribosome to the P (peptidyl site)

c. For each amino acid added, a loaded tRNA molecule is bound to the P site

d. Each new polypeptide bond is formed between the C-terminal end of the growing chain and the α-amino group of the amino acid bound to tRNA in the P site

e. Amino acids are activated by being attached to tRNA, but ATP hydrolysis is also directly needed for peptide bond formation

14. The termination of polypeptide synthesis:

a. Occurs every time a ribosome encounters UAA, UAG or UGA sequences in mRNA

b. Occurs at the stop codons UAA, UAG and UGA

c. Occurs when special tRNA molecules that carry no amino acid recognise stop codons

d. Involves the enzymatic cleavage of the bond joining the N-terminal amino acid in the chain to its tRNA

e. Is followed by separation of the ribosomal subunits, which dissociate from the mRNA; only then does the mRNA become available for translation by another ribosome

15. During collagen formation its peptide chains are subject to chemical modification and transport. Amongst the processes involved are:
(1) tropocollagen is secreted from the cell; (2) some proline side chains are hydroxylated; (3) crosslinks are formed between helices; (4) three chains assemble to form a triple helix. In which order do these processes occur?
    a. 1, 2, 3, 4
    b. 2, 3 ,4, 1
    c. 3, 4, 2, 1
    d. 1, 3, 4, 2
    e. 2, 4, 1, 3

16. In post-translational modification and transport:
    a. Proteins are made in the compartment of the cell in which they are to function
    b. The two polypeptide chains that form insulin are synthesised separately; they then fold and combine to form insulin
    c. Proteins are transported through the nuclear membrane if they carry a signal sequence that is recognised by an SRP (signal recognition particle)
    d. When a newly synthesised signal sequence is recognised by an SRP, the ribosome to which it is attached halts protein synthesis
    e. Proline hydroxylation in the formation of collagen is carried out while the proline is attached to its tRNA molecule

Short essay question

Explain why mutations caused by the insertion of an extra base, or the deletion of a base from a gene, are often much more serious than mutations produced by the change of a single base.

Self-assessment: answers

Single best answer MCQ answers

1. a. **False**. Methionine and tryptophan are each represented by only one codon.
    b. **False**. Isoleucine is the only amino acid represented by three codons.
    c. **False**. Five out of 20 are: alanine, glycine, proline, threonine and valine.
    d. **False**. Serine, leucine and arginine are each represented by six codons.
    e. **True**. For example, all the amino acids with hydrophobic side chains have U as the second base in their codons.

2. a. **False**. The codons are identical in the first and second positions.
    b. **True**. Look at the genetic code table.
    c. **False**. The third position can be any of the four bases.
    d. **False**. The codons are identical in the first and second positions.
    e. **False**. The third position can be any of the four bases.

3. a. **True**. For example, histidine, aspartate, glutamate and lysine.
    b. **False**. It is the bases in the first two positions that are identical.
    c. **False**. It is the bases in the first two positions that are identical.
    d. **False**. The second base is identical too.
    e. **False**. Only the third base differs between the codons.

4. a. **False**. Leucine represented by UUA, UUG, CUA and CUG is one exception (see also arginine).
    b. **True**. There is no exception.
    c. **False**. Nine amino acids are specified by the first two bases and can have any base in the third position.
    d. **False**. Change in the first base often changes the amino acid but there are exceptions, e.g. leucine is coded for by UUA and CUA.
    e. **False**. Sometimes the third base is important, e.g. Met and Trp.

5. b. Val-His-Leu-Thr-Pro is the correct sequence: GUG codes for valine, CAC for histidine, CUC for leucine, ACC for threonine and CCC for proline.

6. a. **False**. They contain three RNA molecules and about 50 proteins.
    b. **False**. One mRNA molecule can have more than one ribosome to form a polysome.
    c. **False**. Eukaryotic ribosomes are larger.
    d. **False**. They are found in the cytoplasm.
    e. **True**. Initiation of a peptide chain involves the binding of the smaller ribosomal subunit to mRNA. Peptide synthesis can only begin when the larger subunit joins the complex.

7. a. **True**. By definition.
    b. **False**. Each codon represents a single amino acid so the code is unambiguous.
    c. **False**. There are 61 codons to represent 20 amino acids so the code is degenerate.
    d. **False**. It is virtually identical for all living organisms.
    e. **False**. mRNA is translated in the 5' to 3' direction.

8. a. **False**. It is anticodons that may contain other bases.
    b. **False**. The genetic code is said to be 'unpunctuated'. Bases are read three at a time from a start codon.
    c. **False**. mRNA has untranslated sequences before the Met codon, which signals the starting point for translation, and after the stop codon.
    d. **True**. There are four possible bases in each of the three positions so there are 64 (4×4×4) possible codons. Three are stop codons.
    e. **False**. There are three stop codons. The start codon also codes for methionine.

9. a. **False**. The bases forming the anticodon are not at the end but on a loop within the tRNA molecule.
    b. **True**. Recognition is achieved by base pairing.
    c. **False**. As for all base pairing, the sequences are antiparallel.
    d. **False**. The base pairing rules are relaxed between the third (3') base on the codon and the third (5') base on the anticodon.
    e. **False**. 'Wobble', the term coined by Crick, describes how one anticodon can recognise more than one codon.

10. a. **False**. Some tRNA molecules can recognise more than one codon.
    b. **False**. Some amino acids need more than one tRNA molecule to recognise all their codons.
    c. **False**. Fidelity of protein synthesis depends on each tRNA being loaded with a single amino acid.
    d. **True**. When they are represented by more codons than one tRNA molecule can recognise.
    e. **False**. Stop codons are recognised by proteins associated with ribosomes.

11. a. **True**. These enzymes are responsible for ensuring that the tRNA molecules are correctly loaded.
    b. **False**. AMP and pyrophosphate are produced from ATP.
    c. **False**. The carboxyl group of the amino acid forms an ester bond.
    d. **False**. Some have associated hydrolases that can cleave any amino acid wrongly attached to the tRNA so that it is not used for peptide synthesis.
    e. **False**. Mismatches usually involve a smaller amino acid with a side chain not excluded from the enzyme's active centre.

12. a. **False**. A promoter is a DNA sequence where RNA synthesis is initiated.
    b. **True**. Formylmethionyl-tRNA^{Met} matches the start codon.
    c. **False**. The 30S (small) ribosomal subunit is the first to bind to mRNA but both subunits are required.
    d. **False**. The 50S (large) ribosomal subunit completes the initiation complex.
    e. **False**. ATP is not directly required.

13. a. **False**. GTP is hydrolysed to GDP and inorganic phosphate.
    b. **True**. To make room for the binding of the next aminoacyl-tRNA.
    c. **False**. Aminoacyl-tRNA binds first to the A site where it is matched to the next codon.
    d. **False**. The latest amino acid in the chain is bound to its tRNA in the A site when the new peptide bond is formed.
    e. **True**. ATP is only involved in aminoacyl-tRNA synthetase action, not directly in peptide bond formation.

14. a. **False**. These sequences only act as stop codons if they are in the reading frame.
    b. **True**. U followed by two purines. UGG, which also matches this pattern, codes for tryptophan.
    c. **False**. Proteins known as release factors are involved, not tRNA molecules.
    d. **False**. The bond cleaved joins the tRNA to the C-terminal carboxyl group of the peptide.
    e. **False**. An mRNA chain can be read by many ribosomes at once following each other along the sequence.

15. e. This is the correct sequence. Proline side chains are hydroxylated, this allows the triple helix to form, the tropocollagen is secreted and, once fibres have been assembled, the molecules are crosslinked.

16. a. **False**. Most proteins are transported to the site where they are to function.
    b. **False**. Insulin is made as a single sequence which folds and is then cleaved selectively.
    c. **False**. An SRP mediates transport through the endoplasmic reticulum.
    d. **True**. It stops temporarily while the complex docks on the endoplasmic reticulum membrane.
    e. **False**. It occurs with proline incorporated in a precursor protein.

Short essay answer

Changing a single base may not even change the amino acid if the change occurs in the third position of a codon. If it does change the amino acid, there is a high probability that the change will introduce an amino acid that is chemically similar; for instance, one non-polar amino acid side chain will be replaced by another non-polar side chain. Unless the amino acid is at a very critical point in the sequence, function of the protein might well be preserved.

Inserting or deleting a single base will alter the reading frame and produce a frameshift mutation. There will be a loss of function of the protein unless the mutation is very close to the C-terminal. Downstream from a frameshift mutation, every codon and every amino acid is altered. Also, insertion and deletion mutations often bring stop codons into the altered reading frame. One way to recognise the true reading frame in a newly determined DNA sequence is the relative absence of stop codons.

15 Molecular aspects of viruses

Overview

Viruses are cellular parasites that have genetic information for their own replication but which rely on the cellular machinery of their host cell to reproduce. Viral genes may be either DNA or RNA. Replication of RNA genes needs processes such as reverse transcription that are additional to those provided by the host. This dependence offers possibilities for chemotherapy to treat infections by some viruses, notably HIV.

15.1 Virus composition and structure

Learning objectives

You should be able to:

- describe the use of viruses for studying the assembly of macromolecular structures, programmed gene expression and the evolutionary strategy of parasites

- describe the composition and nature of viral genomes

- describe the role of proteins in viral structure

- describe the use of host biochemical processes by viruses.

Viruses are subcellular parasites that must infect the cells of other organisms to propagate themselves. Their structures are much smaller and simpler than those of cells and they have a very limited genome; as a result, they rely on their host cell to provide most of the synthetic machinery needed for viral replication. They can be considered as genetic elements that invade a host cell and take over its cellular machinery to replicate themselves before moving on to infect further cells.

Use of viruses as model systems

Viruses are much studied because they are of such medical and agricultural importance. They are also studied because, with their small size and relative simplicity, they can be used as model systems for the study of processes seen in more complex life forms. Many viral genomes are strictly limited in size by the structure of the virus, so, when the complete base sequence of a viral genome is determined, a function can be identified for most parts of the sequence. This is in contrast to the genomes of eukaryotes, where much of the sequence may well have no function.

Examples of processes in which viruses provide useful model systems follow.

Assembly of macromolecular structures
Viruses have very small genomes so they must build their structures with a very limited number of proteins. Study of mutant viruses allows the pathways of virus construction to be explored.

Programmed gene expression
Viruses must express their genes in a time-dependent manner if the infection process is to be successful. Control systems governing the expression of viral genes are model systems for development in higher organisms. Viral control systems capable of switching between different possible life cycles have also been discovered and studied.

Evolutionary strategy and the host–parasite relationship
Successful parasites tend to inflict minimal damage on their hosts so that a flourishing population of hosts remains for the parasite to infect. New strains of a virus that start by being particularly damaging to their hosts evolve to become less virulent. Evolution can be particularly rapid in viruses because of their vast numbers and short generation times. The evolution of viruses is easily studied within the human lifespan. Viruses have

Table 24 Examples of viruses

Type	Example	Genome size (genes)	Host/effects
DNA viruses			
Single-stranded (a few bacteriophage)	Phage M13		*E. coli*
Double-stranded (very common)	Phage λ		*E. coli:* lysogeny or cell lysis
	Herpes	70	Human: cold sores, genital lesions
	Simian virus 40 (SV40)	5	Monkeys: tumors in rodents
	Smallpox virus		Human: smallpox
RNA viruses			
Single-stranded (very common)	Polio	8	Human: infantile paralysis, poliomyelitis
	Tobacco mosaic virus (TMV)	6	Tobacco plant: lesions on leaves
	Human immunodeficiency virus (HIV)	7	Human: acquired immunodeficiency syndrome (AIDS)
	Influenza	12	Human and other animals: respiratory disease
	Rous sarcoma	4	Birds: tumour in chickens
Double-stranded (a few animal viruses)	Reovirus	22	Human: infant enteritis

evolved that can infect a very wide range of living cells: animals, plants and bacteria.

Biochemical studies

Bacterial viruses, also known as *bacteriophage* or *phage*, are widely used in biochemical studies both as objects of study and as tools for gene sequencing, gene transfer, gene expression and gene cloning. Table 24, which shows a short list of much-studied viruses and bacteriophages, illustrates the wide range of hosts used, the varied nature of their genetic material and the range of sizes for viral genomes.

Viral genome

Viruses always contain a genome composed of nucleic acid. The nature and amount of nucleic acid can vary depending on the virus. Virus genomes can contain either DNA or RNA and in each case it may be single-stranded or double-stranded. Plant viruses are all RNA viruses. Usually the nucleic acid forms a single molecule, but in a few cases it is segmented; for example, the genome of the influenza molecule exists as eight RNA molecules. The number of genes in a virus can vary from less than ten to several hundred. For reasons that will be described below, DNA viruses tend to have larger genomes than RNA viruses do.

Viral proteins

The nucleic acid forming the viral genome is covered by a protein coat or capsid. In cylindrical viruses such as

tobacco mosaic virus, the coat is built from many copies of a single protein component arranged in a regular helix around the genome (Fig. 143). In this virus, a single-stranded RNA chain of 6390 nucleotides is packaged by 2130 identical molecules of a protein that contains 168 amino acid residues. Spherical (or more strictly icosahedral, shaped like a solid having 20 faces) viruses build their capsids with as few as three protein components. Some spherical bacteriophages, such as bacteriophage T4, have further protein components forming a tail, which is used to inject the viral genes into the host bacterium during the infection process (Fig. 144). This phage was used in classic experiments to demonstrate that only the DNA need enter a cell for infection to occur. The protein components all remained outside the cell.

Some spherical viruses have a membranous envelope surrounding the capsid. This membrane is derived from the host cell in which the virus was assembled but it also

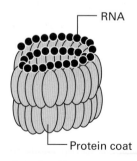

Fig. 143 Tobacco mosaic virus. Only a short section of the long cylinder is shown.

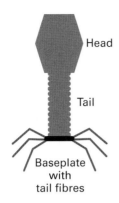

Fig. 144 Structure of bacteriophage T4.

contains virus-specific membrane proteins. A few viruses must carry one or two molecules of an enzyme needed for virus replication.

Use of host functions

Viruses depend on the metabolic pathways of their host cells to provide building blocks, amino acids and nucleotides for building the next generation of viruses. Host cell metabolism also provides ATP for energy since viruses have no way to synthesise it. Viruses provide mRNA, but the host cells provide ribosomes, tRNA and amino acid-activating enzymes for the synthesis of viral proteins. This high dependence on host processes has made viruses difficult targets to attack by chemotherapy. Most drugs that could block viral replication would also block some vital function of the host cell.

15.2 Viral multiplication

Learning objectives

You should be able to:

- describe the processes used by viruses to infect cells

- explain how viruses with RNA genomes may replicate their genomes

- describe the function of reverse transcriptase in retroviruses.

Virus multiplication occurs in three stages: *infection*, *replication* and *release*.

Infection

For a virus to infect its host it must somehow get its nucleic acid into the cell. Different viruses achieve this

in different ways but it generally involves binding of part of the virus to a receptor on the host. This receptor is often a protein with a normal useful function in the host. This is one reason why each virus is only able to infect a limited range of host cells.

Bacteriophage T4, which infects *E. coli*, has a hollow tail with a base plate carrying fibres at its end (Fig. 144). The base plate and fibres recognise and bind to a structure on the bacterial surface. Viral DNA is then injected into the bacteria leaving all the viral protein outside.

Viruses with envelopes may achieve entry by endocytosis, the virus binding to a membrane receptor on the surface of the host. Human immunodeficiency virus (HIV) binds to the CD4 receptor on T lymphocytes. Cells with no CD4 receptors cannot be infected. Viral envelope and cell membrane fuse, releasing the viral capsid, which contains the viral nucleic acid, into the cell.

Replication

A virus must replicate its nucleic acid and also bring about the synthesis of its protein components if it is to multiply and produce more virus particles. DNA animal viruses enter the nuclei of their host cells, which contain all the synthetic machinery and materials used by the host for replication of its own DNA. Some viruses stimulate division of host cells that were not currently dividing, thus increasing their ability to replicate DNA.

Replication of RNA viruses

Host cells have no enzymes that can replicate RNA, so RNA viruses must provide enzymes to do this. Different RNA viruses employ different strategies; these are additional processes (Fig. 145) that modify those outlined in the Central Dogma of Molecular Biology (p. 177). The various strategies for replicating viral RNA can be used to group the viruses into classes (Fig. 146):

Class 1. The single-stranded genome consists of positive-strand RNA, which can be used directly as a messenger in the host cell. To replicate its genome, the virus must use the positive strand as a template to make a negative strand. This is achieved with RNA replicase, an RNA polymerase that uses an RNA template to

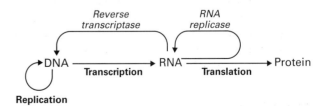

Fig. 145 Information flow in organisms. Either reverse transcriptase or RNA replicase is required for replication of the genome of RNA viruses.

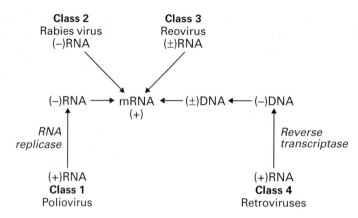

Fig. 146 Replication strategies of viruses with RNA genomes.

specify the base sequence of its product. Once a negative strand is made, it can be used to make more viral RNA. RNA replicase may be part of the viral particle or may be synthesised by the ribosomes of the host using viral RNA as messenger.

Class 2. The single-stranded genome consists of negative-strand RNA, which can be copied to make new viral genomes but must be used as a template for positive-strand synthesis before synthesis of virus-coded proteins can begin.

Class 3. The genome is double-stranded.

Class 4. The single-stranded genome is positive and is replicated by a DNA polymerase, *reverse transcriptase*, which can use RNA as a template (so violating the 'Central Dogma' that information flows from DNA to RNA). The DNA made is incorporated into a chromosome of the host cell and can be transcribed to RNA for use as messenger and to construct new viral particles. Viruses such as HIV that use reverse transcriptase are known as *retroviruses*.

The enzymes that RNA viruses use to replicate their RNA are less accurate than DNA polymerase III since they have no proof-reading ability. RNA viruses are, therefore, much more vulnerable to mutation than DNA viruses and are not able to sustain such large genomes. RNA replication would introduce so many errors into a large genome that viable viruses would rarely be produced.

Release

Virus particles assemble from new viral nucleic acid and virus-coded proteins synthesised within the host cell. They must emerge before they are capable of further infection. Phage λ codes for an enzyme that lyses the host bacterium, releasing the next generation of phage particles and killing the host cell in the process. Synthesis of this enzyme must obviously be carefully timed by the phage since its premature action would destroy the host cell before the new phages could assemble.

Viruses that acquire an envelope leave the host cell by exocytosis, taking part of the plasma membrane with them. This membrane contains virus-coded membrane proteins which the new virus particles use during infection of their next hosts.

15.3 Viruses can coexist with their hosts

Clinical note:
Therapy for retrovirus infection

Since reverse transcriptase is not required by the host cell, it would appear to be a potential target for chemotherapy against HIV and other retroviruses. Inhibitors of reverse transcriptase such as AZT (azidothymidine), a nucleoside analogue, have indeed been used to treat HIV infection. However, its use imposes a strong selection pressure on the virus, which responds by mutation of its reverse transcriptase to produce an enzyme much less susceptible to inhibition by AZT. Long-lasting control of virus multiplication cannot, therefore, be achieved by treatment with this single inhibitor. *Multiple drug* treatment regimens currently offer better prospects for successful therapy.

Learning objective

You should be able to:

• explain how viruses can coexist with their host cells.

Not all viruses multiply themselves immediately after they infect a suitable host cell. More successful strategies are available. One such strategy is that used by phage λ.

By using its so-called *lytic pathway*, phage λ can infect *E. coli*, multiply and produce over 100 copies of itself that emerge about half an hour after infection. A few cycles of infection in this manner would soon exhaust the supply of potential hosts. But phage λ has another pathway, its *lysogenic pathway* (Fig. 147). In this pathway, after the phage has first infected the host cell, the phage DNA, which was injected in a linear form, circularises and then integrates with the circular DNA molecule of its host. Once integrated, it produces a repressor protein that suppresses the synthesis of all phage proteins except the repressor itself. Each time the host cell divides thereafter, another copy of phage DNA is made, still integrated in the bacterial DNA. If conditions for bacterial growth become less than ideal, the stress response by the bacteria may trigger excision of the phage DNA and expression of all the phage genes; in other words, the phage reverts to its lytic pathway.

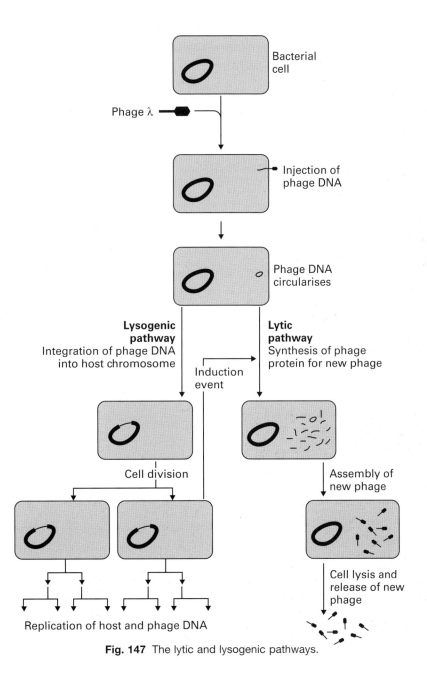

Fig. 147 The lytic and lysogenic pathways.

Self-assessment: questions

Single best answer MCQs

1. Identify the correct statement concerning virus–host relationships.
   a. Viruses can use animal cells and bacterial cells as hosts but not plant cells
   b. Each virus can usually infect a wide range of cell types
   c. Viruses evolve rapidly because of their vast numbers and short generation times
   d. New strains of viruses usually evolve to become more damaging to their hosts
   e. Some bacteriophage have hollow tails through which they inject proteins into their bacterial hosts

2. The genome of a virus can determine how that virus replicates. Which of the following is accurate concerning viral genomes?
   a. Are composed of either RNA or DNA and histone proteins
   b. Can be double-stranded but not single-stranded DNA
   c. In RNA viruses they are usually single-stranded but a few are double-stranded
   d. In RNA viruses they tend to be larger than in DNA viruses
   e. Always consist of a single nucleic acid molecule

3. Which of the following is correct concerning viral structure?
   a. All viruses have a membranous envelope
   b. Viral envelopes are made from host membrane proteins and viral phospholipid
   c. All viruses have a protein coat known as a capsid
   d. Some viruses are cylindrical in shape with a protein core covered by nucleic acid
   e. Viruses always contain nucleic acid but never contain enzymes

4. Which of the following is correct concerning general aspects of viruses?
   a. They halt the metabolic processes of the host cell
   b. They have no metabolism so they do not need ATP
   c. They obtain the building block molecules for their own replication from the cell they have infected
   d. They depend so much on host enzymes that enzyme inhibitors can never be used to control virus replication

   e. They use host cell ribosomes but use viral mRNA and viral tRNA for the synthesis of viral protein

5. RNA viruses:
   a. Need processes not included in the Central Dogma of Molecular Biology
   b. Do not use viral RNA as mRNA to direct the synthesis of viral proteins
   c. Are generally less liable to mutate than DNA viruses
   d. Depend on host cell enzymes for replication of their nucleic acid
   e. Use reverse transcriptase to replicate their RNA

6. Which of the following is correct concerning retroviruses?
   a. They can have DNA or RNA genomes
   b. They use reverse transcriptase
   c. They are scientifically interesting but of no medical importance
   d. They are not pathogenic
   e. They have a low rate of mutation

7. In which order do the following processes occur when a HIV virus infects its host cell? (1) viral proteins, including reverse transcriptase, are synthesised; (2) viral RNA is used as a template to make DNA; (3) viral mRNA is synthesised; (4) DNA synthesised by reverse transcriptase is incorporated in a host chromosome.
   a. 1, 2, 3, 4
   b. 4, 3, 2, 1
   c. 2, 4, 3, 1
   d. 4, 3, 1, 2
   e. 2, 3, 4, 1

8. Which of the following is correct concerning bacteriophage λ?
   a. It infects its host E. coli cell and immediately lyses it.
   b. It injects a circular DNA molecule into its host
   c. It can incorporate its DNA into the DNA of its host
   d. In its lytic pathway it only expresses one gene to make a repressor protein
   e. It is interesting to study but bacteriophages are of no practical importance since they only infect bacteria

Short essay question

Why study viruses?

Self-assessment: answers

Single best answer MCQ answers

1. a. **False**. Some viruses can use plant cells as hosts. All plant viruses are RNA viruses.
    b. **False**. Each virus is adapted to infect and replicate in a very limited range of host cells.
    c. **True**. The rapid evolution of viruses makes them specially dangerous pathogens.
    d. **False**. Both virus and host evolve to make viral infection less damaging.
    e. **False**. This is the way in which phage DNA can enter the host cell. No phage protein enters.

2. a. **False**. Viruses with each kind of nucleic acid are found but they do not have histones.
    b. **False**. The great majority of DNA viruses are double-stranded but some phage have single-stranded DNA.
    c. **True**. The great majority of RNA viruses are single-stranded.
    d. **False**. RNA replication is less accurate than that of DNA so RNA viruses cannot maintain very large genomes.
    e. **False**. Some viral genomes contain more than one nucleic acid molecule; for example, influenza virus has a genome consisting of eight RNA molecules.

3. a. **False**. Not all viruses have an envelope.
    b. **False**. The phospholipid is from the host and the proteins from the virus.
    c. **True**. Viral nucleic acid is always packaged in protein.
    d. **False**. The core is nucleic acid and the coat is protein, e.g. tobacco mosaic virus.
    e. **False**. Many virus particles contain one or two enzyme molecules, e.g. reverse transcriptase in HIV.

4. a. **False**. Viruses rely on the metabolism of their host cells for energy and building blocks.
    b. **False**. Viruses need energy for synthesis of their nucleic acids and proteins.
    c. **True**. For example, amino acids for synthesis of viral protein.
    d. **False**. Viruses present a few targets for control by drugs, e.g. inhibitors of reverse transcriptase and viral protease in HIV.

e. **False**. Viral mRNA is used but the host cell provides the tRNA.

5. a. **True**. The Central Dogma makes no provision for replication of RNA.
    b. **False**. Some have positive-strand RNA which is used as mRNA.
    c. **False**. They are much more likely to mutate; RNA replication is less accurate than that of DNA.
    d. **False**. Host cells do not have enzymes to replicate RNA.
    e. **False**. Reverse transcriptase makes DNA using RNA as a template. Some RNA viruses use an RNA polymerase that uses an RNA template. It is known as RNA replicase.

6. a. **False**. They have RNA that they reverse transcribe to produce DNA sequences.
    b. **True**. This enzyme is by definition found in all retroviruses. It catalyses the reverse of transcription forming DNA from an RNA template.
    c. **False**. HIV, human immunodeficiency virus, is a retrovirus.
    d. **False**. HIV, human immunodeficiency virus, is a retrovirus.
    e. **False**. Reverse transcription is more error prone than DNA replication. HIV is very mutable.

7. c. This the correct answer. (2) viral RNA is used as a template to make DNA; (4) DNA synthesised by reverse transcriptase is incorporated in a host chromosome; (3) viral mRNA is synthesised; (1) viral proteins, including reverse transcriptase, are synthesised.

8. a. **False**. Immediate lysis would be suicidal. The phage needs an intact host and delays lysis until it has replicated.
    b. **False**. The DNA is linear when injected but forms a circle once inside.
    c. **True**. In the lysogenic pathway.
    d. **False**. It is in its lysogenic pathway that phage λ only expresses this gene.
    e. **False**. Phage are important vectors in genetic engineering.

Short essay answer

The following list indicates some reasons:

- medical importance: many diseases are caused by viruses
- agricultural importance: many animal and plant diseases are caused by viruses
- genetic engineering: viruses are widely used as vectors.

In addition, viruses provide excellent model systems for studying the following: gene organisation, control of gene expression, virus capsids as models for the assembly of macromolecular structures, virus entry to and exit from host cells as models for endocytosis and exocytosis.

It has been suggested that benign viruses could be used as vehicles to introduce genes to cells selectively and so alleviate inherited disease. For example, in cystic fibrosis where the inactivity of a chloride channel leads to lung damage, it may be feasible to introduce the missing gene into the cells where its absence is causing disease.

16 Biochemical functions of the liver

Overview

Almost every major metabolic pathway is present in the liver and, clearly, it has a vital role to play in fuel balance, facilitated by its anatomical location and the fact that it receives fuels and metabolites directly from the gut via the portal vein. Liver glycogen is of primary importance for glucose homeostasis in the fed and fasted states. The liver has the ability to process fatty acids to ketone bodies, fuels that are critical to survival during starvation. Almost all plasma proteins are synthesised in the liver. The liver is the principal organ involved in xenobiotic metabolism through its content of mixed-function oxidases. Many products including hormones and bilirubin are processed in the liver as a prerequisite for their elimination from the body. Bile is a product of the liver, thus the liver has a vital role to play in digestion and absorption of our foods. The liver is the only site in the body of the urea cycle, critical for dealing with potentially toxic ammonia. Impaired liver function compromises many functions leading to serious pathology.

16.1 Carbohydrate, lipid and amino acid metabolism

Learning objectives

You should be able to:

- outline the major pathways for carbohydrate, lipid and amino acid metabolism in the liver

- explain how ethanol is handled in the liver and how it can influence gluconeogenesis.

Carbohydrate metabolism

Table 25 contains core information related to carbohydrate metabolism in the liver. The liver has the ability to store glucose in the form of glycogen in the fed state and break down glycogen and make glucose from non-carbohydrate precursors in the fasted state and during exercise (Chs 7 and 10). Fructose and galactose, produced by the digestion of dietary sucrose and lactose, respectively, are both converted to glucose in the liver.

Ethanol metabolism

The liver is an important site for ethanol metabolism. By the action of NAD^+-dependent *alcohol dehydrogenase*, ethanol is converted to acetaldehyde. The oxidation of acetaldehyde yields acetyl-coenzyme A (acetyl-CoA). If a large amount of ethanol is being metabolised, the resultant increase in NADH reduces TCA (tricarboxylic acid) cycle activity and diverts acetyl-CoA to fatty acid and triacylglycerol synthesis. This can contribute to the development of fatty liver (see below). Hypoglycaemia is another potential consequence of ethanol consumption since the NADH produced converts pyruvate to lactate and prevents its conversion to glucose. Another route for ethanol metabolism involves a cytochrome P-450 ethanol-oxidising system, located in the smooth endoplasmic reticulum. The product is again acetaldehyde.

Lipid metabolism

Table 26 contains core information related to lipid metabolism in the liver. Some fat is synthesised in the liver in the fed state; the activity of this pathway depends upon the nutritional status of the subject. People on high-fat diets typical in Western societies have low activity of the key enzymes of fatty acid synthesis. Most of the glucose that they take up in the liver is converted to glycogen. However, fatty acids derived from chylomicron remnants are converted to triacylglycerol (TAG) by a pathway that uses glycerol 3-phosphate derived from glucose metabolism. Any

Table 25 Carbohydrate metabolism in the liver

Activity	Pathways	Control
Maintenance of blood glucose	Glycogenolysis and gluconeogenesis	High glucagon/insulin ratio
Fuel storage	Glycogenesis, fatty acid synthesis	High insulin/glucagon ratio
Ribose phosphate and NADPH generation	Pentose phosphate cycle	
Utilisation of other carbohydrates	Fructose and galactose metabolism	

Table 26 Lipid metabolism in the liver

Activity	Pathways
Production of fatty acids	Fatty acid synthesis from glucose, amino acids
Utilisation of fatty acids	Beta-oxidation
Production of ketone bodies	Mitochondrial synthesis from fatty acids and ketogenic amino acids
Cholesterol biosynthesis	
Production of bile acids	Biosynthesis from cholesterol
Phospholipid synthesis	
Lipoprotein synthesis	
Provision of 25-hydroxy-vitamin D	Synthesis from vitamin D
Storage of vitamin A	

TAG synthesised in the liver is exported as VLDL (very low density lipoprotein). Fatty acids are oxidised to provide ATP in the fasted state and they are also the precursors of ketone bodies. The liver is the major organ involved in cholesterol biosynthesis. The liver also acquires cholesterol when it takes up chylomicron remnants (Ch. 9, p. 132). Bile acid biosynthesis is unique to the liver, and the formation of bile in that organ is critical for lipid digestion. Large amounts of vitamin A are stored in the lipocytes (Ito cells) of the liver. The liver is the site for the synthesis of 25-hydroxy-vitamin D, the precursor of calcitriol (Ch. 17, p. 245), formed in the kidney.

Fatty liver

The accumulation of TAG in the liver is indicative of abnormal function and leads to liver damage. A cause of fatty liver can be failure of normal lipoprotein synthesis caused by a variety of factors. One such is where there is a deficiency of *choline*; hence choline is called a *lipotropic factor*.

Amino acid metabolism

When a person's diet contains protein in excess of requirements for protein synthesis, much of the amino acids produced by protein digestion are catabolised in the liver, where they can be converted to glycogen and TAG or completely oxidised to generate ATP (Table 27). The liver is the only organ in the body with a functional urea cycle. Under fasted conditions, the conversion of amino acid carbons to glucose by the gluconeogenic pathway achieves great significance. Most of the plasma proteins are synthesised in the liver and are discussed in Chapter 19. Key transport proteins for steroid hormones and thyroid hormones are also synthesised in the liver and these are discussed in Chapter 17.

Table 27 Amino acid metabolism in the liver

Activity	Pathways
Energy metabolism	Individual pathways then the TCA cycle and oxidative phosphorylation
Urea synthesis	The liver is the sole site in the body
Glucose/glycogen production	Gluconeogenesis from glucogenic amino acids, e.g. alanine

16.2 Metabolism of xenobiotics

Learning objectives

You should be able to:

- explain what is meant by Phase 1 and Phase 2 metabolism of xenobiotics
- describe the role of the liver in hormone inactivation and the consequences of liver malfunction.

The turnover of many biologically active endogenous compounds (e.g. hormones) and almost all drugs occurs in the liver; the enzymes involved are localised in the smooth endoplasmic reticulum. The enzyme systems are inducible and their activity often determines the duration of action of the drugs they metabolise.

Drug metabolism usually achieves two goals:

- inactivation of the compound
- increased water solubility of the compound.

Increased water solubility facilitates elimination by the kidneys or in bile.

Drug metabolism occurs in two phases.

Phase 1
Initial metabolism often involves members of a gene family called cytochromes P-450, which are *mixed-function oxidases*. These enzymes, which have broad specificity, catalyse oxidations and demethylations of naturally occurring compounds and xenobiotics that are lipophilic. Mixed-function oxidases require NADPH.

Phase 2
These reactions involve polar molecules being added to the products of Phase 1 to produce water-soluble end-products that are finally excreted via the kidney or via bile. For example:

- benzoic acid with glycine
- steroids and phenols with glucuronic acid

Clinical note:
Drug interactions

Some of the cytochromes P-450 are induced by drugs and this can complicate therapy with a second drug that is also a substrate of the induced enzyme. Similarly, in multiple drug therapy or liver disease, there may be competition for the drug-metabolising enzymes. This tends to be most important with drugs with a narrow therapeutic index, e.g. warfarin, digoxin or cyclosporin.

- indoles and steroids with sulphuric acid
- aromatic acids with glutamine.

Hormone inactivation

The liver is responsible for much of the inactivation of hormones, a process essential to the fine control of hormone levels in blood. Examples include:

- metabolism and inactivation of adrenaline (epinephrine) and noradrenaline (norepinephrine) by *monoamine oxidase* and *catechol O-methyl transferase* and conjugation of their products with glucuronic acid
- de-iodination of thyroxine and triiodothyronine
- insulin reduction to separate A and B chains by *insulin–glutathione transhydrogenase*; these separate inactive chains can then be hydrolysed
- metabolism and inactivation of steroid hormones such as cortisol, testosterone, progesterone and oestradiol by double bond reduction and conjugation of hydroxyl groups with glucuronic or sulphuric acids to form very water-soluble products.

16.3 Bile pigment metabolism

Learning objectives

You should be able to:

- trace the metabolic pathways involving the haem component of haemoproteins
- describe the role of the liver in bilirubin metabolism, including mechanisms of uptake, glucuronidation and secretion into bile
- outline major causes of unconjugated and conjugated hyperbilirubinaemia (jaundice).

Bile pigments are hydrophobic metabolites of the haem rings in haem proteins. They are taken into the liver and converted to water-soluble metabolites that are secreted into bile. Problems with uptake, conjugation or secretion of bile pigments lead to jaundice.

Bile pigments are produced from haem in the spleen

Bile pigments are formed from haem proteins, with most being derived from senescent erythrocytes by conversion of the haem of haemoglobin to biliverdin and subsequent reduction to bilirubin in cells of the reticuloendothelial system (RES), predominantly in the

(a) Synthesis of bilirubin in spleen

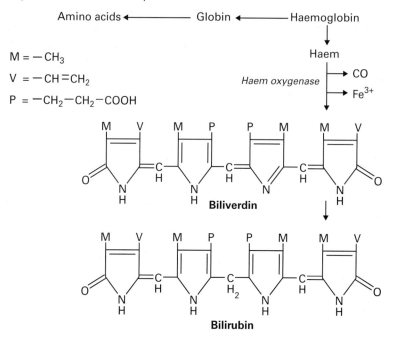

(b) Bilirubin metabolism in liver

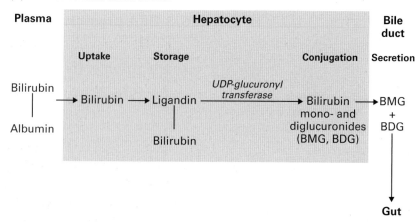

Fig. 148 Bilirubin synthesis in the spleen (a) and its metabolism in the liver (b).

spleen. Other proteins, such as the electron transport chain cytochromes and cytochromes P-450, are also sources of bilirubin; they have a short half-life, whereas haemoglobin has a long half-life because of the long life of erythrocytes. Tissues forming bile pigments contain a highly active enzyme system, *haem oxygenase*, which is associated with the smooth endoplasmic reticulum (Fig. 148). In the presence of oxygen and NADPH, a membrane-bound cytochrome P-450 oxidises one of the carbons that bridges the pyrrole rings and releases it as carbon monoxide. This effectively opens the porphyrin ring to yield the linear tetrapyrrole chain of *biliverdin*. The globin (or other apoprotein portion) is hydrolysed to free amino acids, which will be reconverted in part to

newly synthesized protein. The iron that is released when the haem is cleaved will be almost quantitatively retained for recycling into new haemoproteins. Biliverdin rarely accumulates or escapes from cells because it is acted upon as soon as it is formed by a very active, soluble biliverdin reductase enzyme that also requires NADPH. The product is *bilirubin*, the principal bile pigment found in the body.

Bilirubin is transported to the liver

Bilirubin made in the RES diffuses into the bloodstream where it binds with albumin in the plasma. Upon reaching the hepatic cells, the albumin–bilirubin complex dissociates, and free bilirubin is taken up using *bili-translocase* (Fig. 148). It then becomes bound to a specific carrier protein (ligandin) in the cytosol.

Bilirubin conjugation with glucuronic acid precedes secretion into bile

A major function of the liver is to convert the bilirubin to a water-soluble form by attaching sugar derivatives onto two of the pyrrole rings, a process called *conjugation*. The sugar derivative, glucuronic acid, is added in its activated form, UDP-glucuronic acid; this is derived in the liver by the action of a soluble dehydrogenase upon UDP-glucose. A specific enzyme in the endoplasmic reticulum, *UDP-glucuronyltransferase*, catalyses the addition of glucuronic acid to the two propionyl side chains of bilirubin in ester linkages. The resulting conjugated form of the bile pigment, bilirubin diglucuronide (BDG), has the hydrophilic sugar residues to offset the hydrophobic property of the rest of the molecule.

Bilirubin is secreted into bile

The conjugated and unconjugated bilirubin molecules may then be passed from the hepatic cells into the bile canaliculi, utilising the *ATP-dependent canalicular multidrug resistance-like protein*. They then percolate down the biliary tree to the gallbladder before being released into the intestinal tract. In the intestine, BDG is metabolised to *urobilinogen*, some of which is reabsorbed and is in turn excreted in urine, i.e. we have an enterohepatic circulation of bile pigment metabolites. Urobilinogen that is not reabsorbed is excreted in faeces.

Excess levels of bile pigments cause jaundice

When bile pigments accumulate in the blood and other body fluids, either because of excessive formation or because of inadequate removal in the bile, they may produce an intense yellow coloration of the skin. This condition, termed icterus or *jaundice*, may result from:

- massive breakdown of erythrocytes (haemolysis) leading to overproduction of bilirubin from haemoglobin catabolism
- a defect in the mechanisms by which the liver disposes of the normal flux of bilirubin.

Neonatal jaundice has to be treated

This is really a normal event since the glucuronyltransferase and ligandin system is still immature during the first few days of life. However, premature babies can achieve very high levels of unconjugated bilirubin; if it gets into the central nervous system, leading to *kernicterus*, there is the possibility of a motor disorder. Treatment is usually by phototherapy, where the bilirubin in the skin is converted to a water-soluble (easily excreted) derivative. You can see this treatment in any neonatal unit of a hospital.

Other forms of jaundice

These can be due to:

- defects in bilirubin uptake and glucuronyltransferase (Gilbert's disease)
- absence of glucuronyltransferase activity (Crigler–Najjar disease)
- defective hepatic excretion (Dubin–Johnson syndrome)
- hepatitis/cirrhosis (viral hepatitis or alcoholic cirrhosis)
- biliary obstruction (obstructive jaundice caused by stones, cancer, etc.).

16.4 Liver function tests

Learning objectives

You should be able to:

- describe the major liver function tests and especially those used to measure synthetic ability, cholestasis and necrosis

- explain why prothrombin time is a useful test of the liver's synthetic ability.

It is important to realise that as much as 80% of the liver cells can be damaged or removed with no evidence of abnormality of liver function, i.e. the liver has great reserve activity. In this way, significant liver damage is not usually associated with an abnormal glucose tolerance test, even though we know that much of the glucose is usually metabolised in the liver during such a test.

Liver function tests (LFTs) include:

- the measurement of serum albumin and prothrombin time (PT) of plasma as indices of *synthetic ability* of the liver
- the measurement of alkaline phosphatase as a test for *cholestasis*

- the measurement of aminotransferases [aspartate aminotransferase (AST) and alanine aminotransferase (ALT)] as a test for *inflammation and necrosis*
- measurement of serum bilirubin.

Elevated PT is a very sensitive test for the synthetic capability of the liver and is dependent upon the fact that factor VII, involved in the extrinsic blood coagulation pathway and measured by PT (Ch. 19), is a factor that has a relatively short half-life. Since factor VII is a vitamin K-dependent blood coagulation factor, the vitamin K status of any subject being evaluated has to be considered in interpreting data.

Serum alkaline phosphatase is derived from liver, bone, intestine, placenta and kidney. It is possible to measure the liver isozyme and an increase in its level in serum is associated with obstructive and cholestatic liver disease.

When the liver is damaged, as in viral hepatitis, enzymes present in high concentrations in hepatocytes appear in serum in increased amounts. Of the aminotransferases, ALT is more liver-specific (it is involved in the gluconeogenic pathway from alanine to glucose).

Self-assessment: questions

Single best answer MCQs

1. Identify a correct statement or statements concerning bilirubin metabolism and jaundice.
   a. In Crigler–Najjar syndrome there is a lack of UDP-glucuronyltransferase
   b. An ATP-dependent canalicular multidrug resistance-like protein (CMRP) is involved in the secretion of bilirubin diglucuronide into the bile
   c. Urobilinogen produced in the gut is returned to the liver by enterohepatic circulation thus accounting for its presence in urine
   d. Both a and c are correct
   e. a, b and c are all correct

2. Identify the statement in Column A concerning liver function that is correctly associated with the statement in Column B.

A	B
a. Phase 2 metabolism of drugs	Mixed-function oxidases
b. Phase 1 of drug metabolism	Conjugation with polar molecules
c. Ethanol metabolism	Impaired gluconeogenesis
d. Saturated fatty acids	Gluconeogenesis
e. Ketone bodies	Utilisation as fuels by liver

3. Identify a correct statement or statements concerning liver function tests.
   a. When liver damage is due to hepatitis, the ratio of ALT to AST is greater than 1
   b. An increase in liver-specific alkaline phosphatase (ALP) in serum is consistent with cholestatic jaundice
   c. In a subject with damage to about 40% of their liver one can expect to see both hyperammoniaemia and abnormal handling of glucose
   d. a and b are both correct
   e. a, b and c are all correct

4. Which one of the following accurately describes liver function?
   a. A deficiency of choline can cause fatty liver
   b. LDL is the lipoprotein made in the liver to transport TAG to adipose tissue
   c. Drug inactivation in the liver is based on the principle that the liver converts the drug to a more lipophilic metabolite
   d. Factor VII, one of the coagulation factors made in the liver, has a very long half-life
   e. Metabolism of insulin in the liver results in a product with enhanced biological activity

True/false questions

Are the following statements true or false?

1. The liver has a large reserve capacity in terms of its ability to handle glucose loads.
2. In normal subjects in the fed state, gluconeogenesis in the liver is stimulated.
3. The liver is the site for synthesis of 25-hydroxycholecalciferol.
4. The liver is the site of action of vitamin K metabolism in the body.
5. The source of glucuronic acid for bilirubin diglucuronide synthesis is UDP-glucuronate.
6. Drug-metabolising enzymes in the liver are chiefly located in the mitochondria.
7. Bile acids and bile pigments are both metabolites of the haem ring in haemoglobin and cytochromes.

Short essay questions

1. Explain in a few sentences the reason why the measurement of prothrombin time, a blood coagulation test, provides critical information about protein synthesis in the liver.
2. Discuss neonatal jaundice and research the literature to come up with a description of how it is treated, if necessary.

Self-assessment: answers

Single best answer MCQ answers

1. a. **True**. This is a rare form of unconjugated hyperbilirubinaemia.
   b. **True**. CMRP is involved in this process.
   c. **True**. Urobilinogen is the precursor of the urobilin that gives the straw colour to urine.
   d. Correct, but not the best answer.
   e. The single best answer.

2. a. **False**. Phase 2 is where derivatives of drugs are formed that increase water solubility, thus enabling excretion in bile or urine.
   b. **False**. Phase 1 is where the drug is inactivated by reactions catalysed by mixed-function oxidases.
   c. **True**. Ethanol is rapidly oxidised with the generation of NADH. The high ratio of $NADH/NAD^+$ converts pyruvate (an intermediate in gluconeogenesis) to lactate; therefore gluconeogenesis is inhibited and the subject may have severe hypoglycaemia.
   d. **False**. Saturated fatty acids are oxidised to acetyl-CoA which *cannot* generate a net increase in glucose when metabolised.
   e. **False**. Ketone bodies are made in the liver but they are not utilised there.

3. a. **True**. Except when the damage is due to severe alcoholism, the ALT/AST ratio is greater than 1. ALT is somewhat liver-specific given its role in gluconeogenesis. When the liver is damaged, ALT is released into blood.
   b. **True**. ALP can originate from the bile ducts and levels are elevated when there is obstruction.
   c. **False**. The liver has enormous reserves and the damage has to be much greater than 40% for urea cycle activity or the ability to handle glucose to be abnormal.
   d. **True**. This is the single best answer.
   e. **False**. since c is incorrect.

4. a. **True**. Choline is required for phosphatidylcholine synthesis and phospholipids are required for VLDL formation and lipid transport from the liver.
   b. **False**. VLDL is the TAG transporter made in the liver.

c. **False**. The principle is that a more hydrophilic metabolite is formed.
   d. **False**. Factor VII has a short half-life; this explains the use of the PT as an LFT (see below).
   e. **False**. Metabolism of insulin involves its separation into its A and B chains which are biologically inactive.

True/false answers

1. **True**. This means that glucose tolerance is not a sensitive test of liver malfunction.
2. **False**. Why make more glucose when one has fed?
3. **True**. Cholecalciferol can be made in skin and 25-hydroxylation in the liver gives the precursor of the hormone, calcitriol, which is made in the kidney.
4. **True**. Several vitamin K-dependent proteins involved in blood coagulation, including prothrombin, are made in the liver.
5. **True**. UDP is the 'carrier' for biosynthetic reactions that incorporate carbohydrates and some carbohydrate derivatives into molecules.
6. **False**. Most are located in the smooth endoplasmic reticulum.
7. **False**. Bile acids are formed from cholesterol in the liver; bile pigments are made in the spleen from haem.

Short essay answers

1. Prothrombin time (PT) is used by haematologists as a way of quantifying the activity of the extrinsic pathway of blood coagulation (Ch. 19). The range of normal values is small, which means that even a 2- or 3-second prolongation of the PT can be significant and must be pursued. Factor VII is involved in this pathway and is a vitamin K-dependent factor synthesised in the liver. It is distinguished from most other plasma proteins by having a very short half-life. If a patient has hepatocellular disease, liver protein synthesis will be impaired and this is quickly reflected in a prolonged PT. It is important to recognise that, since factor VII is a vitamin K-dependent factor, a prolonged PT can also be caused by vitamin K deficiency. In such cases, the injection of vitamin K will return the PT value to the normal range.

2. Ligandin and UDP-glucuronyltransferase activities develop slowly such that most full-term neonates have what would be considered elevated levels of unconjugated bilirubin in adults. However, ligandin and UDP-glucuronyltransferase increase within a few days after delivery and the bilirubin levels fall. This is important since there is the danger of the child developing *kernicterus* with some degree of brain damage being caused by the bilirubin. Neonatal jaundice is more prominent in premature children so they almost always have their skin exposed to blue light which causes bilirubin in the skin to be converted to a water-soluble derivative that can then be excreted via the urine.

17 The biochemistry of the endocrine system

Overview

One of the axioms of physiology is the relative constancy of the internal environment of the body, *homeostasis*. The endocrine and nervous systems regulate almost all metabolic and homeostatic activities in humans and these two regulatory systems interact. Most endocrine secretions are influenced directly or indirectly by the brain. Various feedback loops exist to provide a stable internal milieu (ionic or fuel homeostasis) or a coordinated series of actions (growth and reproduction). The classical endocrine system involved secretion of hormones into blood and transport to a distant site where specific effects were brought about. However, we now know that there is a *paracrine* system where hormones are made in cells and then influence neighbouring cells without transport in blood. Other hormones influence their cells of origin and that is the less well-studied *autocrine* system.

17.1 General aspects

Learning objectives

You should be able to:

- explain how the physicochemical properties of hormones affects their transport, activation and mechanisms of action
- describe in outline how polypeptide hormones are synthesised
- describe in outline how thyroid hormones are synthesised
- outline how steroid hormones are synthesised.

The homeostatic role of the endocrine system is usually divided into five major areas (summarised in Table 28).

Chemical nature of hormones

Rather than memorising a particular hormone's detailed chemical structure, it is important to appreciate the nature of its chemical structure since, to a large degree, that is what determines how it is made, how it is transported and how it acts. There are three general chemical classes:

- *Peptides*. These include large complex polypeptides that contain disulphide bonds and may be glycosylated, as well as linear peptides with as few as three amino acid residues.
- *Amino acid derivatives*. These are either made from single amino acids or from the coupling of two amino acids. Examples are the catecholamines, adrenaline (epinephrine) and noradrenaline (norepinephrine) and the thyroid hormones thyroxine (T_4) and triiodothyronine (T_3).
- *Steroids*. Steroid hormones such as cortisol, progesterone, aldosterone, androgens and oestrogens contain an intact steroid nucleus, whereas in calcitriol the steroid nucleus has been disrupted.

Table 28 The scope of endocrine regulation

System	Hormones involved
Ionic homeostasis	
Control of Na^+/K^+ ratios in blood	Aldosterone
Control of $[Ca^{2+}]$ in blood	Parathyroid hormone, calcitonin, calcitriol
Control of water balance	Antidiuretic hormone
Fuel homeostasis	
Control of blood glucose concentration	Insulin in the fed state
	Glucagon, adrenaline (epinephrine), cortisol, growth hormone in the fasting state and during exercise
Basal metabolic rate	Thyroid hormones
Regulation of growth	
Growth of cartilage	Growth hormone, mediated by insulin-like growth factor (IGF-1; somatomedin C)
Growth and development	Growth hormone, thyroid hormones
Regulation of reproduction, sexual differentiation and lactation	
Control of gonadal function	Luteinising hormone (LH), follicle-stimulating hormone (FSH), testosterone, oestradiol
Control of lactation	Prolactin, oxytocin
Pregnancy	Human chorionic gonadotrophin (hCG), human chorionic somatomammotrophin (hCS), progesterone, oestradiol
Gastrointestinal activity	
Pepsin and acid production	Gastrin
Bicarbonate release from pancreas	Secretin
Release of bile from gallbladder	Cholecystokinin
Enzyme release from pancreas	Cholecystokinin

The biosynthesis of hormones

Peptide hormones are coded for by particular genes and synthesised by the standard protein biosynthetic machinery (Ch. 14). There are usually multiple copies of the genes for shorter peptides, and single hormone molecules are derived by post-translational proteolysis. Some hormones may be synthesised as separate subunits, which then associate (e.g. the glycoprotein hormones of the adenohypophysis).

Since peptide hormones are to be secreted from the cells of origin, the mechanism of production is similar to that for other secreted proteins (Ch. 14, p. 207). The classic example of this is insulin, which is synthesised in the pancreatic beta cell as preproinsulin which contains a signal peptide sequence that is removed generating proinsulin. The action of intracellular peptidases on proinsulin yields insulin plus a connecting peptide (C-peptide):

Preproinsulin→Proinsulin→Insulin + C-peptide

Other hormones for which there are large prohormones include growth hormone, parathyroid hormone, ACTH (adrenocorticotrophin), oxytocin, ADH (antidiuretic hormone) and glucagon.

Amino acid derivatives are synthesised by unique pathways, each having several enzymatic steps. There are two groups of this type of hormone.

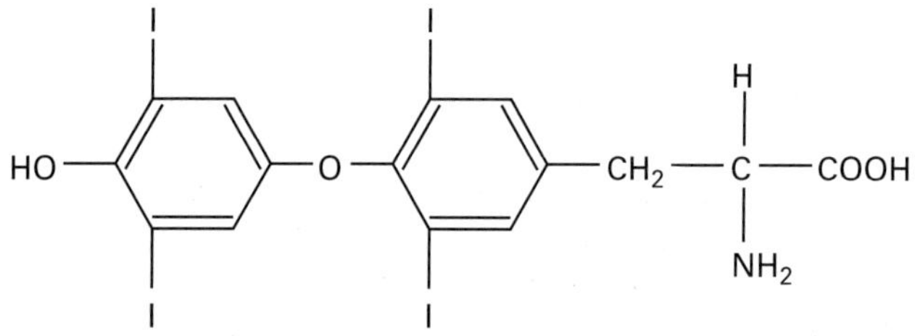

Thyroxine (T_4)

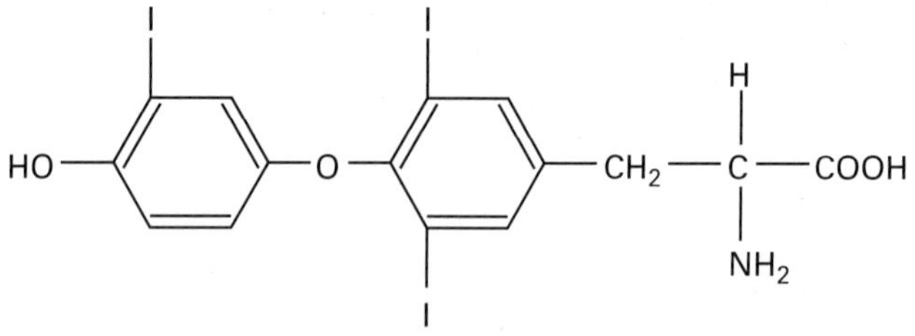

Triiodothyronine (T_3)

Fig. 149 The structures of the thyroid hormones.

Thyroid hormone biosynthesis (Fig. 149) involves the protein thyroglobulin in the follicular epithelial cells of the thyroid gland (Fig. 150). This protein contains a large number of tyrosine residues that can be iodinated. Iodide derived from the diet is taken up by the thyroid as a secondary active process. There is uptake into kidney, gastric and salivary glands too, but the

S

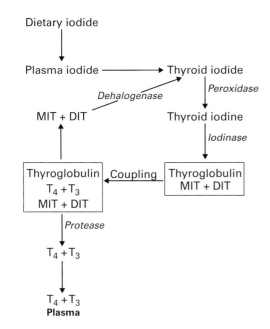

Fig. 150 Thyroid hormone biosynthesis.

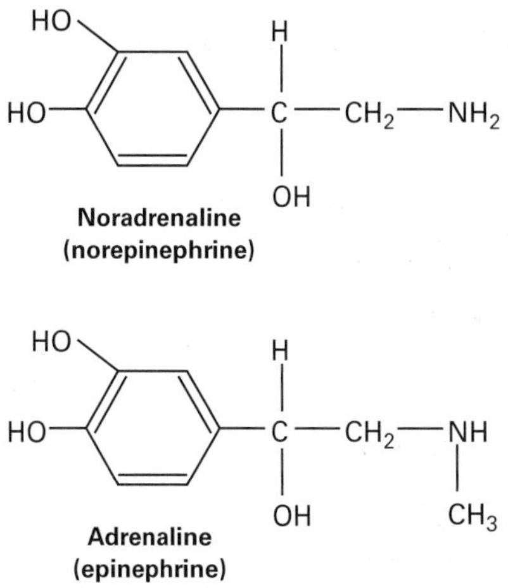

difference is that only in the thyroid is the iodine used to iodinate a protein. A *thyroperoxidase* (TPO) catalyses the oxidation of iodide to iodine as well as the iodination of tyrosyl residues, leading to the formation of monoiodotyrosine (MIT) and diiodotyrosine (DIT) within thyroglobulin. TPO also catalyses the coupling of two DIT residues to form T_4 and a small amount of T_3 is also generated. These reactions occur at the apical membrane of the cell.

Thyroglobulin is an exportable glycoprotein. It is stored in the *colloid* from where it can be internalised by micropinocytosis. When thyroid hormones are required, the internalised thyroglobulin interacts with lysosomes to form secondary lysosomes and the thyroglobulin is digested to its constituent amino acids (including T_4, T_3, MIT and DIT) by the action of lysosomal proteases. T_4 and much less T_3 are then secreted into blood. Much more iodine is present in MIT and DIT than in T_4 and T_3 and that iodine is salvaged by the action of a thyroidal dehalogenase.

Adrenaline (epinephrine) and noradrenaline (norepinephrine) (Fig. 151) are synthesised in the chromaffin cells of tissues such as the adrenal medulla as well as in the brain and in sympathetic nerve endings (Fig. 152). Tyrosine is the precursor and *tyrosine hydroxylase*, a mixed-function oxidase that requires tetrahydrobiopterin as coenzyme, catalyses the rate-controlling step. Dopamine and noradrenaline (norepinephrine) are intermediates, but the presence of *phenylethanolamine N-methyltransferase* (PNMT) allows for adrenaline (epinephrine) synthesis in adrenal medulla. PNMT is induced by high concentrations of glucocorticoid, a situation brought about by the anatomical relationship

Fig. 151 The structures of adrenaline (epinephrine) and noradrenaline (norepinephrine).

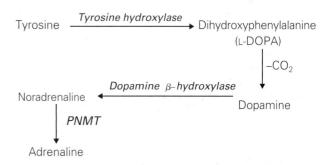

Fig. 152 Catecholamine biosynthesis.

of the adrenal medulla and the adrenal cortex. Adrenaline (epinephrine) is stored complexed to ATP in granules within the chromaffin cells.

Steroid hormones are also synthesised by unique pathways, each having several enzymatic steps. There are many types of steroid hormones but they are all derived from cholesterol, a sterol with 27 carbons. The steroid hormone products depend upon the tissue, but overall the pathway can be described as:

$$C_{27} \rightarrow C_{21} \rightarrow C_{19} \rightarrow C_{18}$$

In the critical first step, cholesterol undergoes side chain cleavage, losing six carbons to give *pregnenolone*, the precursor of all the steroid hormones. The structures of the steroid hormones are shown in Figure 153.

- The C_{21} steroids are progesterone, and the corticosteroids, aldosterone and cortisol.
- The C_{19} steroids are androgens such as testosterone and dehydroepiandrosterone (DHEA).
- The C_{18} steroids are the oestrogens; oestradiol is the most important.

Oxygens are added in the conversion of pregnenolone to the steroid hormones; the oxygens are derived from

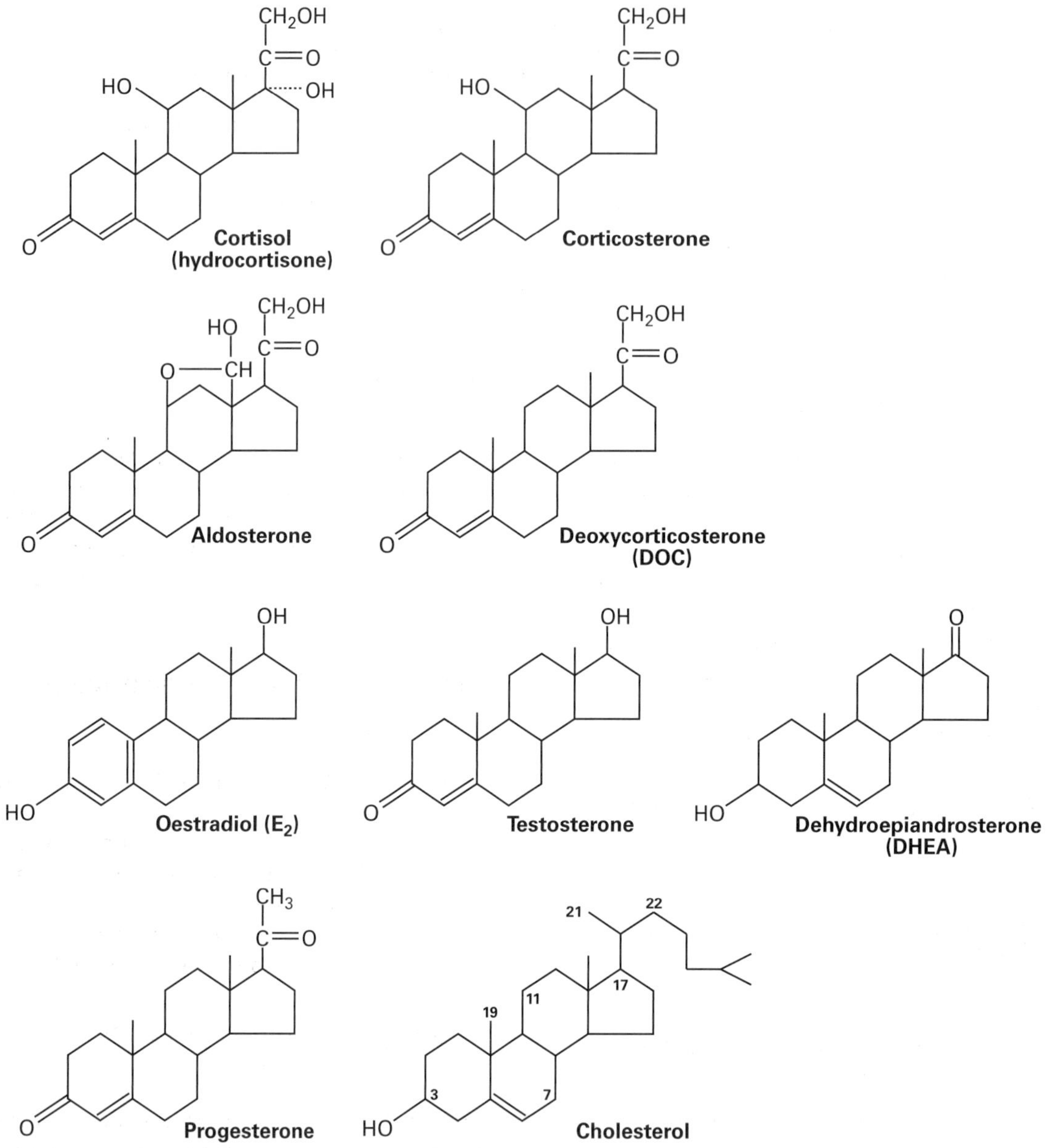

Fig. 153 The structures of steroid hormones and cholesterol.

molecular oxygen in reactions catalysed by a family of haem-containing enzymes called *cytochromes P-450* which require NADPH as cofactor.

Physicochemical properties of hormones

Another classification focuses on the water or lipid solubility of the hormone in question. Hormones in the water-soluble class (peptide hormones and catecholamines) have a number of key differences from the lipophilic hormones (thyroid hormones and steroid hormones) (Table 29).

Water-soluble hormones are transported in the plasma in the free state, have short half-lives (this affects treatment regimens) and, since they do not pass readily through lipid bilayers, they act by binding to specific receptor molecules on the plasma membranes of target cells.

Lipophilic hormones are transported mostly bound to plasma proteins, but it is the free fraction that is biologically active and controlled. The total concentration of a lipophilic hormone will change if the concentration of its transport protein is altered; an understanding of this is important when clinicians interpret hormone assay data on their patients. They have longer half-lives

Table 29 Contrasting properties of hydrophilic and lipophilic hormones

	Hydrophilic hormones[a]	Lipophilic hormones[b]
Transport in blood	Free	Transport protein involved
Half-life	Short	Long
Receptor site	Plasma membrane	Nucleus
Extraglandular activation	Rare	Common
Mechanism of action	Second messsenger	Transcription factor

[a]Proteins and peptides as well as catecholamines such as adrenaline (epinephrine) and noradrenaline (norepinephrine).
[b]Lipophilic hormones have limited water solubility and include all steroid hormones and the thyroid hormones T_4 and T_3.

and can cross lipid bilayers to target receptors normally present in the nuclei of target cells. Some lipophilic hormones, thyroxine and testosterone are examples, undergo extraglandular bioactivation. Thyroxine is converted to the much more active *triiodothyronine* (T_3) in thyroid hormone target tissues. Testosterone, which is secreted from the gonads and elsewhere in the body, is converted to *oestradiol*, a female sex hormone, or to *5α-dihydrotestosterone*, the androgen involved in the development of the secondary male sexual characteristics.

17.2 Hormones of the hypothalamus and pituitary

Learning objectives

You should be able to:

- describe the connection between the hypothalamus and anterior pituitary hormones

- describe the connection between the hypothalamus and posterior pituitary hormones.

The overall importance of the adenohypophyseal and neurohypophyseal hormones is well illustrated by the consequences of *hypophysectomy*:

- atrophy of the gonads, adrenal cortex and thyroid accompanied by decreased secretion of sex hormones, cortisol and thyroid hormones
- interruption of the ovarian (menstrual) cycle
- decreased ability to respond to stress
- inhibition of growth and development in young animals and increased sensitivity to insulin
- temporary diabetes insipidus.

The hormones secreted from the pituitary are listed in Table 30. Those arising from the anterior pituitary are controlled by releasing and inhibitory hormones that are made in the hypothalamus (Table 31); they travel to the pituitary via the pituitary portal veins. Antidiuretic hormone and oxytocin are made in the hypothalamus and travel down nerve tracts that terminate in the posterior pituitary from which these hormones are released into blood.

Hormones of the anterior pituitary

These include:

- large polypeptide hormones: growth hormone (hGH), prolactin (PRL)
- glycoprotein hormones: thyroid-stimulating hormone (TSH), luteinising hormone (LH), follicle-stimulating hormone (FSH)
- small peptides: adrenocorticotrophin (ACTH), melanocyte-stimulating hormone (MSH).

Growth hormone and prolactin

Chemistry
hGH is a single chain polypeptide of 191 amino acid residues with two disulphide bridges made in the somatotrophs of the anterior pituitary. PRL is made in mammotrophs and has 199 amino acid residues and three disulphide bridges.

Control of secretion
Control of hGH secretion is complex. There is a pronounced circadian rhythm, with secretion being elevated during the sleep period. hGH is controlled positively by growth hormone-releasing hormone (GHRH) and negatively by somatostatin, both produced in the hypothalamus. Control of PRL by the hypothalamus is inhibitory.

Biological effects
hGH action on growth is mediated indirectly by insulin-like growth factor 1 (IGF-1). IGF-1 feeds back negatively on the hypothalamus to inhibit GHRH and stimulate somatostatin release. PRL stimulates milk production.

Table 30 Hormones of the pituitary

Hormones	Produced by	Site of action
Adenohypophysis		
Glycoprotein hormones		
Thyroid-stimulating hormone (TSH)	Thyrotroph	Follicular epithelial cells of the thyroid
Luteinising hormone (LH)	Gonadotroph	Ovarian follicle, corpus luteum, Leydig cells
Follicle-stimulating hormone (FSH)	Gonadotroph	Ovarian follicle, Sertoli cells
Large polypeptides		
Growth hormone (GH, STH)	Somatotroph	Liver (IGF-1), adipocytes, general
Prolactin (PRL)	Mammotroph	Mammary gland (possibly other sites)
Small peptides		
Adrenocorticotrophic hormone (ACTH, corticotrophin)	Corticotroph	Adrenal cortex adipocytes
β-Endorphin (β-EP)	Corticotroph and	Brain
β-Lipotrophin (β-LPH)	neuro-intermediary lobe	
α-Melanocyte-stimulating hormone (α-MSH)		Melanocytes
Neurohypophysis		
Small peptides		
Antidiuretic hormone (ADH, vasopressin)	Supraoptic and paraventricular nuclei (SON and PVN)	Kidney
Oxytocin (OT)	PVN and SON	Mammary gland, uterus

Table 31 Hormones of the hypothalamus

Hormone	Chemistry	Target
Thyrotrophin-releasing hormone (TRH, TRF)	Tripeptide pyroGlu-His-Pro-NH$_2$	Thyrotrophs
Gonadotrophin-releasing hormone (GnRH, LHRH)	Decapeptide	Gonadotrophs (LH and FSH)
Growth hormone-releasing hormone (GHRH, GRF)	Peptide (44 amino acid residues)	Somatotrophs
Growth hormone-inhibiting hormone (somatostatin)	Tetradecapeptide	Somatotrophs
Corticotrophin-releasing hormone (CRH, CRF)	Peptide (41 amino acid residues)	Corticotrophs

Hormones of the posterior pituitary

Antidiuretic hormone (ADH) and oxytocin (OT)

Chemistry

Both ADH and OT are nonapeptides made from very large precursors that are synthesised in the supraoptic and paraventricular nuclei of the hypothalamus. ADH controls water balance by action on the kidney and also is a vasopressor. OT is part of the neuroendocrine reflex that allows for 'let down' and therefore release of milk from the mammary glands during breast feeding.

17.3 The hypothalamic–pituitary–adrenal cortical axis

Learning objectives

You should be able to:

• outline the hypothalamic–pituitary–adrenal cortical axis (Fig. 154) in terms of corticotrophin-releasing hormone (CRH), ACTH and cortisol and negative feedback

• describe the control of aldosterone synthesis, especially the role of the renin–angiotensin system.

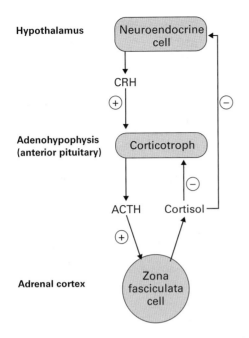

Fig. 154 The hypothalamic–pituitary–adrenal cortical axis.

CRH is a hypothalamic hormone that stimulates ACTH secretion by corticotrophs.

ACTH is a peptide of 39 amino acid residues formed from its precursor, *pro-opiomelanocortin*, in the corticotrophs of the anterior pituitary. ACTH secretion is stimulated by pulses of CRH from the hypothalamus and suppressed by negative feedback by cortisol. Increased secretion of ACTH occurs in stress.

Cortisol (hydrocortisone) is the principal glucocorticoid secreted by the human adrenal cortex. It is derived from cholesterol in the zona fasciculata cells, as outlined in Figure 155. Cortisol secretion is controlled by ACTH. Cortisol is vital in our response to stress and has effects on almost all tissues in the body. Cortisol has a pronounced circadian rhythm. Cortisol can cross the plasma membrane of cells and has the potential to influence the properties of cells provided that they possess glucocorticoid receptors (see section 17.10).

Aldosterone is the principal mineralocorticoid secreted by the human adrenal cortex. Its production is controlled by the renin–angiotensin system; *renin*, made

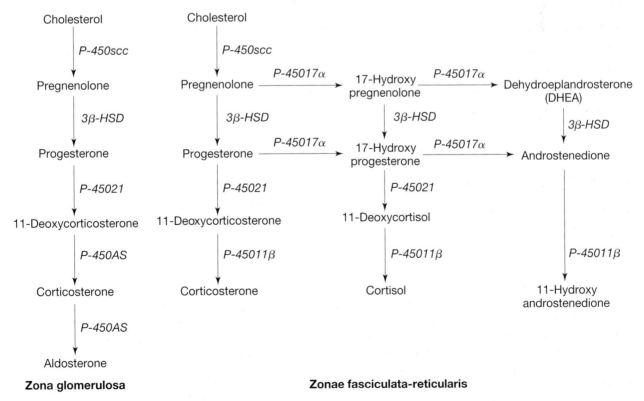

Fig. 155 Steroidogenesis in the adrenal cortex: functional zonation.

in the juxtaglomerular cells of the kidney, is released in response to sodium or volume depletion. In plasma, renin catalyses the formation of angiotensin I from angiotensinogen, a precursor protein made in the liver. In the lungs, *angiotensin-converting enzyme* (ACE) permits conversion of angiotensin I to angiotensin II, with the latter stimulating aldosterone production and secretion by increasing P-450scc activity. High potassium also stimulates aldosterone secretion by a direct effect on zona glomerulosa cells. The enzyme involved in the late pathway for aldosterone synthesis is also a cytochrome P-450. P-450$_{AS}$ catalyses the three steps involved in converting 11-deoxycorticosterone to aldosterone. Aldosterone increases sodium retention and potassium excretion following binding to mineralocorticoid receptors in the distal convoluted tubule and collecting ducts of the kidney. Other tissues affected by aldosterone include sweat, salivary and intestinal glands.

Pathology

As with many endocrine glands, there can be undersecretion or oversecretion of adrenal cortical hormones. Since aldosterone and cortisol secretion are both controlled by other hormones (angiotensin II and ACTH, respectively), adrenal hypofunction and hyperfunction can be either primary or secondary. Diagnosis often relies on suppression and stimulation tests, which depend upon negative feedback control mechanisms.

17.4 The hypothalamic–pituitary–gonadal axis

Learning objectives

You should be able to:

- outline the hypothalamic–pituitary–gonadal axis in terms of negative feedback

- describe the two-cell hypothesis in the ovary accounting for the synthesis of oestradiol and how it relates to FSH and LH

- explain in outline the ovarian cycle

- describe the role of 5α-reductase in the synthesis of dihydrotestosterone.

Complex interactions existing between the components of this system are critical for sexual differentiation, puberty, the ovarian cycle and spermatogenesis. Gonadotrophin-releasing hormone (GnRH) from the hypothalamus controls the secretion of two hormones from the anterior pituitary: luteinising hormone (LH; luteotropin) and follicle-stimulating hormone (FSH); these, in turn, are responsible for the control of the gonads (Fig. 156). The female gonad (ovary) produces the steroid hormones oestradiol and progesterone. The

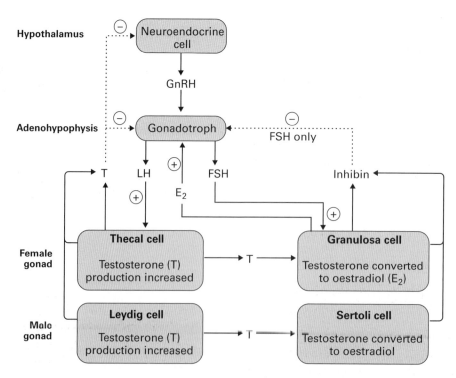

Fig. 156 The hypothalamic–pituitary–gonadal cortical axis.

male gonad (testis) makes testosterone, which has a vital role in male sexual differentiation and the development of the male phenotype. Negative feedback control is an essential feature of this endocrine axis. Hormones produced during pregnancy in the placenta include progesterone, oestrogens and human chorionic gonadotrophin (hCG). The oestrogens are produced from androgens, much of which arises from the fetal adrenal.

Testosterone

In males, the Leydig cells (interstitial cells) produce testosterone from cholesterol under the control of LH. Within the male gonad, testosterone is also a prohormone serving as a precursor for the formation of oestrogen in the Sertoli cells. Testosterone also has an anabolic effect leading to increased size of kidney, heart and skeletal muscle mass; it also has behavioural effects, being largely responsible for the development of the male phenotype. Testosterone is the precursor of 5α-dihydrotestosterone (DHT), which is essential for differentiation of the urogenital sinus and tubercle to prostate and external genitalia. This is an example of testosterone acting as a prohormone. The formation of DHT requires the presence of a steroid 5α-reductase in target tissues. An XY fetus lacking 5α-reductase will be born with ambiguous genitalia and appear to be female.

In females, testosterone serves as the precursor of oestradiol. The latter crucial hormone is made in granulosa cells of the pre-ovulatory ovary from testosterone made in thecal cells. LH stimulates androgen production by thecal cells and FSH stimulates oestrogen production by activating granulosa cell *aromatase*.

Oestrogens and progesterone

They are both synthesised in the ovary and their levels fluctuate during ovarian cycles. A rise in oestradiol secretion near the mid-point of the ovarian cycle leads to increased LH secretion and soon thereafter to ovulation. Progesterone is synthesised from cholesterol and is produced in large amounts by the corpus luteum. Increased oestradiol and progesterone are required for essential proliferative changes in the uterus in the luteal phase of the ovarian cycle.

17.5 The hypothalamic–pituitary–thyroid axis

Learning objectives

You should be able to:

- outline the hypothalamic–pituitary–thyroid axis in terms of negative feedback

- explain the concept of thyroxine as a 'prohormone'
- describe the role of TBG in thyroid hormone transport
- identify hormonal levels in thyroid disease.

The thyroid hormones, thyroxine (T_4) and triiodothyronine (T_3), are iodinated amino acids synthesised in the follicular epithelial cells of the thyroid gland. They have significant effects on almost all tissues in the body. Their production is controlled by thyroid-stimulating hormone (TSH, thyrotrophin) originating in the anterior pituitary. TSH, in turn, is regulated by thyrotrophin-releasing hormone (TRH) secreted from the hypothalamus (Fig. 157). TSH influences all metabolic steps in thyroidal follicular cells, including iodide uptake, iodination and processing of thyroglobulin. Details of thyroxine biosynthesis were presented in section 17.1 and Figure 150.

Important points about the thyroid hormones are:

- T_4 is the major hormone secreted by the thyroid and it serves as the precursor of T_3.
- T_3 is much more active than T_4.
- T_4 and T_3 are bound to a very large degree by plasma proteins; thyroxine binding globulin (TBG) made in the liver is the principal plasma protein involved.

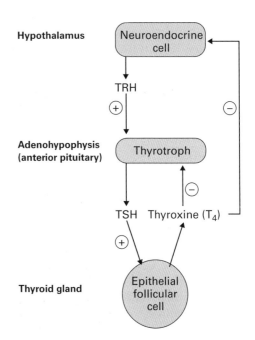

Fig. 157 The hypothalamic–pituitary–thyroidal axis.

Pathology

Thyroid hypofunction and hyperfunction can be either primary or secondary.

Graves' disease is a common form of hyperthyroidism where patients have in their blood thyroid-stimulating antibodies, which bind to TSH receptors and cause thyroid hyperactivity. Serum T_4 and T_3 are elevated, therefore TSH levels in these patients will be much below normal (negative feedback control again).

Primary hypothyroidism can involve congenital defects in thyroid hormone biosynthesis or destruction of the thyroid by thyroid autoantibodies. If hypothyroidism exists in a subject during growth and development, he or she may show mental retardation as well as stunted growth (cretinism). It is now established practice to test newborn children to ensure that they are not hypothyroid. Chronic iodine deficiency leads to goitre (an enlarged thyroid gland), and areas of the world where endemic goitre is common have low iodide in the environment. It is most common in mountainous regions (e.g. Alps, Himalayas and Andes).

17.6 The endocrine control of calcium and phosphate

Learning objectives

You should be able to:

- describe the functions of calcium and phosphate in the body and the importance of tight control of $[Ca^{2+}]_p$

- explain the role of parathyroid hormone in the control of calcium and phosphate metabolism

- outline the pathway for calcitriol synthesis and its role in the body

- describe the source of calcitonin and its role in the body.

Calcium through its presence in bones and teeth is the major mineral in the body but it has many other critical roles. Therefore, it is not at all surprising that calcium levels in the plasma and in the cytoplasm of cells are finely controlled. The control is mainly through the action of parathyroid hormone (PTH) and calcitriol, a hormone derived from vitamin D. Calcium and phosphate are intimately linked in bone but their metabolic roles in cells are quite different.

Functions of calcium ions

- *Intracellular*: muscle contraction; cell motility; secretion phenomena; nerve function; growth and differentiation; second messenger involved in the action of many hormones.
- *Extracellular*: cell adhesion; aggregation of platelets; membrane integrity; blood coagulation.

Functions of phosphate ions

- *Intracellular*: buffering; energy metabolism (sugar phosphates, ATP); component of membranes (phospholipids); component of nucleic acids; modification of many enzymes through cycles of phosphorylation/dephosphorylation; in signal molecules (2,3-BPG, cyclic AMP, inositol triphosphate).
- *Extracellular*: buffering (especially important in urine).

Calcium homeostasis

In any normal individual, there are only very minute fluctuations in plasma calcium ion levels despite variable intake of calcium in the diet and the potential to excrete calcium in urine. This implies close regulation. This is done by the parathyroid glands located behind the thyroid in the neck region. These glands (usually four in number in humans) synthesise and secrete parathyroid hormone, which, in effect, protects against hypocalcaemia by direct actions on bone and kidney and indirect actions on the gastrointestinal tract. Vitamin D (cholecalciferol) is a fat-soluble vitamin that has been known for a long time to be essential for efficient calcium absorption. Lack of vitamin D is classically associated with the development of rickets and osteomalacia in growing children, leading to impaired bone formation and the classical picture of bow legs. It became clear that vitamin D per se could not be directly involved in promoting increased calcium absorption in the gut. We now know that vitamin D is the precursor of *calcitriol*, which is the hormone involved in the control of calcium absorption.

Calcitonin is another hormone potentially involved in calcium homeostasis. Here are key points about the three participants.

Parathyroid hormone (Fig. 158)
- Polypeptide made in the chief cells of the parathyroid gland.
- Secretion is triggered by low plasma calcium ion (Ca^{2+}) levels; high plasma calcium ion levels have the opposite effect.

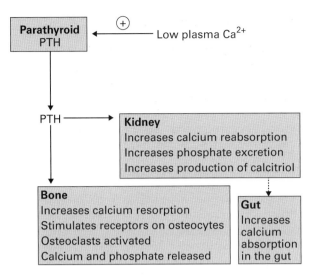

Fig. 158 Actions of parathyroid hormone (PTH).

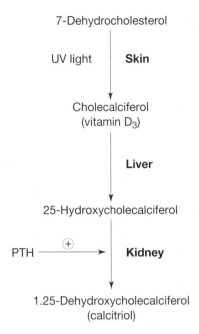

Fig. 159 The synthesis of cholecalciferol and its conversion to calcitriol.

- Action on kidney increases calcium reabsorption and phosphate excretion. It also increases calcitriol production.
- PTH increases bone resorption. PTH is usually described as acting on bone resorption by increasing osteoclastic activity. Osteoclasts produce acid hydrolases and acids that aid in resorption. However, osteoclasts do not possess PTH receptors, so the activation of osteoclasts is indirect via effects on osteoblasts (which do have PTH receptors), which then release factors that stimulate osteoclasts (i.e. it is a paracrine system). The dissolution of bone mineral leads to the release of calcium and phosphate into blood.

Calcitriol (Fig. 159)

- 25-Hydroxycholecalciferol is converted to calcitriol in the kidney proximal tubule by the action of a 1-hydroxylase stimulated by PTH.
- When calcium levels are normal, the 25-hydroxycholecalciferol is converted to inactive 24,25-dihydroxycholecalciferol.
- Calcitriol acts on the gut to increase the synthesis of a calcium binding protein and also to increase phosphate absorption. The calcitriol receptor in the gut is a nuclear protein analogous to those for steroid hormones.
- *Pathology*. Low intake or low production of vitamin D leads to osteomalacia. Impaired bone formation can also occur if there is a lack of 1-hydroxylase in the kidney with renal osteodystrophy being a finding in patients with end-stage renal disease.

Calcitonin

- Calcitonin is a peptide made in the parafollicular cells of the thyroid gland (T_4 is made in the epithelial follicular cells).
- Presumably secreted in response to high plasma levels of calcium ions. However, it is thought to be of little physiological importance in humans, except (possibly) in pregnancy, where it could have a role in promoting loading of calcium into the bones of the mother.
- Calcitonin is very active when administered to humans and has therapeutic uses.
- Calcitonin promotes the laying down of calcium into bone and it inhibits calcium reabsorption in the kidney.

17.7 Hormones of the adrenal medulla

Learning objectives

You should be able to:

- describe the hormones of the adrenal medulla and their role in the body.

The adrenal medulla and cortex are embryologically, anatomically and functionally separate. The medulla receives some of its blood supply from the cortex. It receives a rich nerve supply of preganglionic sympathetic fibres. The adrenal medulla has the ability to synthesise catecholamines such as adrenaline (epinephrine) and noradrenaline (norepinephrine) starting from the amino acid tyrosine (Figs 151 and 152). Adrenaline (epinephrine) is a 'stress' hormone, classically associated with 'fight' and 'flight'.

17.8 Other hormonal systems

Learning objectives

You should be able to:

- explain the roles of erythropoietin and atrial natriuretic factor in the body.

Erythropoietin

The remarkable constancy of the circulating red cell mass in adults suggests that the process of erythropoiesis is rigidly controlled. Exposure to low oxygen tensions increases erythropoiesis, whereas hyperoxia reverses this. The glycoprotein hormone erythropoietin stimulates erythropoiesis and its production in the kidney is sensitive to changes in pO_2. Erythropoietin binds to a cell surface receptor in erythroid progenitor cells in bone marrow.

Atrial natriuretic factor

Atrial natriuretic factor (ANF) is a small peptide that is synthesised in cardiocytes in the right atrium in response to hypervolaemia and hypernatraemia. It has actions at several sites including the kidney, where it increases sodium excretion and inhibits renin secretion. The latter effect will lead to decreased activity of the renin–angiotensin system, lower aldosterone secretion and, again, increased sodium excretion. It also inhibits ADH secretion from the posterior pituitary. The sum of these actions is to counteract any increase in the sodium and water content of the body. It also acts on peripheral resistance arteries by a mechanism involving a receptor with innate guanylate cyclase activity. The resulting increase in cyclic GMP leads to phosphorylation of key proteins.

17.9 Mechanisms of hormone action

Learning objectives

At the end of this section you should be able to:

- outline signal transduction pathways for water-soluble hormones that involve the G proteins G_s, G_i and G_q

- describe the signal transduction pathways involving the tyrosine kinase family of receptors

- describe the signal transduction pathways for lipid-soluble hormones such as thyroid hormones and steroid hormones

- describe the messenger system involving nitric oxide and the role of nitric oxide synthase.

All hormones influence processes in the body by interacting with protein receptors located in target tissues. Since each hormone has a unique chemical structure it should be obvious that a receptor must recognise that unique structure: binding elicits a signal that is transduced in the target cell. The two major subgroups of hormones, water-soluble and lipid-soluble, generate signals that are quite distinct from one another and have receptors that are in the cell plasma membrane or within the cell, respectively.

Transduction of signals from water-soluble hormones

There are three types of signal transduction systems known:

- cyclic AMP
- inositol phosphates and diacylglycerol
- tyrosine kinase family of receptors.

Cyclic 3',5'-AMP and protein kinase A

The discovery of a second messenger in the transduction of signals from adrenaline (epinephrine) and glucagon was a major advance in understanding the transmission of signals within cells. The compound was an adenine nucleotide called adenosine 3',5'-monophosphate (Fig. 160), otherwise known as cyclic AMP. It is produced by the action of the enzyme *adenylate cyclase* on ATP. Cyclic AMP activates a *protein kinase* (protein kinase A; PKA) by binding to and removing inhibitory subunits of the enzyme, thus liberating the active catalytic subunits. PKA then phosphorylates hydroxyl groups on serines or threonines in certain proteins leading to dramatic changes in their activities. For example, the binding of adrenaline (epinephrine) to β-adrenoceptors on skeletal muscle leads to an increase in cyclic AMP, activation of PKA and phosphorylation and activation of phosphorylase kinase; this then converts inactive phosphorylase b to active phosphorylase a with a resultant increase in glycogenolysis in muscle (Ch. 7, p. 99). A similar series of events is associated with the

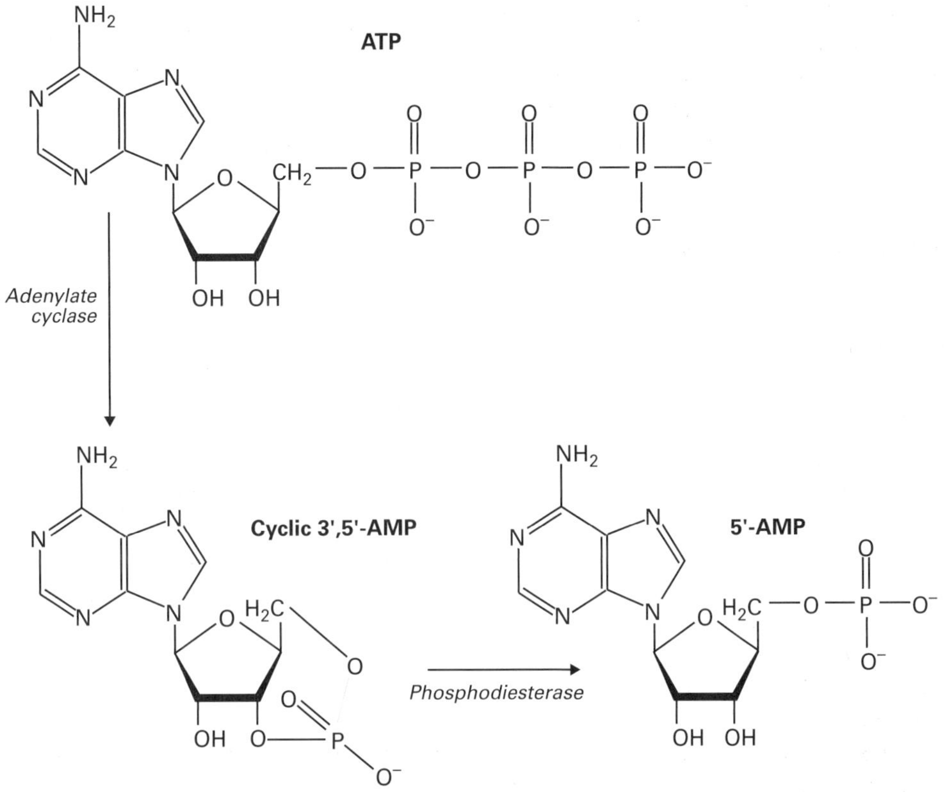

Fig. 160 Cyclic AMP production and metabolism.

activation of liver phosphorylase by the action of glucagon. Cyclic AMP levels are returned to basal levels by the action of a phosphodiesterase, which converts the cyclic AMP to AMP (Fig. 160).

The transmission of the signal from the hormone outside the cell to the adenylate cyclase inside the cell involves G proteins. Following binding of certain hormones to their receptors, GTP binds to the alpha subunit of the G protein ($G_s\alpha$) causing it to dissociate. The $G_s\alpha$-GTP binds to adenylate cyclase, leading to its activation. The signal transduction pathway is shown in Figure 161. Also shown is the switch-off pathway involving a GTPase activity, also present in the $G_s\alpha$ subunit.

Other hormones bind to receptors that are linked to a related G protein, G_i, which suppresses adenylate cyclase activity and thus reduces cyclic AMP levels in target tissues. The mechanism is similar to that seen with G_s in that when the hormone binds to receptor GTP displaces GDP from G_i and $G_i\alpha$-GTP dissociates from the $\beta\gamma$ subunits and binds to adenylate cyclase, leading to its inhibition (Fig. 161). The $G_i\alpha$, like the $G_s\alpha$ subunit, has GTPase activity which is involved in switching off this system. One example of such a hormone is somatostatin interacting with α_2-adrenoceptors. For inhibitory hormones to have an effect, G_s must already be activated by a stimulatory hormone.

Clinical note:
Cholera toxin

Further insight into the details of the pathway involving G_s comes from studies with cholera toxin, the agent in cholera patients that causes massive loss of sodium and water and diarrhoea. Cholera toxin in cells of the gastrointestinal tract uses NAD^+ to bring about the ADP-ribosylation of the $G_s\alpha$ subunit, leading to inhibition of its GTPase. As a result, G_s is permanently activated and large amounts of cyclic AMP are formed and maintained, leading to the gut changes.

Clinical note:
Pertussis toxin

Further insight into the G_i pathway has come from the study of the action of pertussis toxin, the active agent produced by *Bordetella pertussis* involved in whooping cough. Pertussis toxin can ADP-ribosylate the $G_i\alpha$ subunit but only when in its GDP-bound inactive state. GTP cannot exchange for GDP and the net effect is to increase cyclic AMP levels. When this occurs in the respiratory tract, there is excessive secretion of fluid from cells of the airways.

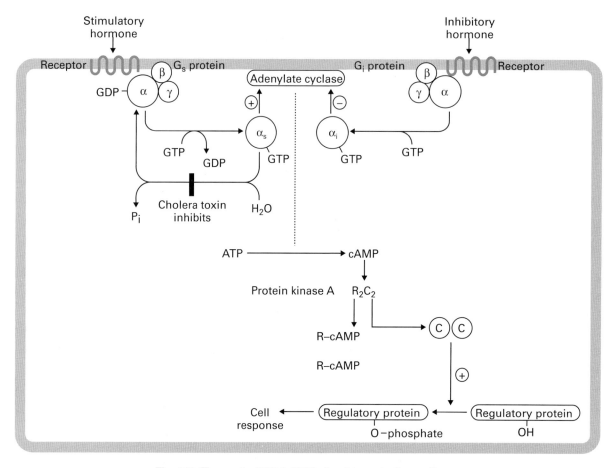

Fig. 161 The cyclic AMP (cAMP) signal transduction pathway.

Clearly, cyclic AMP is a very significant second messenger and its action will depend upon the specific characteristics of the cell in which it is produced. Although most of the initial studies on its effects involved phosphorylation/dephosphorylation of key enzymes in metabolic pathways, it is also involved in the control of gene expression. That mechanism involves a transcription factor, cyclic AMP response element binding protein (CREB), which becomes active upon phosphorylation by PKA and which can bind to a DNA promoter sequence (CRE). Altered gene expression results, leading to the transcription of genes containing such CRE sequences.

It is the balance between adenylate cyclase forming cyclic AMP and phosphodiesterase activity breaking it down that will determine metabolic activity in a target cell (Fig. 161). Drugs present in tea and coffee, theophylline and caffeine, are inhibitors of cyclic AMP phosphodiesterase and they have significant effects upon body functions such as cardiac output and renal diuresis.

Inositol phosphates and diacylglycerol

Several hormones act by changing the intracellular calcium ion concentration, leading to the activation of protein kinase C (PKC). One way in which this occurs is by activation of phosphoinositide-specific phospholipase C (PI-PLC) following binding of such a hormone to its receptor with, in some cases, another G protein, G_q, functioning in the pathway. The substrate for PI-PLC action is phosphatidylinositol bisphosphate (PIP_2), a phospholipid present in the inner layer of the phospholipid bilayer that makes up the plasma membrane. The products are diacylglycerol (DAG) and inositol

Clinical note:
Lithium inhibition of IP_3 metabolism

Some of the IP_3 metabolising enzymes are inhibited by lithium; this may explain how it acts in the treatment of dementia.

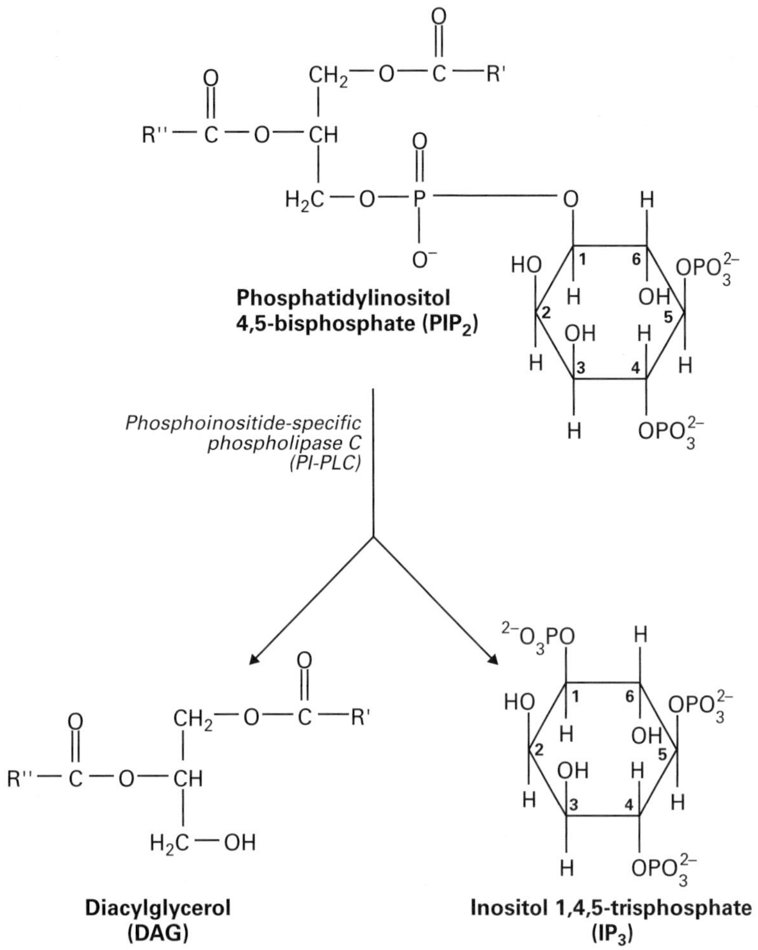

Fig. 162 Generation of two second messengers from PIP$_2$.

1,4,5-trisphosphate (IP$_3$) (Fig. 162), which act as second messengers (Fig. 163). IP$_3$ causes the release of calcium that is sequestered in the endoplasmic reticulum. This leads to activation of several systems including those involving calmodulin (e.g. phosphorylase kinase). DAG is an activator of PKC, which brings about the phosphorylation of serine and threonine residues in other key proteins (that are not substrates for PKA). Examples of hormones that act through this signal transduction mechanism are: angiotensin II, controlling aldosterone secretion in the adrenal cortex; TRH, controlling TSH secretion from the anterior pituitary; and adrenaline (epinephrine), acting through α_1-adrenoceptors to control glycogenolysis in the liver (in muscle, adrenaline (epinephrine) acts through cyclic AMP–PKA systems). Several products of IP$_3$ metabolism have biological activity.

The tyrosine kinase family of receptors

A third type of signal transduction system is involved with the action of insulin and various growth factors on target cells. The details of insulin action with its receptor were described in Chapter 10 and Figure 98.

Other growth factors that have plasma membrane receptor tyrosine kinase receptors include:

- insulin-like growth factor I (IGF-1): the mediator of growth hormone action on cartilage
- epidermal growth factor (EGF): stimulates growth of epidermal and epithelial cells
- platelet-derived growth factor (PDGF): stimulates growth of mesenchymal and glial cells
- transforming growth factor alpha (TGFα): related to EGF.

There is great interest in growth factors given the fact that several oncogene products are growth factors.

Transduction of signals from lipid-soluble hormones

Thyroid and steroid hormones are lipid-soluble and are able to enter many if not all cells in the body and

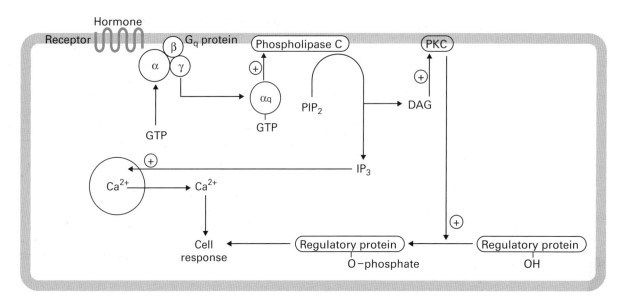

Fig. 163 The inositol phosphate–diacyglycerol signal transduction pathway.

Table 32 The nuclear receptor superfamily

| | Homology compared with the glucocorticoid receptor | |
Receptor for	DNA binding domain	Ligand binding domain
Mineralocorticoids (MR)	94	57
Progesterone (PR)	90	55
Androgens (AR)	77	50
Oestrogens (ER)	52	30
Thyroid hormones (T_3R)	47	17
Calcitriol (VDR)	42	<15
Retinoic acid (RAR)	45	15

influence their function. Their intracellular receptors are members of a superfamily of nuclear receptors. The C-terminal regions, which show the greatest heterology, are the hormone binding domains of these receptors. The DNA binding domain of the receptor consists of two zinc fingers and is highly conserved; for example, the sequence of the glucocorticoid receptor in this region differs only in three residues from that of the mineralocorticoid receptor (Table 32). The N-terminal domain of these receptors is rather variable.

Having entered a target cell, these hormones bind to cytosolic- or nuclear-located receptors which are associated with chaperone proteins (Fig. 164). In the absence of hormone, the chaperones maintain the receptors in an inactive state. Binding of hormone dissociates this complex and the hormone–receptor complex binds to specific DNA sequences termed hormone-response elements (HRE), which are about 15 base pairs long

with a partial palindromic sequence. The outcome is transcription of specific genes and synthesis of specific proteins that bring about the physiological effect of the hormone in question.

It is of interest that cortisol (a glucocorticoid) and aldosterone both bind efficiently to the mineralocorticoid receptor in kidney. Given the fact that the circulating cortisol concentration far exceeds that of aldosterone, the question must be asked, will the receptor not always be fully occupied by cortisol and, therefore, never be responsive to aldosterone. The answer is that, in aldosterone target tissues such as the kidney, the receptor is protected by an enzyme, *11β-hydroxysteroid dehydrogenase type II*, which metabolises any cortisol to its inactive metabolite, cortisone.

Recent evidence has indicated that there are *non-genomic* effects due to steroid hormones, implying that they can interact and affect plasma membrane systems.

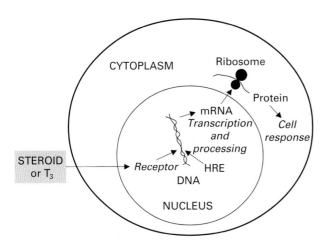

Fig. 164 Signal transduction of steroid and thyroid hormones.

Other messenger systems

Surprisingly, it has been shown that the gas nitric oxide (NO) is an intercellular messenger; it is of particular importance in the blood vessels where it influences their dilation. NO is released by endothelial cells under the influence of changes in intracellular calcium levels. NO is produced by the action of the enzyme *NO synthase* using arginine as substrate, the other product being citrulline. Guanylate cyclase is activated by NO and, as a result, cyclic GMP levels increase. Cyclic GMP stimulates a cyclic GMP-dependent protein kinase that brings about relaxation of smooth muscle.

Nitroglycerine, a substance used to alleviate the pain caused by insufficient blood flow to heart muscle (angina), acts as a vasodilator with the mediator being NO.

17

Self-assessment: questions

Single best answer MCQs

1. From your knowledge of the physicochemical properties of hormones identify the correct statement or statements concerning water-soluble hormones.
   a. Insulin, thyroid-stimulating hormone (TSH), cortisol and thyroxine are all very water-soluble
   b. Their half-lives are longer than those of lipid-soluble hormones
   c. They bind to plasma membrane receptors
   d. a and c are both correct
   e. b and c are both correct

2. Angiotensin II production will be increased as a result of which one of the following?
   a. A decrease in serum potassium concentration
   b. An increase in serum calcium concentration
   c. An increase in plasma renin activity
   d. An increase in serum sodium

3. Which area in the adrenal gland undergoes atrophy after hypophysectomy?
   a. Adrenal capsule
   b. Zona glomerulosa (ZG)
   c. Zona fasciculata (ZF)

4. What cells in the islets of Langerhans respond to elevated levels of blood glucose by secreting insulin?
   a. Alpha cells
   b. Beta cells
   c. Delta cells

5. A decrease of serum calcium (Ca^{2+}) levels would cause one of the following?
   a. A decrease of calcitriol formation
   b. An increase in 25-hydroxycholecalciferol 24-hydroxylase activity
   c. An increase in 25-hydroxycholecalciferol 1-hydroxylase activity
   d. Increased secretion of a hormone from C cells
   e. All of the above are correct.

6. Select the correct statement or statements concerning hormone biosynthesis.
   a. Hypothalamic hormones such as TRH whose amino acid sequence is pyro-Glu-His-Pro-amide are synthesised from large precursors

   b. All steroid hormones produced in the gonads or the adrenal cortex are synthesised from cholic acid
   c. The thyroid gland is one of several glands in the body that can concentrate iodide and then use iodine to iodinate proteins
   d. Both a and b are correct
   e. a, b and c are all correct

7. Demonstrate your understanding of hypothalamic control of the pituitary by identifying the single correct statement.
   a. In Graves' disease caused by a thyroid-stimulating immunoglobulin (TSI), circulating levels of TSH (thyroid-stimulating hormone) are much lower than in normal subjects
   b. Injection of a large dose of cortisol into a normal subject stimulates both ACTH (adrenocorticotrophin) and endogenous cortisol production
   c. Cutting the blood supply from the hypothalamus to the anterior pituitary leads to decreased secretion of all of the anterior pituitary hormones
   d. In a patient with primary hypothyroidism, blood levels of TSH will be very low
   e. The hypothalamic control of growth hormone only involves a releasing hormone (GHRH; growth hormone releasing hormone)

8. Select from the list below the steroid hormone that increases in blood towards the mid-point of the ovarian cycle leading to a surge in LH (luteinising hormone) secretion.
   a. Testosterone
   b. Dehydroepiandrosterone
   c. Oestradiol
   d. Progesterone
   e. Cortisol

9. Identify the single correct statement concerning the endocrine control of calcium and phosphate.
   a. Increasing calcium reabsorption in the kidney is the only mechanism available for increasing $[Ca^{2+}]_p$ in the body
   b. 1,25-Dihydroxycholecalciferol (calcitriol) production in the kidney is stimulated by calcitonin

c. PTH (parathyroid hormone) action on bone occurs via binding of this hormone to PTH receptors on osteoclasts

d. PTH action on the kidney inhibits phosphate reabsorption leading to increased phosphate excretion

e. Both hypophosphataemia and hypocalcaemia lead to decreased production of calcitriol in the kidney

10. Upon binding of glucagon, the glucagon receptor affects its target cell metabolism by:
    a. Causing autophosphorylation of some of its own tyrosyl residues
    b. Interacting directly with the cell's transcriptional machinery
    c. Causing the α-subunit of the membrane-bound complex G_s to dissociate after binding GTP
    d. Causing the membrane-bound complex G_i to be dissociated
    e. Interacting directly with adenylate cyclase to increase cyclic AMP levels in the cell

11. Steroid hormone receptors:
    a. have structural features in common with receptors for thyroid hormones
    b. have a molecular domain that can recognise specific nucleotide sequences in control genes
    c. Are relatively specific in their ability to bind only steroid hormones of a particular class (e.g. oestrogens, glucocorticoids, etc.)
    d. a and c are both correct
    e. a, b and c are all correct

True/false questions

Are the following statements true or false?

1. Destruction of the adrenal cortex in a subject (leading to primary hypoadrenocorticism) will result in pigmentation, which is a useful clinical sign.
2. LH and FSH are controlled by the same hypothalamic releasing hormone.
3. In normal subjects, aldosterone secretion is increased by either sodium depletion or potassium loading.

4. Inositol 1,4,5-trisphosphate (IP_3) and diacylglycerol are hormonal second messengers produced when phospholipase C acts upon the membrane phosphatidylinositol 4,5-bisphosphate (PIP_2).
5. An early consequence of the binding of insulin to its receptor is the phosphorylation of tyrosine residues in the receptor, which then interacts with IRS (insulin receptor substrate) molecules.
6. Erythropoietin production by the kidney is increased by a low pO_2 in the blood supply to the kidney.
7. Cholera toxin interferes with the function of both G_s and G_i.
8. ADH (antidiuretic hormone) secretion is inhibited in normal subjects by water loading.
9. Pregnenolone is the precursor of aldosterone, cortisol and cholecalciferol.
10. Oestrogen production from androgen in Sertoli cells involves the formation of an aromatic ring.
11. Cortisol inhibits the expression of the PNMT (phenylethanolamine N-methyltransferase) gene in the adrenal medulla.
12. The insulin receptor and the adrenaline (epinephrine) β-adrenoceptor have similar structures and employ similar signal transduction mechanisms.
13. Atrial natriuretic factor (ANF) stimulates aldosterone secretion.
14. A defect in steroid 5α-reductase affects the level of dihydrotestosterone in various tissues in the male.
15. Steroids must have a 11β-hydroxyl group to be active as glucocorticoids.

Short essay questions

1. Give an outline of how steroid hormones are synthesised in the body.
2. Describe possible causes for a newborn child having elevated levels of thyroid-stimulating hormone (TSH) in its blood.
3. Write short notes on each of the following:
   a. pertussis toxin
   b. diacylglycerol
   c. phosphodiesterase
   d. hormone-response element
4. Outline the role of the skin, kidney and lung in the endocrine system.

Self-assessment: answers

Single best answer MCQ answers

1. a. **False**. Thyroxine and cortisol are not water-soluble.
    b. **False**. Because they are not protein-bound, they are turned over at a faster rate than lipid-soluble hormones. This affects their use in therapy!
    c. **True**. After binding, a signal is transduced to internal systems.
    d. **False**. a is incorrect.
    e. **False**. b is incorrect.

2. a. **False**. Aldosterone is increased in response to hyperkalaemia. The effect is direct on the zona glomerulosa.
    b. **False**. No known connection between the two.
    c. **True**. Renin stimulates angiotensin II production which leads to AII production through the action of converting enzyme.
    d. **False**. Increased sodium decreases renin which in turn decreases AII.

3. a. **False**. There isn't pituitary control of the adrenal capsule.
    b. **False**. It is the inner zones that are controlled by ACTH; ZG is controlled by the renin–angiotensin system.
    c. **True**. ACTH stimulates ZF growth and cortisol production.

4. a. **False**. They are the source of glucagon.
    b. **True**. These are the cells that respond to hyperglycaemia.
    c. **False**. These are the cells that synthesise somatostatin.

5. a. **False**. PTH (parathyroid hormone) increases in response to hypocalcaemia leading to increased calcitriol formation.
    b. **False**. PTH increases in response to hypocalcaemia; this reduces 24-hydroxylation of 25-hydroxy-vitamin D and stimulates 1-hydroxylation of 25-hydroxy-vitamin D. Normocalcaemia causes an increase in 24-hydroxylation!
    c. **True**. This occurs due to the increase in PTH and calcitriol production increases.
    d. **False**. C cells secrete calcitonin; if anything, calcitonin secretion would decrease in response to hypocalcaemia.
    e. **False**. a, b and d are all incorrect!

6. a. **True**. There is no mechanism for synthesising this tripeptide from three amino acids.
    b. **False**. The precursor is cholesterol.
    c. **False**. It is only in the thyroid where iodination occurs.
    d. **False**. b is incorrect.
    e. **False**. b and c are incorrect.

7. a. **True**. TSI has TSH-like actions on the thyroid so excess thyroxine is produced and this will feedback to inhibit TSH secretion.
    b. **False**. ACTH is inhibited and, as a consequence, cortisol production falls.
    c. **False**. Prolactin *increases* because the control from the hypothalamus is inhibitory and cutting the blood supply removes that inhibitor.
    d. **False**. The impaired thyroid function means that thyroxine levels will be very low and the obvious consequence is elevated TSH in plasma. This finding is diagnostic of primary hypothyroidism!
    e. **False**. Somatostatin is also involved and its action is inhibitory.

8. a. **False**. This is a very unlikely candidate in a woman.
    b. **False**. This weak androgen is adrenal in origin.
    c. **True**. Hormone synthesis in the thecal and granulosa cells combine to give lots of oestradiol and this feeds back *positively* on LH and the surge in LH causes ovulation.
    d. **False**. Progesterone production comes *after* ovulation.
    e. **False**. Another unlikely candidate from the adrenal cortex.

9. a. **False**. Bone resorption is another obvious mechanism; also increased calcium absorption in the gut.
    b. **False**. PTH is the stimulator of calcitriol production in the kidney.
    c. **False**. Osteoclasts are activated but they lack PTH receptors. The PTH receptors are on osteocytes and they communicate with osteoclasts (paracrine!).
    d. **True**. This is the so-called 'phosphaturic' action of PTH.
    e. **False**. Hypocalcaemia increases calcitriol via an increase in PTH. Hypophosphataemia has a direct effect on calcitriol production.

10. a. **False**. That describes insulin mechanism of action.
    b. **False**. All actions are via a second messenger.
    c. **True**. G_s is involved. GTP binds, the α-subunit of G_s dissociates leading to activation of adenylate cyclase and an increase in cyclic AMP.
    d. **False**. It acts through G_s.
    e. **False**. It acts via a G protein system (G_s).

11. a. **True**. The homology is especially high in the DNA binding domain of the receptor.
    b. **True**. This is the DNA binding domain.
    c. **True**. Their specificity resides in the hormone binding domains, which have much reduced homologies.
    d. **True** but not the single best answer.
    e. This is the single best answer.

True/false answers

1. **True**. The inability to synthesise cortisol leads to high secretion of ACTH and it has MSH (melanocyte-stimulating hormone) activity.
2. **True**. Despite a long search for unique separate releasing hormones for LH and FSH, GnRH (gonadotrophin-releasing hormone) appears to function for both.
3. **True**. Aldosterone action is critical to the fine control of both electrolytes. The sodium effect is via the renin–aldosterone system. Potassium effect is direct.
4. **True**. Calcium plays a vital role in the mechanism of action of hormones that work through DAG (diacylglycerol) and IP_3 (inositol triphosphate). Protein kinase C is activated in this pathway.
5. **True**. This is termed 'autophosphorylation'.
6. **True**. This is an attempt to compensate for low pO_2 by increasing red cell production.
7. **False**. Cholera toxin acts through preventing the inactivation of $G_s\alpha$.
8. **True**. This enables water to be excreted in greater amounts to compensate.
9. **False**. Pregnenolone is the precursor of aldosterone and cortisol but it is 7-dehydrocholesterol which is the precursor of cholecalciferol (vitamin D) in the skin.
10. **True**. Oestrogens are the only steroid hormones with aromatic A rings.
11. **False**. Cortisol induces PNMT by increasing transcription of the PNMT gene.
12. **False**. Both receptors are in plasma membranes but are quite distinct structurally. The insulin receptor has tyrosine kinase activity. The adrenaline (epinephrine) receptor has a series of domains that span the plasma membrane seven times.
13. **False**. ANF is part of the system that opposes aldosterone.
14. **True** The prostate is affected and secondary male sex characteristics.
15. **True** Cortisone per se is inactive until reduced to cortisol.

Short essay answers

1. The key points are:

   - Cholesterol (C_{27}) is the precursor of all steroid hormones.
   - Steroid hormone-producing tissues receive the cholesterol from plasma LDL (low-density lipoprotein) through receptor-mediated endocytosis.
   - The initial and rate-controlling reaction is the cleavage of six carbons from the side chain of cholesterol to give pregnenolone. The enzyme involved is cholesterol side chain cleavage cytochrome P-450 (P-450scc), a member of a large gene family.
   - The steroid hormone pathways from pregnenolone then vary according to tissue and cell type.
   - In order for cortisol and androgen to be made, 17α-hydroxylase has to be present. In the adrenal cortex, that activity is restricted to the zonae fasciculata and reticularis, with the former making cortisol, the chief glucocorticoid in the body, and the latter making mainly dehydroepiandrosterone (DHEA) and its sulphate.
   - 17-Hydroxypregnenolone is the precursor of DHEA, which can be converted to testosterone and other androgens; testosterone is made in the granulosa cells of the ovary and Leydig cells of the testes.
   - In the Sertoli cells of the testes and the granulosa cells of the ovary, androgens such as testosterone are aromatised to give oestrogens.
   - In the zona glomerulosa of the adrenal cortex, 17α-hydroxylase is absent but there is another cytochrome P-450, aldosterone synthase, which accounts for that zone's ability to make aldosterone, the principal mineralocorticoid in the body.
   - In the corpus luteum and in the placenta, pregnenolone is converted to progesterone, which has important effects upon the uterus and is necessary for the maintenance of pregnancy.

- The rate-controlling cholesterol side chain cleavage step is controlled by different hormones in different tissues: ACTH (adrenocorticotrophin) controls it in the zonae fasciculata and reticularis of the adrenal; angiotensin II controls it in the zona glomerulosa of the adrenal; LH (luteinising hormone) controls it in ovarian thecal cells and Leydig cells of the testes.
- The cytochromes P-450 that catalyse the hydroxylation reactions involved in steroidogenesis use molecular oxygen and have a requirement for NADPH.

2. The very high levels of TSH (thyroid-stimulating hormone) are diagnostic of primary hypothyroidism. The thyroid is defective in its ability to make T_4 (thyroxine). The molecular basis can be defects in any of the steps of thyroid hormone biosynthesis. The consequence is that TRH (thyrotrophin-releasing hormone) and TSH from the hypothalamus and pituitary, respectively, are secreted in increased amounts. Given the fact that these infants have low thyroid hormone levels and the role that T_4 plays in growth and development, it becomes important for them to start therapy with replacement T_4 as soon as possible. For that reason, and given the fact that they are normal at birth because of the T_4 they have obtained from their mothers, all newborn children should be screened for hypothyroidism by having their TSH measured.

3. a. *Pertussis toxin*. This is the toxin produced by the *Bordetella pertussis*, the bacterium that causes whooping cough. It alters the $G_i\alpha$ subunit of the G_i regulatory protein by a process known as ADP-ribosylation. The altered $G_i\alpha$ cannot exchange GTP for GDP and adenylate cyclase is not inhibited in normal fashion. The end result is enhanced secretion of mucus in various parts of the lung.
   b. *Diacylglycerol* (DAG). This is one of the products of phospholipase A_2 action in the plasma membrane on phosphatidylinositol 4,5-bisphosphate. This hydrolysis participates in the response to several hormones. DAG activates protein kinase C, which, in turn, catalyses the phosphorylation of multiple proteins in target tissues for hormones operating by this mechanism.
   c. *Phosphodiesterase* (PDE). This enzyme is critical to terminating the response to a hormone whose action is mediated by cyclic 3',5'-AMP. It does so by hydrolysing cyclic AMP to 5'-AMP and inorganic phosphate. Clearly, cyclic AMP levels in cells are influenced by the relative activities of PDE and adenylate cyclase. The mechanism of action of many hormones involves cyclic AMP, and PDE can be considered to be involved in 'switching off' the response of the cell to the hormone in question. Caffeine, theophylline and related compounds are inhibitors of PDE.
   d. *Hormone-response element* (HRE). HREs are part of the regulatory DNA region involved in the action of steroid and thyroid hormones (and others) on the transcription of genes in target tissues. This element binds a hormone–receptor complex and is usually located a few hundred nucleotides upstream from the transcription initiation site.

4. *Skin*. Vitamin D (cholecalciferol) is synthesised in skin by the action of ultraviolet light on 7-dehydrocholesterol. Cholecalciferol is the precursor of 25-hydroxycholecalciferol (made in the liver), which in turn is converted to the hormone calcitriol in the kidney as part of the defence against hypocalcaemia.
   Kidney. The kidney produces several endocrine factors:

- *Erythropoietin* (EP) is synthesised in the kidney in response to low oxygen tension in blood. The increased red cell synthesis that occurs, stimulated by EP, accounts for the polycythaemia observed in individuals who live at high altitude.
- *Calcitriol* is synthesised in the kidney from 25-hydroxycholecalciferol, stimulated by parathyroid hormone (PTH). PTH is secreted in increased amounts in response to hypocalcaemia. Calcitriol contributes to restoring calcium in blood by increasing calcium absorption in the gut.
- *Renin* is produced in the kidney in response to decreased pulsing pressure through the renal artery and/or reduced filtered sodium. Its role is to produce angiotensin I from angiotensinogen in blood; the angiotensin I is converted to angiotensin II, which by increasing aldosterone production causes increased sodium reabsorption.

The kidney is also the target for several hormones and responds by altering its activity.

- The kidney is a target for *parathyroid hormone* (PTH), with the response being increased calcitriol formation, increased calcium reabsorption and increased phosphate excretion.
- The kidney is also a target *for antidiuretic hormone* (ADH), where the response is to increase water reabsorption.

- The kidney is *the site of action of aldosterone*, the response being increased sodium reabsorption and increased potassium excretion.
- *Atrial natriuretic factor* (ANF) is part of the system that responds to increased blood pressure and volume. It inhibits renin release from the kidney, reducing aldosterone production and sodium reabsorption in the kidney.

Lungs. *Converting enzyme*, which catalyses the conversion of angiotensin I to angiotensin II, is localised to the lung. ACE inhibitors are effective in the treatment of various forms of hypertension where angiotensin II levels should be lowered.

18 Nutrition

Overview

There are multiple examples of nutritional deficiency that often lead to life-threatening disease. The practising doctor needs to know about these conditions and the fundamental aspects of nutrition that pertain to their patients. Examples of nutritional deficiencies include: protein deficiency causing *kwashiorkor*; protein-energy malnutrition causing *marasmus*; vitamin A deficiency leading to *xerophthalmia* (night blindness); vitamin B_{12} deficiency, the cause of *pernicious anaemia*; folate deficiency, which results in megaloblastic anaemia and is now implicated in neural tube defects such as *spina bifida*; iron deficiency, the leading cause of anaemia; and thiamine deficiency resulting in *beri-beri*. Nutritional disease also occurs when there are defects in supply of essential amino acids and fatty acids, and when there is inadequate supply of other vitamins, as well as macronutrient metals such as sodium, potassium, calcium and magnesium and trace elements such as iron, iodine and selenium. Nutritional excess (obesity) is emerging as one of the major health problems in Western society.

18.1 General aspects

Learning objectives

You should be able to:

- define body mass index
- describe how body fat is measured.

It is essential that you have knowledge of functional nutrition; this should include knowing the nutrients in the food that we eat and how they contribute to our well-being, growth and health. Important nutrition issues relate to: growth and development; the relationship between excess fat and coronary heart disease and diabetes mellitus; pregnancy; and malnutrition.

A major impetus for the study of body composition in the population as a whole is the relationship between diet and mortality. Governments are obliged to give advice on diets, and during the past two years there has been an 'order of magnitude' change in the 'Food Guide Pyramid' prepared by the US Department of Agriculture. Advice given in 1992 was oversimplified. The errors arose mainly from the overemphasis on minimising fats in the diet. The old pyramid seemed to encourage the intake of carbohydrates and, by so doing, it ignored the connection between carbohydrate intake and diabetes. Potatoes were included under 'vegetables' and they clearly are not. Also, the old pyramid failed to recognise that all fats are not bad. For details on the new pyramid the following article is essential reading: Willett, W.C. and Stampfer, M.J. (2003) Rebuilding the food pyramid. *Scientific American* January: 64–71.

Fortunately, nutrition is now a major topic in the media and doctors need to know even more than their patients do, especially in an age when obesity and diabetes mellitus are epidemic.

Body composition

Body weight and height are the most commonly used parameters related to body composition; the term body mass index (BMI) is weight in kilograms divided by the square of the height in metres. Normal ranges have been established for adult males (20–25) and women (18–24) and it is clear that values about 20% above or below this range are associated with increased relative mortality. Of particular concern in developed countries is the increased mortality seen in those who are obese, i.e. have very large amounts of body fat. The following are some of the principal facts and questions related to body composition:

- It is important to be able to determine how much fat a subject has. *Lean body mass* is calculated by methods that measure the gamma rays emitted by the naturally occurring potassium isotope (^{40}K) or by measuring neutron-activated ^{15}N. *Total body water* is measured by administering deuterium-labelled water and measuring it in body fluids.

- Given the fact that fat tissue (0.9 g/cm^3) is less dense than lean tissue (1.1 g/cm^3), a measure of body fat can be obtained by measuring body density. Weight is easy to measure and body volume is obtained by weighing a person in air and water with the differences in kilograms being the volume in litres (this is Archimedes' principle). Another way to gain information on the extent of body fat is to measure skinfold thickness at various sites in the body using skinfold callipers.

- Average data for a 70 kg man is 17% adipose tissue, 45% lean body mass, 25% extracellular water and 13% extracellular solids. However, if one calculates the energy stored in adipose tissue, it is about 100-fold greater than the energy stored in the lean body tissue. The values for fat, carbohydrate and protein are about 440, 4.3 and 34 MJ, respectively, in a 70 kg person. For adult women, there is significantly more adipose tissue compared to men.

- Changes occur during life: adults compared with newborn have a lower percentage of their body as brain, skin and abdominal viscera but show an increase in muscle and bone. The human fetus is quite lean and there are big increases in fat and protein late in fetal development. Premature babies have many problems because of this late development, with the lower protein levels being especially critical. Less protein means fewer enzymes and less metabolic activity.

18.2 Macronutrient requirements

Learning objectives

You should be able to:

- outline positive and negative aspects of carbohydrates in our diet

- explain the importance of monounsaturated fats and the essential fatty acids in terms of health

- define protein quality and how it affects nitrogen balance.

There are six essential nutrients that must be included in our daily diet:

- carbohydrates
- proteins
- fats (lipids)
- water
- vitamins
- minerals.

Carbohydrates, fats and proteins are the major nutrients (fuels) in our diet and in the body. Carbohydrates and fats are the principal sources of energy but proteins can also be used and are especially important during fasting.

The dietary fuels

Carbohydrates

At the present time there is ongoing debate about the amount of carbohydrates that should be included in our diet. The popularity of high carbohydrate/low fat diet is on the wane and the success of the Atkins diet, where carbohydrates are severely restricted, demands reassessment of the overall guidelines. The high *glycaemic index* of refined carbohydrates has to be paid attention to, especially in view of the rapid explosion of type 2 diabetes mellitus in the world. The usual advice is that most of the carbohydrates we eat should be in the form of complex carbohydrates, but some starches have a high glycaemic index. The result is a large release of insulin, which can lead to hypoglycaemia and then hunger and therefore overeating and obesity.

Other complex carbohydrate known as dietary fibre is also present in our diet and there is evidence that it is beneficial in reducing the incidence of diverticular disease of the colon, cancer of the colon and coronary heart disease. Another major dietary carbohydrate is sucrose. Overindulgence in sucrose can cause dental caries, probably because bacteria living in the mouth efficiently use the glucose moiety to make dextrans, sticky polysaccharides that adhere to the teeth, building up dental plaque. High sucrose intake is also implicated in heart disease. Lactose, the disaccharide sugar found in milk, is the third significant dietary carbohydrate. Although it is very well handled in infants and young children, many people in Asia, Africa and South America have the tendency to develop *lactose intolerance* owing to falling levels of lactase in the gut (see p. 76).

Fat

Fat contributes 35–40% of the total calorie intake in a typical Western diet, but the long-term public health aim until now has been to reduce that towards 30%. That advice was based upon the connection between saturated fat and a high incidence of coronary heart

It is recognised that a high fat intake in Western society is correlated with an increased incidence of cardiovascular disease. Cholesterol is especially important (p. 132), but total fat is also a concern. Although smoking is the greatest risk factor in terms of cardiovascular disease, excess fat intake and excess weight (as fat tissue) are also significant risk factors, but not as problematic as presented in the popular press.

disease (CHD) in Western societies. However, even that advice is coming under scrutiny especially when comparisons are made between various ethnic groups and different countries.

The Mediterranean diet with its high intake of monounsaturated fatty acids (oleic acid in olive oil) is now recognised as being vastly superior to low-fat diets high in saturated fat. Table 33 compares percentage of calories from fat with the incidence of coronary heart disease (CHD) in men from Eastern Finland who consume a diet high in saturated fat intake, men in Japan, where there is a traditional low-fat diet, and men from the Greek island of Crete, where there is also a relatively high fat diet but one based on olive oil (containing the monounsaturated fatty acid, oleate).

The high intake of monounsaturated fat and fish by men on Crete was beneficial. Total fat tends to be emphasised, but clearly we need to consider the type of fat. The rates of CHD were much higher in Eastern Finland than in Crete despite the equivalent intake of calories as fat. Remarkably, the men in Crete had much lower incidence of CHD than the men in Japan despite the much lower percentage calories from fat in the Japanese men.

Fat has high energy value and when in our food has satiety value. It is the source of the essential fatty acids *linoleate* and *linolenate*, which are precursors of compounds such as prostaglandins, thromboxanes, leukotrienes and prostacyclin (Ch. 9, p. 138). There is solid evidence that

diets with a lot of ω-3 fatty acids are protective against CHD. In summary, doctors need to keep informed in this area and stay ahead of their patients.

Dietary fat consists mainly of triacylglycerol, but there can also be significant amounts of cholesterol as cholesteryl esters (Ch. 9, p. 132).

Margarine is the oldest example of a fat manufactured to simulate a natural product: butter. Some natural oils (e.g. fish and soybean) have melting points that are too low for the formulation of many products. This is due to the high degree of unsaturation of the constituent fatty acids. Catalytic hydrogenation is used to overcome the problem as it reduces the number of double bonds. One consequence of the hydrogenation is an increase in the number of *trans* double bonds. However, there are concerns about the safety of *trans* unsaturated fatty acids produced during hydrogenation because of the growing evidence that they have cholesterol-raising properties. Manufacturers of margarine have used fractionation techniques to overcome this problem and *trans* fatty acids are gradually being removed from the food chain.

Protein

Dietary proteins vary with diet. Dietary carbohydrate has a protein-sparing action that is significant, especially in undeveloped countries. From a nutritional point of view it is vital that dietary protein contains an adequate complement of *essential amino acids* (Ch. 8, p. 116) and that they are available in sufficient quantity to meet the protein synthesis requirements of the body. If a person's diet does not contain enough of each essential amino acid then that person will go into *negative nitrogen balance*, where more nitrogen is excreted than is ingested. Protein quality is an important concept describing whether or not a particular dietary protein provides all of the essential amino acids. Egg and milk proteins are very rich in essential amino acids. Meat proteins also have the full complement of essential amino acids. Plants contain less protein and one has to eat a lot of cereal if one is to satisfy the requirement for essential amino acids. Clearly, one should eat a *mixed diet* and avoid 'food fads'.

Table 33 Dietary fat intake and heart disease

Country	Percentage calories from fat in traditional diet	Incidence of CHD per 10 000 men over a period of 10 years
Japan	10	500
Eastern Finland	38	3000
Crete	40	200

Data from Willett, W.C. and Stampfer, M.J. (2003) Rebuilding the food pyramid. *Scientific American* January: 64–71.

18.3 Vitamins

Learning objectives

You should be able to:

- list the various fat-soluble vitamins and describe their source, absorption, transport and function as well as the dangers of excess intake

- list the various water-soluble vitamins and describe their source and role in the body, especially their involvement as precursors of coenzymes

- describe the water-soluble vitamin deficiency states

- describe how vitamin B_{12} and folate are absorbed in the gut.

Vitamins are required to be present in our diet. Human diseases are caused by vitamin deficiencies and there has been a long history describing disorders related to diets deficient in vitamins, including reports from China around 2000 BC (beri-beri) and Greece around 500 BC (night blindness). Even in developed countries they can occur in vulnerable groups. Vulnerable groups need to receive special consideration in their diets (e.g. women for iron and calcium; children, pregnant women and lactating women for many vitamins and minerals; the elderly, who can have inefficient absorption; post-surgical patients).

Vitamins are divided into two categories depending upon their water-solubility.

The fat-soluble vitamins (Table 34)

The absorption of the fat-soluble vitamins from the gut follows the same path as fat. Fat malabsorption states can lead to deficiency of fat-soluble vitamins. They are stored mostly in the liver, although vitamin E is also stored in adipose tissue. Significant quantities are stored so that the manifestation of deficiencies is slower than for the water-soluble group of vitamins. Another consequence of storage is that excess intake can be toxic; this is well established for both vitamins A and D. The vitamin activity of each is not confined to a single substance. They are mainly heat-stable.

Vitamin A

Vitamin A (retinol) is the most important of the fat-soluble vitamins (Fig. 165). It was the first to be discovered. We derive most of our vitamin A from β-carotene, which is present in carrots, spinach, broccoli and apricots. The other source is vitamin A itself, which is present in liver, fish oil, eggs, kidney and dairy products.

Transport and metabolism
Dietary retinoids are transported from the intestine as retinol esters in chylomicrons for storage in the liver. Transport from the liver is with the retinol bound to retinol binding protein (RBP). RBP binds to *transthyretin*. In retinoid-dependent epithelial tissues, retinol binds to cellular retinol binding protein (CRBP) and is converted to *retinoic acid*. As shown in Figure 165, retinol exists in three oxidation states: as an alcohol (retinol), an aldehyde (retinal) and as an acid (retinoic acid). Retinal is formed from retinol by a dehydrogenation reaction that is reversible. Retinoic acid is produced from retinal by oxidation and that reaction is irreversible.

Function
The most well-defined function of vitamin A is in the visual process (Fig. 166). Retinoic acid behaves like a steroid hormone. The retinoic acid receptors (RARs) are members of the thyroid hormone/steroid hormone receptor superfamily (Ch. 17, p. 250). Effects include roles in growth and differentiation of epithelial tissue. There are effects on steroid hormone biosynthesis, synthesis of glycosaminoglycans, gametogenesis and differentiation of keratinocytes.

Hypervitaminosis A
Excess intake of vitamin A causes loss of appetite, abnormal skin pigmentation, loss of hair and dryness of

Table 34 The fat-soluble vitamins

Symbol	Name	Human disease	Intake (µg per day)	Source
A	Retinol	Blindness, abortion, defects in epithelium	750	Fish oils, liver, dairy products
D	Calciferol	Rickets	25	Fish oils, milk, eggs, action of sunlight on skin
E	Tocopherol	Infertility		Vegetable oils, milk, wheat germ
K	Phylloquinone	Bleeding (infants)		Gut flora, vegetable oils

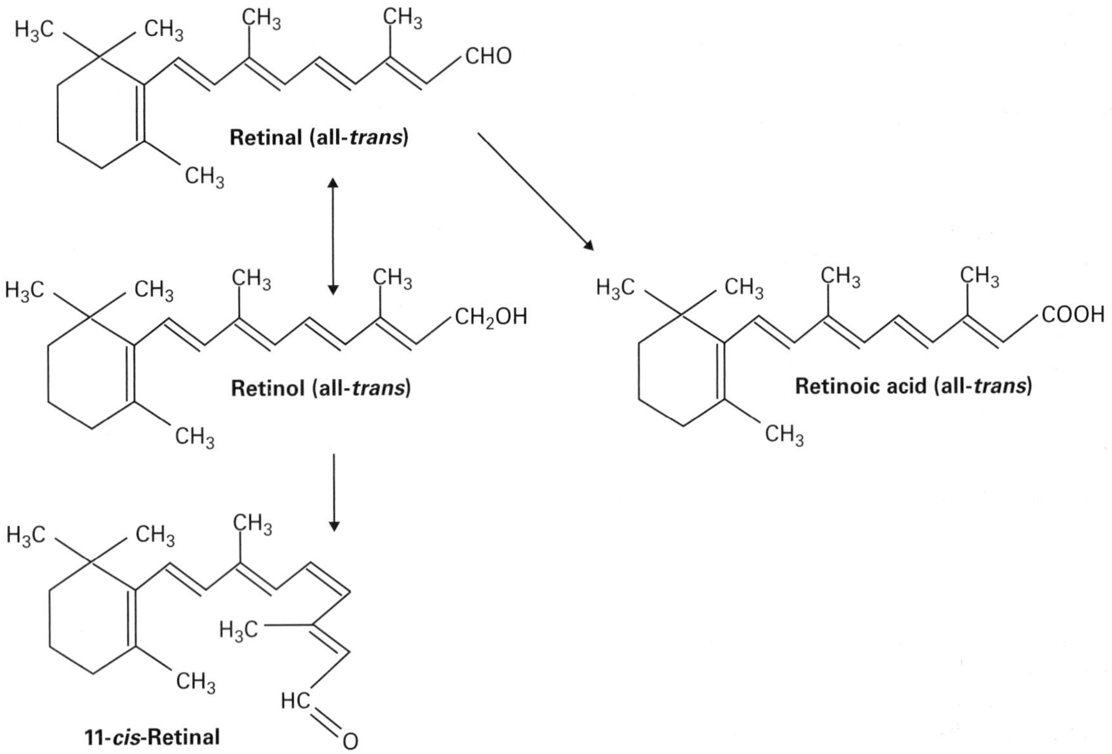

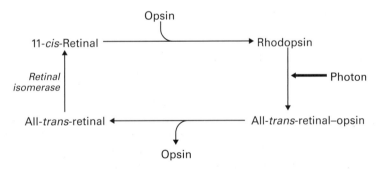

Fig. 165 Vitamin A forms. 11-*cis*-Retinal is the chromophore of rhodopsin, the photoreceptor of the rod outer segments in sthe eye.

Fig. 166 Retinal and the visual cycle.

skin, pain in the long bones and bone fragility and very high doses can be lethal.

Vitamin E

The chief role of vitamin E (α-tocopherol; Fig. 167) is to participate in the protection of cells against oxygen free radicals. It is an antioxidant and functions in a complex system that includes the trace element selenium and the tripeptide glutathione. If our diet contains lots of polyunsaturated fatty acids (PUFA), then there is an increased demand for vitamin E. Under these condi-

tions, a vitamin E deficiency results in haemolysis of red blood cells.

Vitamin K

Vitamin K is an anti-haemorrhagic factor (Ch. 19, p. 278) since it is required as a coenzyme for the production of several of the blood coagulation factors, including prothrombin, factors VII, IX and X and proteins C and S. We are not solely dependent upon our diet as vitamin K is manufactured by colonic bacteria. A deficiency of vitamin K can occur in neonates, leading to

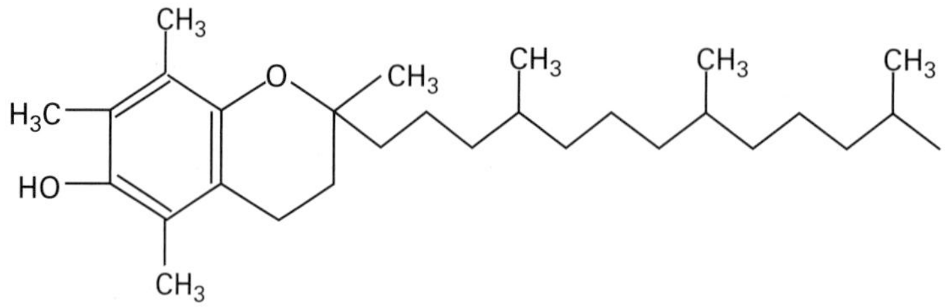

Fig. 167 The structure of α-tocopherol (vitamin E).

haemorrhagic disease of the newborn. All newborn babies should receive vitamin K by injection as a preventive measure.

Vitamin D

Vitamin D is involved in the control of calcium metabolism in the body (Ch. 17, p. 245). It can be formed in skin that is exposed to UV light and is a prohormone, being the precursor of calcitriol.

The water-soluble vitamins

Many of the water-soluble vitamins are components of coenzymes or prosthetic groups for important enzymes in metabolism (Table 4, p. 74). Knowledge of the participation of specific vitamins in metabolism has practical (clinical) significance when one is treating subjects with inherited defects in critical pathways. Megadose vitamin therapy is useful as a therapeutic approach to the treatment of some inborn errors of amino acid catabolism.

Thiamine, riboflavin, nicotinamide, pyridoxine, pantothenic acid and biotin are water-soluble vitamins that are widely distributed in foodstuffs. There is no particularly good source of folic acid other than liver, but grains are now enriched with this vitamin. Vitamin B_{12} is also found in liver. Fruits and vegetables are rich in ascorbic acid (vitamin C). Structures of several of the water-soluble vitamins are shown in Figure 168.

Thiamine

Its coenzyme form is *thiamine pyrophosphate* (TPP). Key points about thiamine and TPP include:

- TPP is required for the conversion of pyruvate to acetyl-CoA by the pyruvate dehydrogenase complex (PDC) and of α-ketoglutarate to succinyl-CoA in the tricarboxylic acid (TCA) cycle as well as the metabolism of α-keto acids derived from the three branched-chain amino acids.
- TPP is also the coenzyme for transketolase in the pentose phosphate pathway.

- Because of the integral involvement of TPP in the metabolism of glucose and fatty acids, the daily requirements of thiamine are linked to the total energy expenditure of any individual.
- *Deficiency* of thiamine leads to *beri-beri*, where the impairment of oxidative metabolism of glucose leads to altered nervous system and cardiac muscle function. Thiamine deficiency is not uncommon in alcoholics.

Nicotinamide (niacin)

Nicotinamide is found in the key coenzymes NAD^+, $NADP^+$, NADH and NADPH. Key points about nicotinamide and its coenzyme forms include:

- NAD^+ and $NADP^+$ are vital for oxidation–reduction reactions in metabolism catalysed by dehydrogenases.
- NADPH is involved in reductive biosynthesis.
- The daily requirements for nicotinamide are also linked to the total energy expenditure of any individual.
- *Deficiency* of niacin leads to *pellagra*, where there are obvious skin lesions as well as cheilosis (cracked lips) and glossitis (inflamed tongue).
- *Sources* of niacin are in the diet, but it is also formed from the amino acid tryptophan by a pathway that has several steps, which are dependent upon adequate pyridoxine being present. Pellagra-like symptoms are occasionally seen in *Hartnup's disease*, an inherited disorder where tryptophan (and other neutral amino acids) absorption is impaired.

Vitamin B₂ (riboflavin)

Riboflavin is important in energy metabolism. The nucleotides containing this vitamin are FAD and FMN. Key points about riboflavin and these nucleotides include:

- FAD is present in flavoprotein enzymes involved in oxidation–reduction reactions of intermediary metabolism.

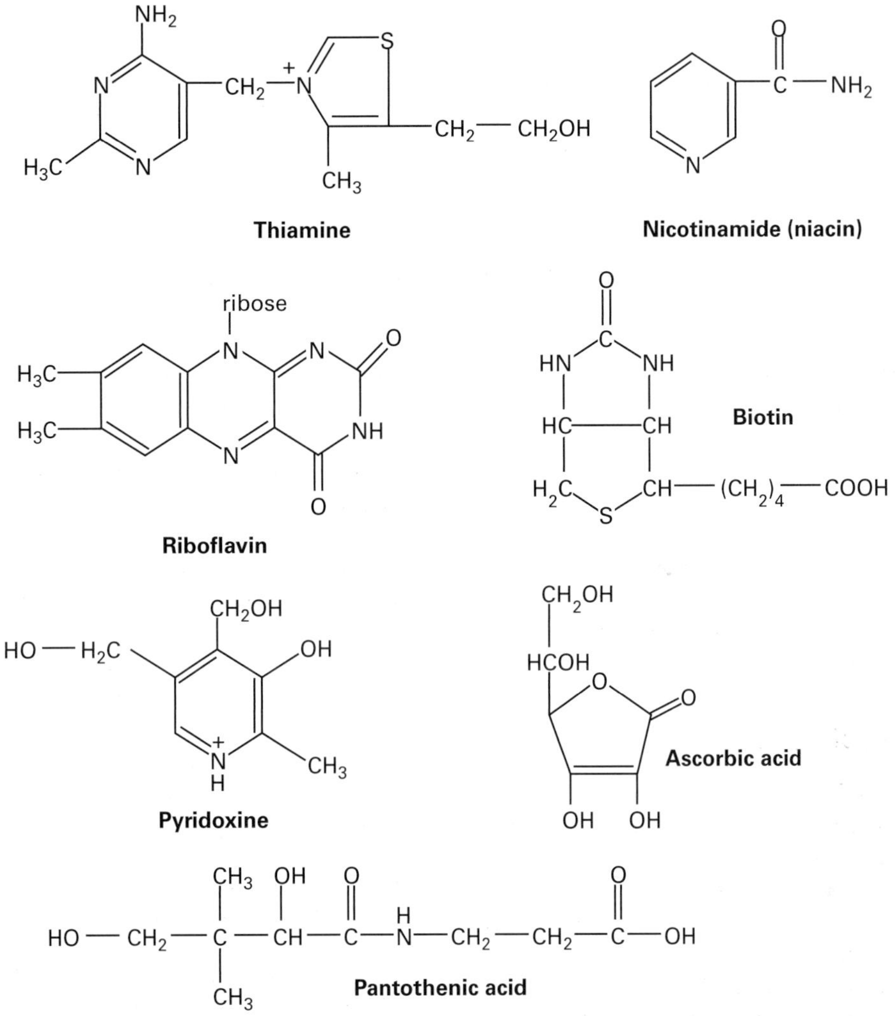

Fig. 168 Structures of some water-soluble vitamins.

- FAD is involved in pyruvate and α-ketoglutarate dehydrogenase complexes, succinate dehydrogenase, fatty acyl-CoA dehydrogenase, the glycerol 3-phosphate shuttle; FMN is involved in the electron transport chain.
- *Deficiency* of riboflavin affects epithelial tissues, leading to cheilosis, angular stomatitis, glossitis and photophobia.

Vitamin B_6 (pyridoxine)

Pyridoxine exists in three oxidation states: pyridoxine (an alcohol), pyridoxal (an aldehyde) and pyridoxamine (an amine); all three are equally potent. It is as pyridoxal phosphate (PLP) that this vitamin participates in metabolism. Key points about pyridoxine and PLP include:

- PLP participates in essential enzymatic reactions of amino acid catabolism (Ch. 7), including transamination and decarboxylation.

- Glycogen phosphorylase has PLP linked to it through the ε-amino group of a lysine.
- *Deficiency* is rare but can occur in alcoholics.

Pantothenic acid

Although deficiency of pantothenate is very rare, the importance of pantothenic acid becomes clear when one recalls the role of acetyl-CoA in intermediary metabolism. Pantothenate is also part of acyl carrier protein (ACP) involved in fatty acid synthesis (Ch. 9, p. 128). Pantothenate contains a thiol group (derived from cysteine) through which acyl groups are bonded in both coenzyme A and ACP. Coenzyme A is involved in:

- pyruvate and α-ketoglutarate dehydrogenase complexes
- fatty acid beta-oxidation and fatty acid synthesis
- the catabolism of branched-chain amino acids.

Biotin

Biotin is the prosthetic group for four carboxylases. The biotin is covalently attached through the ε-amino group of a lysine. The pathways of intermediary metabolism include:

- gluconeogenesis (pyruvate carboxylase)
- fatty acid synthesis (acetyl-CoA carboxylase)
- odd-numbered fatty acid oxidation (propionyl-CoA carboxylase)
- amino acid catabolism (propionyl-CoA carboxylase and β-methylcrotonyl-CoA carboxylase).

Biotin is derived from the diet but is also made by gastrointestinal flora.

Biotin deficiency in humans has been found only when diets included large amount of raw egg white. The latter contains a heat-labile glycoprotein, *avidin*, which binds biotin tightly. Rare disorders have been reported in enzymes of the biotin cycle, including failure to synthesise the biotinylated holocarboxylases.

Vitamin C (ascorbic acid)

Vitamin C exists in two forms: ascorbic acid and dehydroascorbic acid. Ascorbic acid is a donor of reducing equivalents. Key points about ascorbate include:

- It is critical for the biosynthesis of collagen, where it is the coenzyme for both *proline hydroxylase* and *lysyl hydroxylase*.
- Vitamin C is required for wound healing and bone formation.
- It is important in iron absorption in the gut since it is a reducing agent that can reduce ferric (Fe^{III}) iron in the diet to the absorbable ferrous iron (Fe^{II}).
- Ascorbate is involved in the reaction catalysed by *dopamine β-hydroxylase* in the catecholamine biosynthetic pathway.
- High concentrations are present in the adrenal cortex, where it may be important in preserving the cytochromes P-450 involved in steroid hormone biosynthesis.
- **Deficiency** leads to scurvy, an early sign of which is swollen bleeding gums.
- Diets that include fruits, fruit juice and vegetables provide the high levels that are consistent with good health.

Folic acid

Folate is a complex compound comprising a pteridine ring, *p*-aminobenzoic acid and one or more glutamic acid residues. Tetrahydrofolate (FH_4) is the coenzyme

---

Clinical note:
Spina bifida

Evidence is accumulating that adequate folate intake by pregnant women can prevent spina bifida. The folate is required early in pregnancy to prevent neural tube defects. Adequate folate also may be beneficial in heart disease by lowering homocysteine levels.

derived from folate. Key points about folate and FH_4 include:

- FH_4 is vital in one-carbon metabolism (Ch. 8, p. 118).
- Sulphonamide antibiotics work by inhibiting the incorporation of *p*-aminobenzoic acid (part of the folate structure) during bacterial folate synthesis.
- **Deficiency** of folic acid results in megaloblastic anaemia due to defects in stem cells.
- **Neural tube defects** may be prevented by adequate folate in the diet early in pregnancy. Indeed, in the USA since the government began requiring food manufacturers to fortify cereal, pasta, bread and flour with folic acid, severe brain defects and spinal birth defects have dropped 27%.
- Folate is of use in the treatment of some of the symptoms of pernicious anaemia but it has no effect on the neurological symptoms. Indeed, its overuse by someone with pernicious anaemia may *mask* the neurological symptoms of that disorder.

Vitamin B₁₂ (cobalamin)

Vitamin B_{12} is the anti-pernicious anaemia factor. It has a complex structure that includes a haem-like corrin ring with four pyrroles; the pyrrole nitrogen atoms are bound to a central *cobalt* atom (hence the name cobalamin) and a side chain consisting of a phosphoribo-5,6-dimethylbenzimadozolyl group. Key points include:

- It is synthesised by microorganisms and is found in meats, animal products and sea foods. It is not present in plants or yeasts and strict vegans may develop B_{12} deficiency and therefore anaemia.
- **Deficiency** causes pernicious anaemia, characterised by a macrocytic anaemia. It is most commonly the result of defective absorption of vitamin B_{12} from the gut.
- B_{12} absorption requires the presence of a gastric secretory mucoprotein called *intrinsic factor* (IF) secreted by gastric parietal cells. B_{12} is released from ingested proteins by stomach acid. The B_{12} binds to haptocorrin at the acid pH, but later, when acid is neutralised, B_{12} is released, binds to IF and then the IF–B_{12} complex is absorbed in the ileum by receptor-mediated endocytosis.

B_{12} is involved in only two reactions in the body:

- Methylcobalamin is the coenzyme for methionine synthase. If vitamin B_{12} is deficient (or ineffective), then much of the folate taken in from the diet becomes trapped as methyl-FH_4 (see Ch. 8, p. 118); it is then unavailable for one-carbon metabolism and this impairs nucleotide synthesis.
- Adenosylcobalamin is the coenzyme for a mutase in the pathway from propionyl-CoA to succinyl-CoA. That pathway is involved in the catabolism of odd-numbered fatty acids and of the amino acids methionine, threonine, valine and isoleucine. One indicator of B_{12} deficiency is methylmalonic aciduria.

18.4 Minerals

Learning objectives

You should be able to:

- describe the macrominerals and trace elements, and their source, absorption and roles in the body.

As well as energy, protein and vitamins, we require some other nutrients. The most obvious, apart from water, are the major structural elements: calcium, phosphorus, sodium, potassium and magnesium. Some of these elements are essential in structural components such as bones and teeth. Some are important in osmotic phenomena of fluids. Others are important in acid–base equilibrium. In addition, we require trace amounts of other elements, which are found as prosthetic groups in enzymes and carriers. The most important are iron, selenium, zinc, copper and iodine. In developed societies, mineral deficiencies are rare, although they do exist. Only iron and calcium (and possibly iodine) are likely to be deficient in the developed world, but deficiencies can also be common in certain types of patients.

Calcium

Most (99%) of body calcium is present in the skeleton (*hydroxyapatite* in bone). Calcium ions are needed by all cells. They are involved in almost all processes in the body and the plasma concentration of ionic calcium is subjected to exquisite control (Ch. 17, p. 244).

Daily requirements

We need about 1 g of calcium per day in our diet, but pregnant and lactating women require more. Sources of calcium include milk (cow's milk contains four times that of human milk), cheese and other dairy products. There are low levels in vegetables. Hard water is an important source.

Absorption

Dietary calcium is absorbed by an active process requiring transport proteins whose synthesis is controlled by calcitriol; about 70–80% is still excreted in faeces. Several compounds present in our food complex calcium and hinder its absorption. These include *phytic acid* (found in cereals), *fatty acids* (significant in fat malabsorption states) and *oxalic acid* (found in rhubarb).

Deficiency

Calcium deficiency results in osteomalacia (rickets). It is caused by lack of vitamin D in the diet or insufficient production in the skin (owing to lack of sunlight).

Phosphorus

Phosphorus is required by all cells and its many functions have been described in Chapter 17 (p. 244).

Daily requirements

The average daily intake of dietary phosphorus is about 1.5 g.

Absorption

Phosphorus absorption is controlled by calcitriol action in the gut.

Defective phosphate metabolism (hypophosphataemia) can also lead to rickets. The clearest example is in *X-linked hypophosphataemia*, where renal reabsorption of phosphate is impaired.

Magnesium

The whole body contains about 25 g of magnesium. It is essential in neuromuscular transmission and serves as a cofactor for many key enzymes: for example, the kinases involved in phosphate group transfer in several reactions of glycolysis, acyl-CoA synthetase of fatty acid oxidation and glutamine synthetase of amino acid metabolism.

Magnesium is found in bones and teeth; deficiency occurs in starvation and alcoholism.

Sodium and potassium

Sodium is the principal cation of the extracellular fluid, while potassium is the principal cation of intracellular fluid. This ion gradient is maintained by the sodium pump (Na^+/K^+-ATPase) present in all cells and a major user of ATP. Sodium is involved primarily with the maintenance of osmotic equilibrium and body fluid volume, while potassium is involved primarily with cellular enzyme function. Sodium/potassium balance in the body is under the fine control of aldosterone.

Sodium is present in most foods and sodium chloride is added during food processing. Requirements increase in hot weather, fever and during heavy work. Potassium is also widely distributed in foods.

Chlorine, as chloride

Chloride is required to maintain fluid and electrolyte balance and hydrochloric acid production in the stomach. The chloride shift is important in carbon dioxide transport in blood (Ch. 5, p. 65). Chloride is supplied by many foods and also common salt.

Trace elements

Iron

The major requirement for iron is in haemoglobin and cytochrome synthesis, thus this element has to be discussed in the context of anaemia. Iron deficiency results in deficiency of haemoglobin and is one of the most common forms of anaemia. Deficiency results in a microcytic, hypochromic anaemia. Liver is a very good source of iron. Meat sources are absorbed much more efficiently than plant sources of iron. Milk and milk products are low in iron. Iron is not the only nutrient involved in red blood cell production; also required are folic acid, vitamin B_{12}, protein, pyridoxine, ascorbic acid and copper.

Absorption
Since iron is not actively excreted, iron balance in the body has to be controlled at the level of the intestinal mucosal cell. Crypt cells of the duodenum *sense* the amount of iron in the circulation. Key points about iron absorption include:

- The size of the body's iron stores regulates the efficiency of iron absorption in the gut. Iron deficiency leads to enhanced iron absorption.
- It is Fe^{II} that is absorbed; efficient iron absorption depends upon reduction of dietary ferric to ferrous iron aided by reducing agents such as ascorbic acid. Iron is transported in blood in the form of *transferrin*.

- *Non-haem iron* in the diet is less efficiently absorbed than haem iron. Stomach acid is critical for the release of Fe^{III} from non-haem iron, which is then absorbed into duodenal villus enterocytes using a *divalent cation transporter*.
- *Haem iron* is absorbed by duodenal epithelial cells as an intact metalloporphyrin. Within the cell iron is released by the action of haem oxygenase (see Ch. 16, p. 228). Fe^{III} is reduced to Fe^{II} and enters the same pool as derived from non-haem iron.

Deficiency
Iron deficiency is common. In adults, deficiency can be caused by occult blood loss from the gastrointestinal tract. In children and adolescents, deficiency mainly results from poor nutrition.

Iodine

Forty per cent of the total body iodine is concentrated in the thyroid, where it can be used to iodinate a protein (thyroglobulin) leading to the production of the thyroid hormones (Ch. 17, p. 236). Some geographic locations have low iodine in the water supply and in plant products produced there. Iodine supplementation of common salt (76 μg/g salt) helps prevent iodine-deficiency goitre.

Copper and zinc

These metals are important components of enzyme systems; for example, zinc is the prosthetic group of *carbonic anhydrase* and copper is a prosthetic group of *cytochrome oxidase*. As with iodine, seafoods are good sources of these metals as are liver and kidney.

Selenium

Selenium is the prosthetic group in *glutathione reductase* and is critical for overall antioxidant activity in cells.

Fluorine as fluoride

Although not an essential element, it appears beneficial to have fluoride in the diet since it reduces the incidence of dental caries by making teeth more resistant to acid (formed by bacteria in the mouth) by substituting for hydroxyl groups in hydroxyapatite.

Self-assessment: questions

Single best answer MCQs

1. Which one of the following trace elements is an integral part of the vitamin B_{12} molecule?
   a. Zinc
   b. Iron
   c. Copper
   d. Cobalt
   e. Molybdenum

2. In connection with the identification of overweight individuals and the fat content of diets:
   a. BMI (body mass index) values greater than 30 in an adult male are always indicative of excess body fat
   b. A subject on the 'Mediterranean diet' will have an overall fat intake much lower (half) than that usually seen in 'Western' diets
   c. A large decrease in total circulating cholesterol is one benefit of increasing one's intake of saturated fat
   d. The Mediterranean diet contains a high proportion of δ-9 fatty acids
   e. There are health (cardiovascular) benefits associated with a diet high in *trans* fatty acids

3. Deficiency of pyridoxine in the diet (and hence deficiency of pyridoxal phosphate in the cell) will directly impair the catalytic function of:
   a. glutamate dehydrogenase
   b. glutamine synthetase
   c. glutaminase
   d. alanine aminotransferase
   e. γ-glutamyltranspeptidase

4. Identify the B vitamin in Column A that is aligned with its correct function in Column B.

A	B
a. Niacin	Carboxylation reactions
b. Riboflavin	Transamination reactions
c. Thiamine	Transketolase
d. Pantothenic acid	Oxidation–reduction
e. Pyridoxine	Transmethylations

5. Identify the mineral in Column A that is aligned with its correct function in Column B.

A	B
a. Calcium	Blood coagulation
b. Iron	Antioxidant
c. Copper	Kinases
d. Iodine	Cytochrome oxidase
e. Magnesium	Osmotic equilibrium

6. Identify the single correct statement about the vitamin whose deficiency results in the disorder, pernicious anaemia.
   a. Its absorption in the gut is promoted by achlorhydria
   b. It is absorbed in the gut as a combination with folic acid
   c. It is synthesised in the parotid glands
   d. It forms a complex with a product of gastric parietal cells and is then absorbed in the ileum
   e. Because of its presence in plants it is found in large amounts in the diets of vegans

7. Identify the single correct statement about vitamins A and D.
   a. Both A and D are found in chylomicron remnants and both are toxic when taken in supraphysiological amounts
   b. Retinol binding proteins (RBP) protect retinoids in the gut
   c. Retinoic acid receptors are located to the plasma membranes of target cells
   d. It is the plasma vitamin D concentration in plasma that is used as an index of the vitamin D status of a subject
   e. Calcitriol, the hormone derived from 25-hydroxy-vitamin D in the kidney, is produced in increased amounts in the kidney in response to hypercalcaemia

8. Which one of the following statements about vitamins E and K is correct?
   a. Vitamin E within cell membranes increases the oxidation of polyunsaturated fatty acids (PUFA) in these membranes
   b. Vitamin E uptake by extrahepatic cells involves a special (unique to E) receptor-mediated endocytosis pathway
   c. Total vitamin K excretion over a period of weeks in a normal subject is significantly greater than the total dietary intake of vitamin K over that period
   d. Treatment of subjects with warfarin activates the post-translational modification of glutamate residues in the blood coagulation factors II, VII, IX and X
   e. The production of the atherogenic oxidised form of LDL (low density lipoprotein) is promoted by vitamin E

9. A 44-year-old male patient arranges a visit to your office because of his development of a severe form of exfoliative dermatitis. Since he had never had this problem before you do a thorough physical and take a detailed history. Finally, you elicit from him that he had for the past few weeks had a diet that included a dozen raw egg whites each day as his major source of protein. You are able to tell him that his dermatitis was due to a rare disorder where a protein in egg white, avidin, was binding to which of the following vitamins and preventing its absorption?
   a. Pantothenic acid
   b. Niacin
   c. Biotin
   d. Riboflavin
   e. Vitamin A

10. Which of the following vitamins can be synthesised in the liver by a pathway that involves pyridoxal phosphate and an aromatic amino acid?
   a. Vitamin K
   b. Vitamin D
   c. Thiamine
   d. Niacin
   e. Folate

True/false questions

Are the following statements true or false?

1. Thiamine deficiency in an alcoholic can be recognised by measuring transketolase activity in his/her red blood cells.

2. The Reference Nutrient Intake for thiamine, niacin and riboflavin is based upon the age and sex of individuals.
3. Increased intake of folate by pregnant women reduces the incidence of spina bifida.
4. Iron in vegetables is more readily absorbed than iron in liver.
5. Retinoic acid is the precursor of the all-*trans*-retinal required for vision.
6. It is only the protein intake of an individual that determines whether or not they will be in positive nitrogen balance.
7. Tyrosine is an essential amino acid in normal subjects.
8. A deficiency in a single essential amino acid in the diet of a subject leads to a positive nitrogen balance.
9. Fat-soluble vitamins tend to be stored in the body and high intake can lead to toxicity.

Short essay questions

1. Discuss the role of vitamins in:
   a. Carbohydrate metabolism
   b. Fatty acid metabolism
   c. Amino acid metabolism.
2. Prepare a table that highlights the roles of the various fat-soluble vitamins in the body and their active forms.

Self-assessment: answers

Single best answer MCQ answers

1. a. **False**. Zinc is found in carbonic anhydrase.
    b. **False**. Iron is found in cytochromes and other haem proteins.
    c. **False**. Copper is found in cytochrome oxidase and tyrosinase.
    d. **True**. It is present in the corrin ring of B_{12}.
    e. **False**. Molybdenum is found in xanthine oxidase.

2. a. **False**. Many athletes have BMI values greater than 30 and have low body fat.
    b. **False**. The total fat intakes are almost equivalent. However, the Mediterranean diet emphasises olive oil, not saturated fats.
    c. **False**. The opposite occurs. High saturated fat intake leads to hypercholesterolaemia.
    d. **True**. The principal fatty acid is oleate.
    e. **False**. Intake of *trans* fatty acids is positively associated with CHD (coronary heart disease).

3. a. **False**. NAD^+ or $NADP^+$ are the coenzymes involved with glutamate dehydrogenase.
    b. **False**. ATP is required but not PLP.
    c. **False**. This enzyme catalyses a simple hydrolysis.
    d. **True**. PLP is involved a lot in amino acid catabolism.
    e. **False**. γ-Glutamyltranspeptidase is involved in amino acid transport.

4. a. **False**. Niacin is involved in oxidation–reduction coenzymes.
    b. **False**. Riboflavin is involved in oxidation–reduction coenzymes.
    c. **True**. Thiamine in TPP is the coenzyme for transketolase.
    d. **False**. Pantothenic acid is involved in acyl transfer.
    e. **False**. *S*-Adenosylmethionine is the source of methyl groups.

5. a. **True**. The coagulation pathway cannot function normally without Ca^{2+}.
    b. **False**. If anything, iron generates oxygen free radicals.
    c. **False**. Copper is found in cytochrome oxidase.
    d. **False**. Iodine is required for thyroid hormone biosynthesis.
    e. **False**. Magnesium is required by many kinases, including hexokinase.

6. a. **False**. Stomach hydrochloric acid releases B_{12} from dietary protein.
    b. **False**. It is absorbed in combination with intrinsic factor.
    c. **False**. Animals and humans cannot synthesise B_{12}.
    d. **True**. Parietal cells are the source of intrinsic factor that binds B_{12} and the complex is absorbed in the ileum by receptor-mediated endocytosis.
    e. **False**. Plants per se do not contain B_{12}; microorganisms manufacture B_{12}.

7. a. **True**. The fat-soluble vitamins are absorbed along with dietary fat and appear in chylomicrons. Overdosing with A and D is dangerous.
    b. **False**. RBP protect retinoids in the circulation.
    c. **False**. They are hydrophobic and retinoic acid receptors are in the nucleus.
    d. **False**. It is the level of 25-hydroxy-vitamin D that is a guide to sufficiency of vitamin D.
    e. **False**. Calcitriol production is stimulated by parathyroid hormone, which is secreted in increased amounts in response to hypocalcaemia.

8. a. **False**. Vitamin E protects against oxidation of PUFA.
    b. **False**. Fat-soluble vitamins can readily cross cell membranes.
    c. **True**. This is because vitamin K is also synthesised by colonic bacteria, complementing that in the diet.
    d. **False**. Carboxylation of glutamate residues is inhibited by warfarin through interference with the regeneration of dihydro-vitamin K.
    e. **False**. A benefit of vitamin E is prevention of LDL oxidation. Remember that E is an antioxidant!

9. a. **False**. Avidin does not affect pantothenate absorption.
    b. **False**. Avidin does not affect niacin absorption or synthesis.
    c. **True**. Avidin binds biotin preventing its absorption.
    d. **False**. Avidin doesn't affect riboflavin absorption.
    e. **False**. Avidin doesn't affect vitamin A absorption.

10. a. **False**. Vitamin K can be synthesised by colonic bacteria.
    b. **False**. Vitamin D can be synthesised in skin from 7-dehydrocholesterol when exposed to UV light.

c. **False**. Thiamine is only derived from the diet.
d. **True**. A small percentage of our daily requirement for niacin is synthesised in the body from tryptophan.
e. **False**. Folate is derived only from the diet.

True/false answers

1. **True**. TPP (thiamine pyrophosphate) is the coenzyme for transketolase and, of course, red blood cells are easy to obtain from patients.
2. **False**. The recommended intakes depend on the total energy expenditure of the individual; that is, we need more if we are using more fuel to support more energy expenditure. A middle-aged female who is very active in sport will need more of these vitamins than a young male 'couch potato'.
3. **True**. It may also help in reducing the incidence of cleft palate.
4. **False**. The efficiency is greatest from meat, especially liver; the low efficiency from vegetables explains why some vegans develop iron-deficiency anaemia.
5. **False**. Retinol is the precursor of retinal. Retinal to retinoic acid is an irreversible step.
6. **False**. The quality of the protein is important but also whether or not the individual is receiving enough calories (from carbohydrate and fat). If not, they use protein as a fuel and may be in negative nitrogen balance.
7. **False**. Normal individuals are able to make tyrosine from phenylalanine.
8. **False**. A deficiency of any of the essential amino acids leads to negative nitrogen balance.
9. **True**. Hypervitaminoses A and D are potential problems for those taking large doses of these fat-soluble vitamins. Water-soluble vitamins, in contrast, are not toxic; many people take grams of vitamin C daily.

Short essay answers

1. a. *Carbohydrate metabolism*. Nicotinamide (niacin) is part of the cofactors NAD^+, NADH, $NADP^+$ and NADPH. NAD^+ is the cofactor for dehydrogenases involved in glycolysis, pyruvate dehydrogenase complex (PDC) and the tricarboxylic acid (TCA) cycle. Lipoate is also required by PDC as is pantothenate (part of coenzyme A). NADH is required for gluconeogenesis from pyruvate as is biotin. $NADP^+$ is required by both dehydrogenases in the pentose phosphate pathway and NADPH is a product of that pathway. Thiamine is part of a coenzyme, thiamine pyrophosphate (TPP), which is involved in PDC and also α-ketoglutarate dehydrogenase of the TCA cycle. It also functions in the pentose phosphate cycle where it is the coenzyme for transketolase. Riboflavin is part of the cofactors FAD and FMN. FAD is a cofactor in the PDC and is also the coenzyme for succinate dehydrogenase of the TCA cycle. FMN is a component of the electron transport chain. Pyridoxal is part of the coenzyme pyridoxal phosphate, which is an integral part of glycogen phosphorylase.

   b. *Fatty acid metabolism*. Pantothenate is critical for fatty acid oxidation and synthesis because of its contribution to coenzyme A and acyl carrier protein. Nicotinamide and riboflavin are involved in fatty acid oxidation through the participation of NAD^+ and FAD in the beta-oxidation of fatty acids and the TCA cycle. Also, NADPH is required for fatty acid synthesis. Vitamin B_{12} participates in the metabolism of the propionyl-CoA, formed from odd-numbered fatty acids.

   c. *Amino acid metabolism*. The most important vitamin related to amino acid catabolism is pyridoxal, given the role of pyridoxal phosphate in amino acid transamination and decarboxylation. It is also required for other reactions of amino acid metabolism. Nicotinamide and riboflavin are also important because of their role in branched-chain ketoacid dehydrogenase and enzymes of the TCA cycle. Folate and vitamin B_{12} function in one-carbon metabolism, especially with the amino acids serine and histidine.

2. Table 35 describes the roles of the fat-soluble vitamins.

Table 35 The role of the fat-soluble vitamins

Vitamin	Active form	Function
A	Retinal, retinoic acid	Vision, growth and development
D	Calcitriol	Calcium absorption in gut
E	Hydroquinone	Antioxidant
K	Dihydro-vitamin K	Coenzyme for γ-carboxylation of blood coagulation factors

19 Biochemical functions of blood

Overview

Blood samples are easily obtained from patients, and analyses carried out on blood provide critical information about body functions with the number of blood analyses routinely requested expanding every year. The most abundant plasma protein, albumin, is the major contributor to plasma oncotic pressure as well as being a transporter of hydrophobic molecules including drugs. Other plasma proteins have specific functions, including those required for the formation of blood clots. Plasma immunoglobulins are vital participants in the immune system. Red blood cells are key players in oxygen and carbon dioxide transport, and their metabolic pathways are limited but vital to normal function.

19.1 Plasma proteins

Learning objectives

You should be able to:

- outline the functions of albumin, haptoglobin and α_1-antitrypsin
- describe how plasma enzyme assays can yield information on tissue damage.

The plasma proteins have several critical functions:

- maintenance of oncotic pressure
- transport
- buffering
- immunity
- enzymatic
- blood clotting.

Many of the plasma proteins are synthesised in the liver, including albumin, α- and β-globulins, lipoproteins and the proteins of blood coagulation. Their breadth of function is illustrated in Table 36. Immunoglobulins function as antibodies and are made in B lymphocytes (see below). The plasma proteins involved in hormone transport have been discussed in Chapter 17, those involved in lipid transport in Chapter 9 and those involved in blood coagulation are described in detail later in this chapter.

Clinical biochemists obtain measurements of the major classes of plasma protein in a patient's serum by carrying out protein electrophoresis on cellulose acetate or agarose gel. The major classes are pre-albumin, albumin, α_1- and α_2-globulins, β-globulins and γ-globulins, as shown in Figure 169. Plasma protein electrophoretic analysis is of particular use in the diagnosis of nephrotic syndrome, hypogammaglobulinaemia, cirrhosis, α_1-antitrypsin deficiency and paraproteinaemia (high levels of an immunoglobulin made by a single clone of B lymphocytes).

Albumin

Albumin, a 66 kDa protein, is the most abundant plasma protein, being present at a concentration of about 4.5 g/dl in normal adults. About 14 g/day are made in the liver; its synthesis is stimulated by insulin. Serum albumin levels are low in liver disease. Normal serum albumin levels are an indication of good nutrition in patients. The most important functions of albumin are:

- to provide about 80% of the plasma oncotic pressure, which prevents loss of vascular fluid into tissues. It draws back into the venous ends of capillaries water that was forced through the arterial capillary walls by the hydrostatic pressure exerted by heart function
- to bind hydrophobic molecules. It has low affinity but, because of its high concentration in plasma, it has high capacity. Examples of ligands bound by albumin include fatty acids, bilirubin, calcium, thyroid hormones and many drugs including aspirin.

Table 36 The functions of plasma proteins

Plasma protein	Role
Albumin	Maintenance of plasma oncotic pressure
α_1-Antitrypsin	Protease inhibitor
Haptoglobulin	Complexes extracorpuscular haemoglobin
All plasma proteins	Buffering
Transport proteins	
Albumin	Hydrophobic compounds and Ca^{2+}
Caeruloplasmin	Copper
Transferrin	Iron
β-Lipoproteins	Fat
Corticosteroid-binding globulin (CBG)	Cortisol
Thyroxine-binding globulin (TBG), transerythretin (pre-albumin)	Thyroid hormones (T_4 and T_3)
Hormone-related activity	
Angiotensinogen	Angiotensin I precursor
Insulin-like growth factor-1	Mediator of growth hormone action
Blood coagulation	
Fibrinogen, factors V, VIII, XI, XII	Non-vitamin K-dependent
Prothrombin, factors VII, IX, X	Vitamin K-dependent
Immunity	
γ-Globulins, especially IgG and IgA	Antibodies

1. Apply mixture of proteins (e.g. plasma)

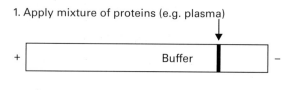

2. Proteins migrate in electric field; rate depends on molecular size and charge

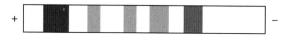

3. After electrophoresis, proteins can be detected optically to produce an electrophoretogram

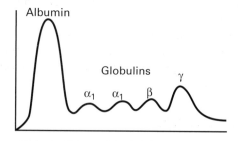

Fig. 169 Separation of plasma proteins by electrophoresis. Peaks indicate relative amounts of the different classes of protein; globulin peaks contain large mixtures of proteins.

Haptoglobulin

Haptoglobulin is an α_2-globulin, molecular weight 90 000. Its chief role is to bind any free haemoglobin in the circulation, thus preventing it appearing in the glomerular filtrate in the kidney. The haptoglobin–haemoglobin complex is then cleared by cells of the reticuloendothelial system.

α_1-Antitrypsin

α_1-Antitrypsin has a molecular weight of 52 000. Various serine proteases are inhibited by being complexed with α_1-antitrypsin. It is especially important as an inhibitor of leucocyte elastase in the lower respiratory tract. Low levels of α_1-antitrypsin are found in about 5% of cases of emphysema.

Enzymes in blood

Enzymes that function in blood include those required for blood coagulation (see below). Low concentrations of other enzymes are present in plasma arising from cell breakdown with release into blood of cellular contents. When tissues are damaged by a disease process, large amounts of tissue enzymes are released and their measurement is used to aid diagnosis, e.g. creatine kinase and lactate dehydrogenase for heart disease, amylase for pancreatitis, alanine aminotransferase in liver disease.

19.2 Immunoglobulins

Immunoglobulins (antibodies) belong to one of the systems that combat invasion of the body by foreign, potentially pathogenic, organisms present in the environment. Antibodies have the ability to bind to antigens on pathogens and this facilitates their removal by phagocytes.

Classes of antibodies

Immunoglobulins are a family of proteins and are divided into five classes, with each class having a distinct set of functions. They are all glycoproteins with variable proportions of carbohydrate in each class.

IgG
- major antibody of the secondary immune response
- can cross the placenta.

IgM
- this antibody is made by the fetus in utero
- the predominant early antibody in response to an antigen.

IgA
- predominant immunoglobulin in secretions such as saliva, colostrum, human milk, tears and gastrointestinal and respiratory secretions.

IgD
- occurs on cell surfaces; precise function unknown.

IgE
- found on mucosal surfaces
- triggers histamine release when antigen binds to it
- is a defence against worm parasites.

Antibody structure

IgG (γ-globulin) has a typical antibody structure (Fig. 170). There are pairs of larger ('heavy'; H) and smaller ('light'; L) chains. Each L chain has a molecular weight of 25 000 and is common to all classes of immunoglobulin. The H

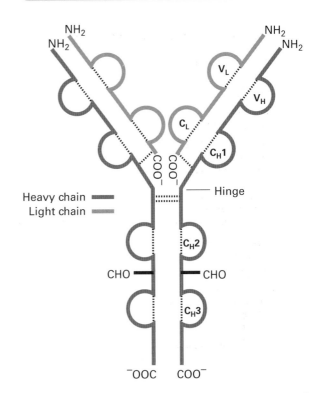

Fig. 170 Schematic representation of an immunoglobulin G (IgG) molecule. Light (L) and heavy (H) chains are shown with their constant (C) and variable (V) regions. The dotted lines represent disulphide bonds.

chains vary for each class and each has a molecular weight of 50 000–70 000. The chains are linked by disulphide bonds that are both intra- and interchain. Important aspects of immunoglobulins include:

- Each L chain has one variable (V) and one constant (C) domain.
- Each H chain has one variable and three constant domains in IgG.
- The two H chains are linked to each other through two interchain disulphide bonds at the 'hinge' region. The hinge allows for flexibility and thus there are two antigen binding sites per IgG molecule.
- Variable regions of both L and H chains are at the N-terminal end of IgG. This is the site for antigen to bind to antibody.
- Located within the variable domains of the L and H chains are hypervariable regions through which the paired HV and LV contribute to the antigen binding site of the IgG.

Antibody diversity

Antibodies are made by B lymphocytes and it is important to recognise that all of the antigen binding specificities are present in the various clones of B cells *before* they encounter the antigen. There are tens of millions of antigen specificities, which exceed the number of genes in the human genome. Gene shuffling allows a limited number of genes to give rise to the vast number of antigen binding specificities:

- A gene coding for the variable region of an L chain is made by shuffling 300 V_L genes so that one of them can finish attached to any one of four joining genes (J_L) which link the variable construct to the single gene coding for the constant region of the L chain. There will be at least 1200 possible V_L/J_L constructs.
- Similar shuffling occurs for H chain variable region but there is an extra class of genes involved. Therefore, any one of about 200 V_H genes can be attached to any one of 12 D (diversity) genes, which in turn can be next to any one of four J_H genes, which join the variable region construct of the H chain to the constant region. As a result, there can be at least $200 \times 12 \times 4$ (i.e. 9600) V_H gene constructs.
- Since an antigen binding site will be composed of the L chain variable region and the H chain variable region, there will be at least $1200 \times 9600 = 11.52$ million antigen binding specificities.

19.3 Blood coagulation

Learning objectives

You should be able to:

- describe the role of platelets in clotting
- explain how fibrinogen is converted to stable fibrin
- outline the extrinsic and intrinsic pathways and their interactions
- explain the role of vitamin K and calcium ions in blood coagulation
- describe how warfarin and heparin act as anticoagulants.

Blood coagulation is a process that results in the formation of a fibrin clot, which seals a damaged or injured blood vessel. Blood coagulation must be:

- on demand, initiated by injury to a blood vessel
- rapid and controlled
- localised at the site of injury to the vessel
- temporary.

The following series of events occurs after injury to a vessel:

1. Local vasoconstriction occurs within a few seconds to limit blood loss, with endothelin being secreted by endothelial cells.
2. Next there is *platelet plug formation*. Disruption of the endothelium exposes collagen and subendothelial elements to which platelets adhere. The platelet plug formed temporarily stops the flow of blood. For the platelets to aggregate and form the plug, a plasma protein known as the *von Willebrand factor* (vWF) is required. It forms a bridge between the platelet and the subendothelium. This is accomplished by binding of vWF to specific receptors (glycoprotein Ib/glycoprotein IX) on the surface of the activated platelets as well as to the subendothelium.
3. The coagulation cascade and fibrin formation are initiated by exposure of negatively charged phospholipids such as phosphatidylserine on the surface of activated platelets or damaged cell membranes. A series of events is triggered at the site with control being achieved by a multiple enzyme cascade that amplifies the early events. The critical step occurs when insoluble fibrin is made from soluble fibrinogen, and the fibrin molecules are crosslinked to increase the tensile strength of the clot.
4. The transient nature of the clot is attested to by the early elaboration of platelet-derived growth factor (PDGF) for permanent tissue repair and the initiation of fibrinolysis.

The blood coagulation cascade

The key feature of blood coagulation is that inactive coagulation factors are present in blood and that they are activated in a stepwise fashion (Fig. 171). By international agreement, roman numerals are used for each well-characterised clotting factor (Table 37) and a lower case letter 'a' is added to the numeral to indicate the active form of a coagulation factor (e.g. Xa). Blood coagulation schemes always appear rather complex, but we will dissect the system shown in Figure 171 by starting from the end-product, a tough fibrin clot, and work backwards to describe the entire system.

Thrombin acts on fibrinogen to produce fibrin

Fibrinogen consists of two pairs of three non-identical polypeptide chains (α, β and γ) joined by disulphide bonds. The subunit structure is usually denoted as $(A\alpha B\beta\gamma)_2$. The presence of many negative charges in the A and B portions of the alpha and beta chains prevents aggregation of fibrinogen. However, when these are

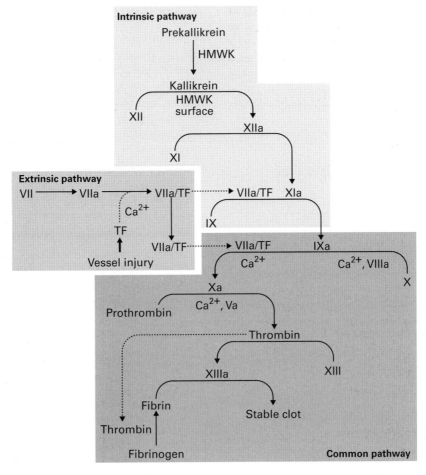

Fig. 171 The traditional blood coagulation scheme showing the reactions of the intrinsic and extrinsic pathways. TF, tissue factor; HMWK, high molecular weight kininogen.

removed by the action of the protease *thrombin*, the fibrin molecules formed can aggregate, become insoluble and form a clot of weak tensile strength as they surround the platelet plug.

Covalent bonds stabilise the clot

Stabilisation occurs through formation of bonds between lysine and glutamine residues in alpha and gamma chains in adjacent fibrin molecules. These reactions are catalysed by the active form of factor XIII (XIIIa), which is a *fibrin transamidase*. Another action of thrombin is to convert factor XIII to XIIIa.

Thrombin is made from prothrombin, factor Xa is required

The above scheme would cause clotting to occur whenever fibrinogen, thrombin and factor XIII were present and this would be disastrous. Since fibrinogen is always present in normal individuals, then the enzymes must

Table 37 Nomenclature for coagulation factors

Number	Factor
I	Fibrinogen
II	Prothrombin[a]
III	Tissue factor
IV	Calcium
V	Proaccelerin
VII	Proconvertin[a]
VIII	Antihaemophilic factor
IX	Christmas factor[a]
X	Stuart factor[a]
XI	Plasma thromboplastin antecedent
XII	Hageman factor

[a]Vitamin K-dependent factor.

not be active under normal conditions. They exist as proenzymes (zymogens) which must be modified to become active when a clot is required to plug up a damaged vessel. Thrombin is generated in the process of coagulation from its precursor in plasma, *prothrombin*. Thrombin is produced from prothrombin by the action of factor Xa and everything must now hinge on the formation of Xa.

Factor X is activated by extrinsic and intrinsic pathways

Two principal pathways have been defined:

- the *intrinsic pathway* in which all of the components are found in plasma (Fig. 171)
- the *extrinsic pathway*, which is activated by tissue factor (TF), a transmembrane protein that is not present in plasma and is contributed by tissue at the site of vessel injury (Fig. 171)
- these two pathways are followed by a common pathway, which is the reactions occurring following the activation of factor X.

Both pathways are required because of tissue factor pathway inhibitor

A defect in one pathway will give a bleeding disorder even if the other pathway is unaffected; for example, a defect in factor VII, a component of the extrinsic pathway, causes a bleeding disorder despite all of the factors of the intrinsic pathway being present. The extrinsic pathway appears to be very active when assayed in vitro and it has always been difficult to understand why the intrinsic pathway plays any role under normal circumstances. That is now understood better since a factor has been identified which after a short period of time inhibits the extrinsic pathway (*tissue factor pathway inhibitor*; TFPI), making it necessary for the intrinsic pathway to function.

The current model links the extrinsic and intrinsic pathways

When a vessel is damaged, it is factor VIIa/TF that activates both factor X to Xa and IX to IXa. Also, thrombin produced through the action of Xa can activate factors IX and VIII, thus continuing the process after TFPI inhibits the action of VIIa/TF. With this model, factor XII, high molecular weight kininogen (HMWK) and prekallikrein play only a minor role. However, when blood is placed in a test tube it will clot through the complete intrinsic pathway.

Two non-enzymic factors are required

These are factors V and VIII, so-called 'positioning factors'. Thrombin action on them gives the more active forms Va and VIIIa. Factor VIII in plasma is stabilised by vWF. The low levels of vWF found in von Willebrand's disease lead to low factor VIII levels and the potential for bleeding (this is *secondary* factor VIII deficiency). Thrombin also activates protein C which digests the active forms of factors Va and VIIIa in the presence of protein S. This latter action of thrombin is important in achieving balance and limiting blood clotting to the site of the damaged vessel. Both protein C and protein S contain Gla residues and are vitamin K-dependent factors (see below).

Clinical note:
Haemophilias

Haemophilia A
This results from deficiency of factor VIII and is the most common of the hereditary deficiencies of blood clotting. The inheritance is X-linked so females are carriers and male descendants of these carriers can be affected. Spontaneous mutations in the factor VIII gene can also occur. An affected subject has impaired intrinsic pathway activity, resulting in prolonged activated partial thromboplastin time (aPTT) but normal prothrombin time (PT). Bleeding time, which is a measure of platelet plug formation, is normal in haemophilia A. Therapy now involves the use of factor VIII made by recombinant DNA techniques to prevent HIV transmission.

Haemophilia B (Christmas disease)
This results from factor IX deficiency. Inheritance is also X-linked and recombinant factor IX is now available for therapy. aPTT is abnormal but PT and bleeding time is normal.

von Willebrand's disease (vWD)
In this disease, levels of von Willebrand factor (vWF) are low. Since vWF is necessary for platelet adhesion, affected subjects have prolonged bleeding times. vWF also stabilises factor VIII so, in this disorder, factor VIII levels can be low, leading to prolonged aPTT as well as prolonged bleeding times. vWD is the most common inherited bleeding disorder. Inheritance is autosomal dominant.

The vitamin K-dependent factors

Vitamin K (Fig. 172) deficiency leads to defects in blood coagulation. Dihydro-vitamin K is the coenzyme for a carboxylase that brings about post-translational modification of prothrombin and factors VII, IX and X (Fig. 173). An extra carboxyl group is added to several glutamates in these factors forming γ-carboxyglutamate (Gla)

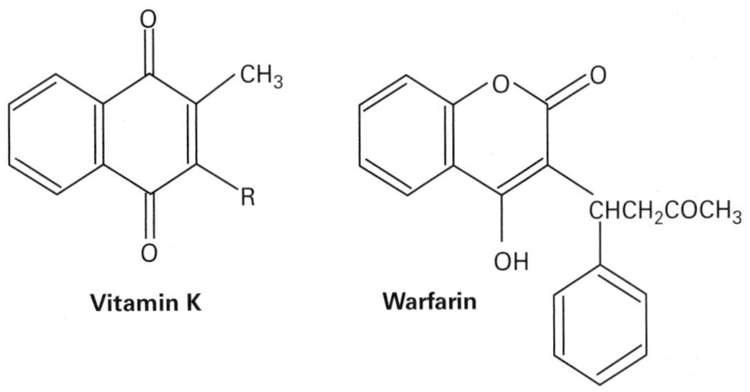

Fig. 172 The structure of vitamin K (R is an alkyl side chain that varies in different vitamin K derivatives) and warfarin.

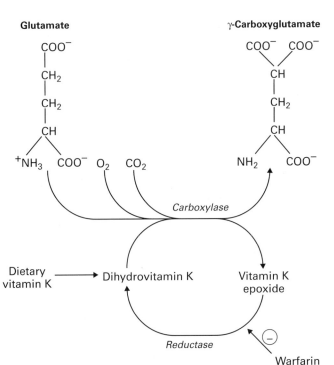

Fig. 173 The role of dihydro-vitamin K in the formation of γ-carboxyglutamate residues in prothrombin and factors VII, IX and X, and the site of action of warfarin, an anticoagulant.

residues. The regeneration of dihydro-vitamin K from the 2,3-epoxide involves two reductions catalysed by enzymes that are inhibited by coumarin anticoagulants such as *warfarin*. Factors with Gla residues bind calcium at least ten times more effectively than the same factors with glutamate residues. The binding of these factors to phospholipid surfaces through calcium localises them at the site of injury to a blood vessel where platelet plug formation has occurred and an active phospholipid surface has been made available.

Anticoagulants

Calcium chelators
Citrate, EDTA (ethylenediamine tetraacetic acid) and oxalate act by complexing ionic calcium, which is required in several steps in the blood coagulation cascade. Citrated blood is used in blood transfusions. Calcium chelators are added to blood to prepare plasma to carry out tests for blood clotting activity. Following centrifugation to sediment all the cells, the clear plasma remains on the top layer. After the plasma is prepared it can be recalcified and the rate of formation of clots can be measured following activation of the system. Serum is prepared by letting blood clot in a tube and then centrifuging at high speed to sediment down all the cells, leaving the serum as the top layer. Serum is depleted in fibrinogen and coagulation factors relative to plasma.

Heparin
This sulphated glycosaminoglycan is made in mast cells and inhibits clotting at several points by increasing several hundred-fold the activity of antithrombin III. Antithrombin III is a serum proteinase inhibitor that inhibits thrombin and also IXa and Xa (but not VIIa). Heparin is used clinically as an acute anticoagulant.

Warfarin
This coumarin-related compound is an inhibitor of dihydro-vitamin K regeneration (Fig. 173) and is used for chronic anticoagulation of patients. In contrast to heparin, it has no effect when added to a blood sample (a person and his/her liver is needed for warfarin to be effective!). Also, warfarin is a rat poison.

Fibrinolysis

In order for a damaged blood vessel to undergo repair, the clot must be dissolved; this is accomplished by fibrinolysis. Tissue-type plasminogen activator (tPA) is in vascular tissues and binds to fibrin clots. It brings about the activation of plasminogen (also bound to clots) to plasmin, a serine protease that dissolves the clot. Recently, tPA has been used successfully to treat patients who have suffered a stroke or a heart attack due to the formation of a clot in a cerebral or coronary artery.

19.4 Red cell metabolism

Learning objectives

You should be able to:

- describe the limited metabolic machinery in mature erythrocytes
- outline the roles of the glycolytic pathway in erythrocytes
- outline the roles of the pentose phosphate pathway in erythrocytes
- explain the problems caused by glucose-6-phosphate dehydrogenase deficiency.

The red cell is notorious for having limited biochemical apparatus. One critical difference between erythrocytes and their precursors, erythroblasts and reticulocytes, is the absence of mitochondria, which are lost within 24 hours of reticulocytes entering the circulation. The consequence of this is that ATP synthesis has to occur via an anaerobic pathway: glycolysis. The other limitation applies to pathways for the generation of NADPH, with only the pentose phosphate pathway being available. Clearly, glucose is the key fuel in the mature red cell.

Roles of glucose metabolism in erythrocytes

The glucose metabolic pathways in red cells are reviewed in Figure 174. The importance of other metabolic intermediates has been discussed in other chapters:

- ATP is required for ion pumps (p. 51).
- NADH is required to maintain the iron in haemoglobin as Fe^{II}. Interaction of the Fe^{II} of haemoglobin with superoxide and other oxygen free radicals can form methaemoglobin (Fe^{III}), which

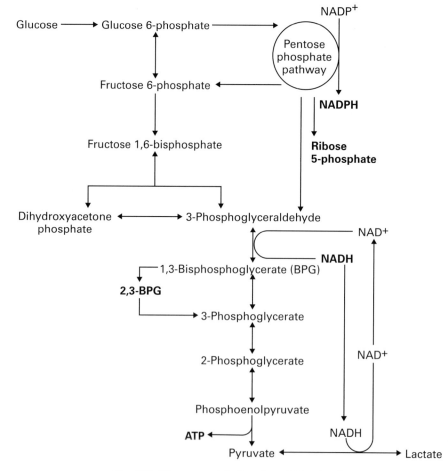

Fig. 174 Glucose metabolism in red blood cells.

Glucose-6-phosphate dehydrogenase deficiency (favism)

This is estimated to affect 400 million people worldwide. Inheritance is X-linked. Highest frequencies are found in tropical Africa, in the Middle East, in tropical and subtropical Asia, in some areas of the Mediterranean and in Papua New Guinea. It leads to impaired generation of NADPH in affected tissues. Since catalase and glutathione (via glutathione peroxidase) are essential for the detoxification of hydrogen peroxide, the defence of the cell against this compound depends ultimately and heavily on glucose-6-phosphate dehydrogenase. The most common clinical manifestations are jaundice and acute haemolytic anaemia. The acute haemolytic anaemia can be triggered by drugs, by infections, or by the ingestion of fava beans (hence, favism). Affected individuals need to be alerted to the medications they must avoid. Epidemiological data indicate strongly that absence or low activity of the enzyme can confer relative resistance against *Plasmodium falciparum* malaria.

Pyruvate kinase (PK) deficiency

This is the most common deficiency of the glycolytic pathway in erythrocytes. The inheritance is autosomal recessive and leads to non-spherocytic haemolytic anaemia. ATP synthesis is compromised since PK catalyses a step leading to ATP synthesis. The PK deficiency also results in increased levels of 2,3-bisphosphoglycerate (2,3-BPG) in erythrocytes as can be deduced from Figure 174. The increase in 2,3-BPG helps compensate for the anaemia since it will shift the oxygen dissociation curve to the right.

cannot bind oxygen. Red blood cells contain *methaemoglobin reductase* to prevent significant methaemoglobin formation. This reductase requires reduced cytochrome b_5, the level of which is dependent upon adequate NADH.

- 2,3-Bisphosphoglycerate (2,3-BPG) is the most important negative modulator of oxygen–haemoglobin association (Ch. 5, p. 62).
- NADPH is required to maintain adequate levels of reduced glutathione, which protects against oxygen free radicals.
- Ribose 5-phosphate contributes to the maintenance of AMP (ATP) levels.

Self-assessment: questions

Single best answer MCQs

1. Identify from the following list of plasma proteins the one that is the major contributor to the plasma oncotic pressure and is also the major transporter of hydrophobic molecules in plasma.
   a. Thyroxine binding globulin (TBG)
   b. Transferrin
   c. VLDL (very low density lipoprotein)
   d. Fibrinogen
   e. Albumin

2. Match the plasma proteins in Column A with functions listed in Column B and identify the only correct match.

A	B
a. α1-Antitrypsin	Activator of leucocyte elastase
b. Haptoglobin	Binds extracorpuscular haemoglobin
c. VLDL	Major transporter of cholesterol
d. Transerythretin	Transport cortisol in blood
e. Albumin	Elevated in the nephrotic syndrome

3. Identify the correct statement or statements concerning antibodies.
   a. Antibodies of the IgG class are the major immunoglobulins in plasma
   b. Antibodies of the IgG class cannot cross the placenta
   c. Antibodies of the IgM class are smaller than IgG
   d. Both a and b are correct
   e. a, b and c are all correct

4. Which of the following are direct actions of the factor VIIa–tissue factor complex in blood coagulation?
   a. X→Xa
   b. IX→IXa
   c. Prothrombin→thrombin
   d. Both a and b are direct actions
   e. a, b and c are all direct actions

5. The final step in blood coagulation is the formation of a stable fibrin clot. Identify the single correct statement about this overall process.
   a. Thrombin acts on fibrinogen to remove small peptides that are enriched in lysine and arginine
   b. Factor XIIIa catalyses a reaction in which a type of peptide bond is formed between fibrin monomers

   c. The clot will not be formed in blood from which red cells have been removed
   d. The process can be blocked in vitro by the addition of warfarin to blood
   e. Cannot occur in a plasma sample in a test tube

6. Which one of the following accurately describes the chemistry or function of factor VIII?
   a. It has proteolytic activity similar to thrombin
   b. It is a participant in the extrinsic pathway
   c. It binds calcium ions in a similar fashion to factor IX
   d. Its levels are low in blood in von Willebrand's disease
   e. Its levels are very low in haemophilia B

7. Accurately match the anticoagulants listed in Column A with the statements in Column B concerning their action.

A	B
a. Citrate	Used as a fuel by mature erythrocytes
b. Oxalate	Removes the heat-labile clotting factors
c. Heparin	Activates antithrombin III
d. EDTA	Removes vitamin K-dependent factors

8. If you had a patient with haemolytic anaemia due to pyruvate kinase deficiency in their red blood cells, would you feel most confident about the diagnosis with which one of the following findings?
   a. Low erythrocyte [2,3-BPG]
   b. High erythrocyte [ATP]
   c. Low erythrocyte [ATP]
   d. High erythrocyte [2,3-BPG]
   e. High ratio of 2,3-BPG to ATP in erythrocytes

9. One of your friends returns from a 4-week business trip to the Congo and tells you that after 2 weeks he felt unusually weak and that his colleagues had noticed yellow coloration in his sclera. He saw a local physician who explained to him that his problems were due to the antimalarial that he had been taking regularly. You were able to tell your friend that he had low levels of which one of the following erythrocyte enzymes?
   a. Transketolase
   b. Hexokinase
   c. Glucose-6-phosphate dehydrogenase
   d. 3-Phosphoglyceraldehyde dehydrogenase
   e. Phosphofructokinase-1

True/false questions

Are the following statements true or false?

1. You would expect to find many aspartate or glutamate residues in the A and B portions of the Aα and Bβ chains of fibrinogen.
2. The concentration of fibrinogen would be identical in plasma and serum samples prepared from the same subject.
3. All of the plasma proteins are made in the liver.
4. There are identical numbers of constant domains in the heavy chains and light chains of IgG.
5. Gene shuffling results in there being a small number of antigen specificities in B lymphocytes.
6. If a patient has a prolonged prothrombin time (PT), in order to fully understand this finding one has to measure PT again a few days after giving the patient an injection of vitamin K.

Short essay questions

1. Write an account of the changes that occur when fibrinogen is converted to fibrin.
2. Explain the ability of warfarin to serve as an anticoagulant.
3. Describe how you would prepare plasma and serum and any differences that exist between them.
4. Discuss the findings you would expect in a subject with pyruvate kinase (PK) deficiency.
5. Explain the biochemical consequences to a patient of having a defect in erythrocyte glucose-6-phosphate dehydrogenase.
6. List three plasma proteins synthesised in the liver that have a role in transporting compounds in blood and in each case write a few sentences that explain the significance of the role.

Self-assessment: answers

Single best answer MCQ answers

1. a. **False**. TBG is the transporter of thyroid hormones in plasma.
   b. **False**. Transferrin is the transporter of iron in plasma.
   c. **False**. VLDL is a transporter of triacylglycerol in plasma.
   d. **False**. Fibrinogen is the protein used to form a fibrin clot.
   e. **True**. Albumin is the major plasma protein in amount.

2. a. **False**. α_1-Antitrypsin inhibits leucocyte elastase.
   b. **True**. Binding occurs prior to clearance of haemoglobin by the reticuloendothelial system.
   c. **False**. The major lipid in VLDL is TAG.
   d. **False**. Transerythretin is another plasma protein that transports thyroxine.
   e. **False**. Albumin levels are very low in nephrotic syndrome due to loss in urine.

3. a. **True**. They can be readily seen in plasma electrophoresis.
   b. **False**. They can and give the fetus some protection from antigens to which the mother has been exposed.
   c. **False**. They are five times larger!
   d. **False**. b is incorrect.
   e. **False**. b and c are incorrect.

4. a. **True**. This reaction continues the extrinsic pathway.
   b. **True**. This is the connection between the two pathways.
   c. **False**. You are looking for a 'direct' action.
   d. This is the single best answer.
   e. **False**. c is incorrect.

5. a. **False**. The fibrinopeptides released are enriched in Glu and Asp (negatively charged).
   b. **True**. The reaction between the amide of Gln and the ε-amino group of Lys forms an isopeptide bond (strong!).
   c. **False**. The clotting machinery is in plasma!
   d. **False**. Warfarin only acts in vivo on someone and their liver.
   e. **False**. The clotting tests are run in tubes!

6. a. **False**. It is a positioning factor.
   b. **False**. It is in the intrinsic pathway.

c. **False**. It doesn't have Gla residues.
   d. **True**. Although VIII is synthesised in vWD, it is labile when vWF is low.
   e. **False**. VIII levels are normal in haemophilia B but IX levels are low.

7. a. **False**. Citrate cannot be used as a fuel (they have no mitochondria) but it can bind Ca^{2+}.
   b. **False**. It binds Ca^{2+}.
   c. **True**. It increases antithrombin III activity several hundred-fold.
   d. **False**. It binds Ca^{2+}.

8. a. **False**. [2,3-BPG] would be high.
   b. **False**. [ATP] would be low.
   c. **False**. Although [ATP] is low, the normal range is large.
   d. **False**. Although [2,3-BPG] is high, the normal range is large.
   e. **True**. The high [2,3-BPG] and low [ATP] when combined establish the diagnosis.

9. a. **False**. Transketolase is normal.
   b. **False**. Hexokinase is normal.
   c. **True**. The defect results in low production of NADPH and therefore low reduced glutathione levels. Thus protection against oxygen free radicals is low. The end result is that erythrocyte membranes rupture.
   d. **False**. Glycolysis is normal.
   e. **False**. Glycolysis is unaffected.

True/false answers

1. **True**. Glutamate and aspartate are dicarboxylic acids and it is the concentration of negative charges in the A and B fibrinopeptides that prevent fibrinogen from aggregating to form a clot.
2. **False**. Serum is prepared by letting a blood sample clot; this means that the serum has low concentrations of fibrinogen compared with plasma prepared by centrifuging blood that is prevented from clotting by the addition of heparin or the removal of calcium ions.
3. **False**. Whereas most are made in the liver, including the most abundant one albumin, many are not, including the immunoglobulins and enzymes released as a result of normal cell turnover throughout the body.
4. **False**. The heavy chains have three and the light chains have one.

5. **False**. On the contrary, gene shuffling accounts for the enormous diversity of antibodies that can be generated in response to antigens.
6. **True**. PT depends upon Factor VII which is a vitamin K-dependent factor with a short half-life. Prolonged PT can be due to K deficiency as opposed to liver malfunction.

Short essay answers

1. Fibrinogen is present in plasma at relatively high concentrations (about 350 mg/dl) and is very water-soluble. It consists of three non-identical pairs of polypeptide chains (α, β and γ) which are linked by disulphide bonds. The critical structural feature is that the N-terminal portions of the alpha and beta chains have many negative charges provided by aspartate and glutamate. When these are removed in the form of fibrinopeptides A and B by the action of thrombin, the fibrin monomers that remain have binding sites exposed that allow them to aggregate to form a low-tensile-strength clot. The aggregated fibrin is held together by non-covalent bonds. Isopeptide bonds are formed between ε-amino groups of lysines and amide groups of glutamines in neighbouring fibrin molecules to give a stable fibrin clot with high tensile strength. This reaction is catalysed by activated factor XIII (formed from XIII by thrombin action).

2. Several blood coagulation factors (prothrombin, factors VII, IX and X) are modified in the liver by having several of their glutamate (Glu) residues carboxylated to form γ-carboxyglutamate (Gla) residues. This gives these proteins a greatly increased ability to bind calcium. The coenzyme for the carboxylase involved in Gla formation is dihydro-vitamin K. In the reaction, dihydro-vitamin K is converted to a 2,3-epoxide and the latter has to be converted back to dihydro-vitamin K if there is to be efficient formation of the Gla-containing factors. The reductases involved in the conversion are inhibited by coumarins such as warfarin. Warfarin is used for chronic anticoagulation of patients. It is frequently described as a 'blood thinner'.

3. To prepare plasma, one has to prevent clotting of the blood sample. This can be done by adding heparin to inhibit multiple steps in the blood coagulation cascade or by complexing calcium ions by use of compounds such as oxalate, citrate or EDTA. The treated blood sample is then subjected to centrifugation at sufficient speed (g) to sediment down all formed elements in blood, including red cells, leucocytes, neutrophils, etc. Lying above the cell layer is plasma. It is plasma that is used for PT and aPTT assays, which are used to evaluate the extrinsic and intrinsic pathways, respectively.

To prepare serum, a blood sample is allowed to clot, usually in a tube standing on ice. The sample is then centrifuged and serum will appear as a clear liquid phase above the formed elements plus clot, which centrifuge to the foot of the tube. Serum will have low levels of fibrinogen and other clotting factors compared with plasma.

4. Red cell metabolism is much impaired in subjects with PK deficiency since red cells are dependent upon glycolysis for ATP synthesis and PK catalyses the step in glycolysis in which net ATP formation is achieved. Red cell lysis will occur and the subject will be anaemic. Increased red cell turnover will lead to increased bilirubin synthesis, which, if it overwhelms the liver's capacity to handle it, will lead to hyperbilirubinaemia (jaundice). Since PK activity is low, glycolytic intermediates that precede it will accumulate, including 2,3-BPG. An increase in the red cell ratio of 2,3-BPG to ATP will help establish the diagnosis.

5. Glucose-6-phosphate dehydrogenase (G-6-PDH) catalyses the first step in the pentose phosphate pathway, which has a principal role of generating NADPH and ribose 5-phosphate. In subjects with a G-6-PDH deficiency, it is red blood cells (RBCs) that are especially at risk since they have a limited number of metabolic pathways available to them (they lack mitochondria) and have no other source of NADPH. A principal role of NADPH in RBCs is to maintain levels of glutathione, which plays a key role in the response of cells to oxidative stress. RBCs in someone with G-6-PDH deficiency will tend to haemolyse, especially when the person takes drugs or foodstuffs (e.g. fava beans) that generate lots of oxygen radicals. In these circumstances, RBC turnover is enhanced because of increased lysis. Oxygen delivery to tissues will be less efficient. In addition, the ability of the body to deal with bile pigments, metabolites of the haem part of haem proteins, is exceeded, leading to jaundice.

6. Three plasma proteins could be albumin, thyroxine binding globulin (TBG) and transferrin.
Albumin. This major plasma protein is the most prominent transporter of hydrophobic molecules in plasma. Examples of such molecules are free fatty acids, unconjugated bilirubin, aspirin and aldosterone. Fatty acids are important fuels for muscles, especially cardiac muscle, and they have to

be transported from their storage site in adipose tissue through an aqueous medium. Albumin also binds calcium: this is of clinical importance as the total calcium in blood will be altered if albumin concentrations are altered.

TBG. The major plasma protein binding thyroxine and triiodothyronine, the thyroid hormones, is TBG. The extent of binding is very high and, clearly, if the level of TBG changes then the total amount of these hormones will change. Knowledge of this is important when one is examining thyroid hormone levels in patients. The level of TBG is increased by oestrogen and this will happen if one treats a subject with oestrogen or if the patient is pregnant.

Transferrin. This protein is responsible for transporting ferric iron in the body. All cells with mitochondria require iron for their cytochromes. Iron is required for haemoglobin synthesis and for cell division and growth. Clearly, iron has to be delivered to cells and this is the function of transferrin. Other proteins are involved in controlling the actual uptake of iron from transferrin into cells.

20 Biochemical genetics and inborn errors of metabolism

Overview

Over 3000 diseases probably have a genetic basis. Many chronic diseases have a genetic component, and genetic predispositions to at least some forms of cancer have been found. Rapid progress has been made recently in understanding the molecular basis of many inherited diseases. Modern techniques of molecular genetics can be used to find the genes involved and to follow these genes from one generation to another. Biochemistry can link a genetic condition and its associated disease. It may then provide the basis for rational treatment. These advances have put diagnosis of genetic disease and genetic counselling on a secure footing and may ultimately enable 'gene therapy'.

20.1 Introduction

Learning objective

You should be able to:

• explain in general terms the human genetic make-up.

The concept of inherited disease was first recognised by Garrod from his studies of four families in which 11 individuals had the relatively harmless disorder *alkaptonuria*. In this condition the subject's urine turns black on standing and there is arthritis in later life. The biochemical basis was accumulation and excretion of homogentisic acid resulting from lack of an enzyme that breaks down a metabolic product of the aromatic amino acids phenylalanine and tyrosine.

Human genetic make-up and mutation

Genes are arranged on chromosomes at *loci*, sites where each particular gene is to be found. If the loci on maternal and paternal chromosomes carry identical versions of a gene, the individual is said to be *homozygous*. If the genes are different, the individual is *heterozygous*.

In the human body most cells are diploid, containing 23 pairs of chromosomes (22 autosomes plus XX or XY sex chromosomes). In each pair of chromosomes one is of maternal origin and the other of paternal origin. Maternal and paternal germ cells are haploid (only one copy of each chromosome per cell, i.e. 22 autosomes plus X or Y). Females have two X chromosomes, but the X chromosome is unpaired in males.

The role of genes in controlling protein structure and function is discussed in Chapters 12 and 14. Table 38 lists the patterns of inherited diseases. New mutations in germ cells are passed on to succeeding generations. New somatic cell mutations are not, but may be important (e.g. in the development of cancer).

20.2 Patterns of inheritance

Learning objectives

You should be able to:

• differentiate between the various patterns of inheritance

• interpret family pedigrees.

Knowledge of Mendelian inheritance is important in investigating inherited disease. Different patterns of inheritance will be seen, depending upon whether the mutant gene is dominant or recessive and whether it is on an autosome or a sex chromosome.

Table 38 Gene changes that can cause disease

Type	Change	Example
Chromosome duplication	Three copies instead of two for one chromosome	Chromosome 21 in Down's syndrome
Amplification	Duplication of a section of DNA, particularly triplet repeats	Myotonic dystrophy
Translocation	Movement of a section of DNA within a chromosome or between chromosomes	Burkitt's lymphoma
Point mutations	Single base change, may or may not affect function (p. 202)	Beta-thalassaemia
Deletions/Insertions	Will result in a frameshift (p. 202)	Alpha-thalassaemia
Mitochondrial DNA changes	Affects mitochondrially coded proteins	Familial mitochondrial encephalomyopathy
Multifactorial polygenic changes	A clear genetic change which may affect several genes but in addition an environmental factor is involved	Diabetes mellitus
Disorders of the mechanism protecting against genome damage	Gene changes have an indirect effect in that the body cannot repair somatic gene damage	Hereditary non-polyposis colon cancer

Autosomal recessive disorders

- Mutant gene must be in one of the 22 autosomes.
- Only in the homozygous state will the clinical condition be apparent.
- Pedigree shows horizontal pattern.
- Both sexes equally affected.
- Affected person's offspring are all unaffected unless the other parent is a carrier.
- Examples include alkaptonuria, cystic fibrosis, Tay–Sachs disease and phenylketonuria.
- Autosomal recessive formerly meant that one in four would be affected in more or less the same way (age of onset, manifestations, severity). With DNA diagnosis, rather than strict pedigree logic, we now know that the severity of clearly related homozygotes varies to degrees not accounted for by the specific mutant alleles they have in common.

Autosomal dominant disorders

- Heterozygotes will manifest the disease, i.e. the subject has one abnormal and one normal gene.
- Pedigree shows vertical pattern.
- Both sexes equally affected and able to pass the defective gene on.
- Examples include familial hypercholesterolaemia and Huntington's disease.
- Lack of penetrance may be an indication that exogenous or environmental factors are involved in the expression of phenotype, e.g. acute intermittent porphyria.

X-linked recessive disorders

- The abnormal gene is on the X chromosome.
- The disorder is almost completely confined to males.
- The pattern is oblique.
- Males have unaffected parents but do have affected uncles.
- Transmitted only by female carriers.
- Examples include haemophilia A and B, and Duchenne's muscular dystrophy.

20.3 Inborn errors of metabolism

Learning objectives

You should be able to:

- identify the enzyme defects in disorders of carbohydrate, amino acid and fat metabolism

- explain in depth phenylketonuria and how methods have been developed to allow for its detection in the newborn

- outline the various approaches to the management of genetic disease.

Mutations can affect biochemical pathways

Figure 175 shows the possible consequences of a deficiency in an enzyme involved in a metabolic pathway. Given that there are thousands of inborn errors of metabolism, it will only be possible to discuss a few of them here. Those that are presented illustrate important aspects of diagnosis and therapy.

Amino acid metabolism

There are many disorders in amino acid metabolism, some of which are summarised in Table 39. Phenylketonuria has had great significance in terms of testing procedures and therapy.

Carbohydrate metabolism

Glycogen storage diseases

There are several glycogen storage diseases (Table 40); in each case there are excessive levels of glycogen in liver or muscle. In several of these it is easy to predict the outcome from knowledge of the significance of the metabolic pathway that becomes impaired:

- hepatic glucose-6-phosphatase deficiency will lead to hypoglycaemia, given the critical role of this enzyme in glucose production by either glycogenolysis or gluconeogenesis
- muscle phosphorylase deficiency will affect the ability to support a high level of muscular contraction given the key role that glycogen serves as the fuel supporting such work.

Other disorders

Other disorders in carbohydrate metabolism are listed in Table 41. Because of the severity of the form of galactosaemia involving defective galactose-1-phosphate uridyltransferase, blood samples from newborn infants are screened for high levels of galactose. The condition is treated by withdrawing lactose (and galactose) from the diet.

Lipid metabolism

Familial hypercholesterolaemia (FH) and sphingolipidoses are discussed in Chapter 9.

Management of genetic diseases

Biochemical approaches

Understanding the biochemical nature of the defect can greatly aid the management of genetic diseases. Here are some successful strategies:

- Control of metabolite levels: e.g. limit uptake of precursors which might undergo toxic accumulation (used in phenylketonuria).
- Supply the missing metabolite: e.g. give thyroxine to treat thyroid insufficiency caused by defects in thyroid hormone synthesis.

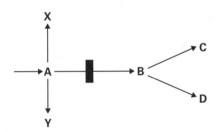

Fig. 175 A defect in a pathway enzyme will have effects: A↑, X and Y (minor metabolites) ↑, B, C and D ↓. In addition, changing levels of components of the pathway may influence other systems.

Table 39 Inborn errors of amino acid metabolism

Amino acid	Name of disorder	Enzyme affected
Phenylalanine	Phenylketonuria (PKU)	Phenylalanine hydroxylase Dihydropteridine reductase
Tyrosine	Tyrosinaemia I Tyrosinaemia II	Fumarylacetoacetate hydrolase Tyrosine aminotransferase
Methionine	Homocystinuria	Cystathionine synthase in the methionine salvage pathway
Branched-chain amino acids	Maple syrup urine disease	Branched-chain keto acid dehydrogenase
Phenylalanine and tyrosine	Alkaptonuria	Homogenistic acid oxidase
Tyrosine	Albinism	Tyrosinase
All amino acids	Hyperammonaemia	Urea cycle defect, e.g. ornithine transcarbamylase

Clinical note:
Phenylketonuria

Phenylketonuria (PKU) is an example of an autosomal recessive disorder. If it is not diagnosed at birth, the phenotype includes mental retardation, neurological seizures and diluted pigmentation of hair and skin.

Biochemical basis
The deficiency of phenylalanine catabolism occurs because phenylalanine 4-hydroxylase is absent or greatly reduced. The enzyme converts phenylalanine into tyrosine, the precursor of dopamine, noradrenaline (norepinephrine), adrenaline (epinephrine) and thyroid hormones (Fig. 176). Phenylalanine 4-hydroxylase is a mixed-function oxidase with a requirement for reducing power, so that the complete system is rather complex (Fig. 177). Clearly, low rates of conversion of phenylalanine to tyrosine can also occur if the tetrahydrobiopterin (THBP) coenzyme is not regenerated owing to defective dihydropteridine reductase. THBP is also required in the biosynthesis of the neurotransmitters dopamine, noradrenaline (norepinephrine), adrenaline (epinephrine) and serotonin. Treatment of PKU caused by defective THBP metabolism involves the addition of DOPA (dihydroxyphenylalanine) and 5-hydroxytryptophan to the diet in addition to restriction of phenylalanine.

Genetic basis
In the classic form of PKU, most mutations are point mutations in either a splice site (40%) or the coding region (single amino acid change: 20%).

Clinical effects
Although the phenylalanine 4-hydroxylase enzyme is present in the liver, the effects are far more wide-ranging, i.e. a defect in one tissue may give clinical symptoms in another tissue. The block in conversion of phenylalanine causes elevated levels of this amino acid in blood and urine. It is the resultant hyperphenylalaninaemia that impairs brain development leading to mental retardation. The term phenylketonuria was coined because a minor catabolic pathway was increased in PKU resulting in the excretion of large quantities of phenylpyruvic acid (a phenylketone). Phenylpyruvic acid is not the cause for the clinical abnormalities. Since phenylalanine is a competitive inhibitor of tyrosinase in melanocytes, there is reduced melanin formation in these subjects. Also, tyrosine levels can be low in PKU.

The diagnosis of PKU is made in neonates
Children with PKU cannot be recognised at birth by physical examination since they have been protected from defective phenylalanine metabolism by their mothers. However, when they consume and metabolise protein they will develop hyperphenylalaninaemia and only a few months' exposure to this will cause reduced mentation (5 IQ points lost per month). Every newborn in the UK is screened for hyperphenylalaninaemia by the Guthrie test, which is a microbiological assay carried out on a dried spot of blood taken (ideally) after the baby is about 5 days old and has had several meals containing protein. The aim is to identify newborn children with the defect in order that dietary therapy can be instituted, by restricting phenylalanine intake in the diet. However, enough phenylalanine must be included since it is one of the essential amino acids. PKU testing is also done in some clinical laboratories using a 'tandem mass spectroscopy' methodology. This allows for as many as 40 inborn errors to be tested on the dried spot of blood samples.

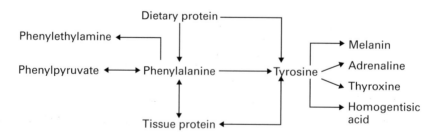

Fig. 176 Phenylalanine and tyrosine metabolism.

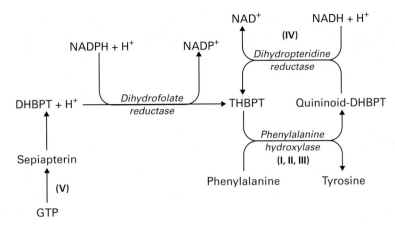

Fig. 177 Phenylalanine hydroxylase and its coenzyme requirement. Defects in phenylalanine hydroxylase result in types I, II and III PKU; defects in regeneration of the tetrahydrobiopterin (THBPT) coenzyme result in type IV PKU; and deficient production of the THBPT precursor causes type V PKU.

Table 40 The glycogen storage diseases

Type	Enzyme affected	Tissues affected	Symptoms
I	Glucose-6-phosphatase	Liver, kidney, intestine	Large liver and kidney, stunted growth, acidosis, hypoglycaemia, hyperlipidaemia
II	Lysosomal glucosidases	All organs	Cardiomegaly, hepatomegaly
III	Debranching enzyme	Liver, muscle, heart	Hepatomegaly, normal lipids and glucose
IV	Branching enzyme	Generalised	Hepatosplenomegaly, ascites, cirrhosis, liver failure
V	Muscle phosphorylase	Skeletal muscle only	Weakness and cramping of skeletal muscle on exercise, no rise of blood lactate
VI	Liver phosphorylase	Liver	Hepatomegaly, normal spleen, no hypoglycaemia, lipaemia or acidosis
VII	Phosphofructokinase-1	Skeletal muscle, red blood cells	Weakness and cramping of skeletal muscle on exercise

Table 41 Disorders in carbohydrate metabolism

Disorder	Defective enzyme
Essential fructosuria	Fructokinase
Hereditary fructose intolerance	Fructose-1-phosphate aldolase
Galactosaemia	Galactokinase or galactose-1-phosphate uridyltransferase
Haemolytic anaemia	Pyruvate kinase, glucose-6-phosphate dehydrogenase

- Use drugs to alter metabolite levels: e.g. to assist in clearance of an accumulating metabolite (use of cholestyramine complexes to increase cholesterol excretion in FH) or to modulate an enzyme activity (inhibition of cytosolic HMG-CoA reductase, the control step of cholesterol biosynthesis, in FH).

- Replace affected organ(s) by transplant: e.g. cystic fibrosis could be treated by a lung or heart/lung transplant; FH homozygotes need a liver transplant to survive; and adult polycystic kidney disease is treatable by kidney transplant.

- Supply the missing protein: this is easy if blood is the tissue affected (factor VIII injections in haemophilia A). There has also been success in replacing defective enzymes with notable success achieved in the treatment of Gaucher's disease and Fabry's disease.

Gene therapy: potential and problems

The aim of gene therapy is to replace the mutated gene with a good copy of the cloned sequence. In practice, there have been many problems and at this time there has been no success. Several therapies have been stopped because of unforeseen negative effects on patients.

20.4 DNA analysis and inherited disease

Learning objectives

You should be able to:

- explain how modern methods are used to detect genetic disorders

- define the terms: cloning, restriction enzymes, restriction mapping, restriction fragment length polymorphisms, polymerase chain reaction; and describe how they are used in modern medicine

- give examples of the use of recombinant DNA technology to prepare proteins of therapeutic value.

Diagnostic methods

Accurate and early diagnosis is needed for successful management and treatment of inherited disease. As well as carrying out diagnosis in existing individuals and making a prognosis for them, we also need to advise them on the prospects for any children they may have. In addition, we need the ability to make antenatal diagnosis to advise parents of the likely prognosis for any baby they have conceived.

Diagnosis can be biochemical or DNA-based. While the latter is more modern, the former is still very useful for some conditions. Normally it is done at 12–16 weeks of gestation by amniocentesis, with a positive diagnosis being followed by counselling. Amniotic cells can be cultured for chromosome and biochemical tests. An enzyme assay carried out on amniotic cells for hexosaminidase A is used to screen for Tay–Sachs disease (p. 138), which causes cerebral degeneration/death at age 3–4 years. Carriers for Tay–Sachs disease have been screened for in Jewish populations; this allows for appropriate counselling for couples who are both heterozygotes for this autosomal recessive disorder. Amniocentesis is risky and it is done at a relatively late stage of development of the fetus. Chorionic villus sampling to obtain fetal cells can be done as early as 6–8 weeks. DNA is extracted from the samples for DNA analyses.

Genetic approaches to inherited disease

Human molecular genetics has revolutionised the detection and monitoring of the mutant genes that cause inherited diseases. The major advantage of DNA analysis for antenatal testing is that the technique is not limited to proteins that the amniocytes express. It is the DNA of the fetal cell that is analysed and that reflects the DNA in every other cell in the body.

Molecular genetics has provided routine techniques:

- for extracting DNA from samples
- for amplifying parts of its sequence to produce enough DNA for other techniques
- for cleaving it at sites where specific short sequences occur
- for determining the length of cleavage fragments
- for determining the sequence of DNA chains hundreds of nucleotide units in length
- for isolating fragments containing sequences of interest
- for locating the positions of sequences of interest on specific chromosomes
- for detecting differences between almost identical sequences
- for expressing sequences that specify the amino acid sequences of proteins.

The following is a summary of biochemical methods now common in medical genetics.

Cloning

Amplification of DNA can be carried out by cloning. The DNA to be amplified is cleaved into fragments, typically thousands of base pairs in length, which are inserted into the DNA of a suitable bacteriophage or other vector that is used to infect bacteria growing in a dish of solid medium. Each phage particle, carrying its unique inserted sequence, produces a plaque on the dish, which contains thousands of new phage, all identical to the original. Phage from each plaque is then propagated in a bacterial culture and harvested.

Polymerase chain reaction

Amplification of DNA sequences may also be achieved by means of the polymerase chain reaction (PCR). In this technique, samples of DNA are used as a template for the in vitro synthesis of new chains (Fig. 178). The whole process is made more convenient by the availability of purified DNA polymerase from thermophilic bacteria which is not destroyed by the high temperatures needed to separate the DNA strands. Repeated cycles of duplication can be performed with a single reaction mixture by programmed temperature changes between the temperatures needed for separation of the DNA chains, for annealing the primers, which are added in excess at the start, and for DNA synthesis.

Restriction enzymes

Specific cleavage of DNA molecules is carried out using *restriction endonucleases* or restriction enzymes (Fig. 179). These enzymes, which are part of a bacterial system for preventing phage infection, recognise specific short (typically six, but sometimes four or eight) base pair sequences within a DNA double helix and cleave both chains at this site. The cleavage sequences are often palindromic, reading the same from left to right or from right to left. Both chains may be cut between neighbouring base pairs to produce blunt ends or the cuts to the two chains may be offset producing sticky ends. Since 4^6 or 4096 different six base sequences are possible, an enzyme that recognises such a sequence will cleave DNA into fragments with an average length of 4096 base pairs. Many such enzymes, each specific for its own cleavage sequence, have been identified and isolated. The enzymes are named after the strain of bacteria in which they occur, e.g. *Eco*R1 from *E. coli*, *Bam*H1 from *Bacillus amyloliquefaciens*. The polynucleotides produced from DNA by treatment with restriction enzymes are known as *restriction fragments*.

Fragment separation by gel electrophoresis

Restriction fragments may be separated from one another and their lengths measured by electrophoresis on agarose gels. All polynucleotides are negatively charged, carrying one negative charge on the phosphate of each nucleotide unit. Their electrophoretic migration rate towards the positive electrode depends only on their length and not on their base composition or sequence. Because of the sieving action of the gel, short fragments migrate faster than long fragments. A mixture

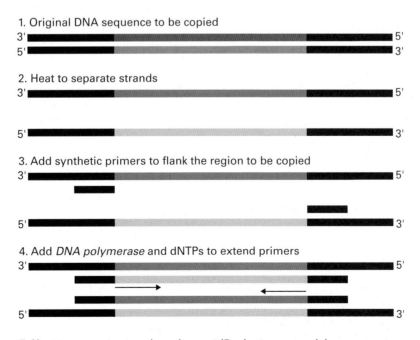

1. Original DNA sequence to be copied

2. Heat to separate strands

3. Add synthetic primers to flank the region to be copied

4. Add *DNA polymerase* and dNTPs to extend primers

5. Heat to separate strands and repeat (5 minutes per cycle)

Fig. 178 The polymerase chain reaction for amplification of specific DNA sequences.

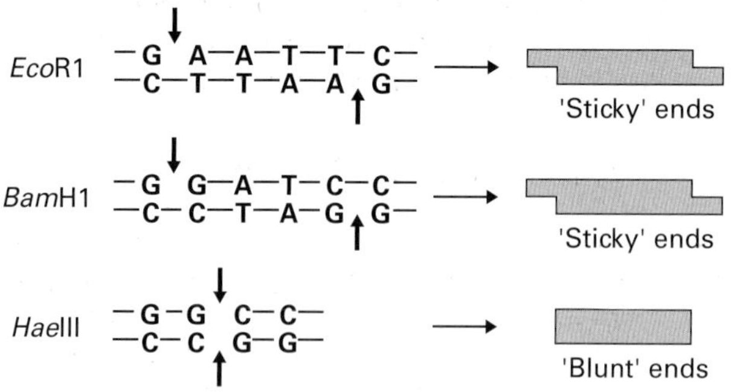

Fig. 179 Examples of restriction endonucleases.

of fragments can thus be separated and the lengths of individual fragments determined by running the mixture on a gel together with marker fragments of known length.

Restriction mapping

Regions of DNA can be mapped by a combination of cleavage with restriction enzymes and measurement of fragment lengths. The restriction map produced in this way is a physical map of the DNA showing the distances between the various restriction sites. Such a map is the basis for a complete base sequence determination of the region.

Restriction fragment length polymorphisms

Mutations occasionally lead to creation of a new cleavage site or removal of a former one. A mutation may thus alter the lengths of restriction fragments produced from a particular region of the DNA. Two fragments may no longer be separated and thus appear as a single fragment with a length of the two combined. Alternatively, a single fragment may have a new site created within it and appear as two shorter fragments. These fragment patterns, which are known as restriction fragment length polymorphisms or RFLPs, behave like Mendelian genes and can be traced from parents to offspring. More importantly, they can be mapped on the chromosomes and provide much more useful markers than conventional genes.

RFLPs in the diagnosis of inherited disease

Mapping restriction sites and locating genes on chromosomes provide powerful and incisive tools for studying the inheritance of mutant genes responsible for inherited diseases. Because crossing over events are rare between sites or genes that are close together on a chromosome, following the inheritance of an RFLP gives very strong evidence about whether a neigh-

bouring gene, perhaps one involved in an inherited disease, has been passed on or not.

DNA sequencing

DNA fragments up to several hundred base pairs long can be sequenced directly by the Sanger 2,3-dideoxy method.

Southern blotting

DNA fragments containing known sequences can be located after gel electrophoresis by the process of Southern blotting. After electrophoretic separation, the fragments are converted to single chain form by treatment with alkali and transferred, or blotted, from the gel to a sheet of nitrocellulose. If the sheet is then probed with short lengths of DNA of known sequence, the probes, which are usually radioactively labelled for easy detection, will anneal with those separated fragments that have a complementary sequence. After excess probes have been washed away, only probes that have annealed will remain on the sheet. Detection of their radioactivity reveals the positions of the required fragments.

Locations of genes on chromosomes can be revealed using a similar technique. Probes, short lengths of DNA carrying either a radioactive or fluorescent marker, can be annealed with suitable chromosome preparations, thereby showing on which chromosome and where within the chromosome sequences complementary to the probe are located. This provides a much more powerful method than conventional genetics for finding gene loci on chromosomes.

Production of proteins of therapeutic value by recombinant DNA technology

A fragment of DNA that codes for a protein can be inserted into a suitable vector that has a promoter sequence near the point of insertion. Expression of the DNA sequence, i.e. transcription to mRNA and translation to protein, may then be achieved by introducing the vector into a host cell. Notice that direct transfer of eukaryotic DNA fragments into bacteria will not work since bacteria cannot deal with any introns the DNA may contain. Better to isolate the relevant RNA from eukaryotic tissue and make so-called cDNA by copying this RNA sequence into DNA using reverse transcriptase. Another problem is that bacteria are incapable of carrying out any post-translational modification the manufactured protein may require. Expression vectors that can use eukaryotic hosts have been developed.

Examples of the use of this methodology are:

- Preparation of factor VIII for treatment of haemophilia A. Previously, haemophiliacs were treated with blood products enriched with this factor. However, some blood used for the preparation was HIV-contaminated and many treated haemophiliacs developed AIDS.
- Preparation of growth hormone, which is used to treat children who are deficient in this hormone. Several growth hormone preparations proved to be contaminated and Creutzfeldt–Jacob disease (CJD), a fatal encephalopathy, developed in some treated subjects. Human growth hormone is now manufactured by recombinant DNA technology. This eliminates the risk of CJD and also produces growth hormone in much larger quantities than were previously available.

- Insulin that had previously been prepared from the pancreas of animals is now produced by recombinant DNA technology; the product is not antigenic.

The Human Genome Project

The Human Genome Project has succeeded in characterising the complete human genome, including its 25 000–30 000 coding units. It is an enabling technology for molecular medicine. Molecular medicine will enable the early detection of diseases and powerful analytical approaches to determine the biochemical nature of diseases. The project was an enormous task given that the human genome is 3×10^9 base pairs (equivalent to a DNA molecule 5 feet long). Most of the DNA (>90%) is non-coding (introns/intergenic sequence/junk DNA) and only 10% is coding.

Self-assessment: questions

Single best answer MCQs

1. You are evaluating a patient who you suspect may have an inborn error of metabolism where the inheritance is known to be autosomal recessive (AR). Which one of the following fits with such a mode of inheritance?
   a. The pedigree would shown a vertical pattern
   b. Both parents would be carriers for the defect
   c. Only male siblings would be affected
   d. Only female siblings would be affected
   e. The mutant gene would be on either X or Y chromosomes

2. You are evaluating a patient who you suspect may have an inborn error of metabolism where the inheritance is known to be autosomal dominant (AD). Which one of the following fits with such a mode of inheritance?
   a. The pedigree would show a horizontal pattern
   b. Only in the homozygous state would the clinical condition be apparent
   c. Only females would be affected
   d. Only males would be affected
   e. Heterozygotes will manifest the disease

3. Identify the inborn error in Column A that is aligned correctly with the defective enzyme causing the disorder listed in Column B.

A	B
a. Phenylketonuria	Tyrosinase
b. Haemolytic anaemia	Pyruvate dehydrogenase
c. Glycogen storage disease I	Muscle glycogen phosphorylase
d. Maple syrup urine disease	Branched-chain ketoacid dehydrogenase
e. Alkaptonuria	Phenylalanine hydroxylase

4. Identify the single statement that applies to sphingolipidoses.
   a. The inheritance is invariably autosomal dominant
   b. The defective enzymes are involved in the synthesis of sphingolipids
   c. In Tay–Sachs disease the defective enzyme is hexosaminidase A

   d. The defective enzymes are located in mitochondria
   e. The sphingolipids that accumulate all contain carbohydrate moieties

5. Identify the only pair in which cause and disease are linked correctly:
   a. Glucose-6-phosphate dehydrogenase (G6PD) deficiency and favism
   b. Homocystinuria and tyrosine metabolism
   c. Niemann–Pick disease and ganglioside accumulation
   d. Defective tetrahydrobiopterin biosynthesis and phenylketonuria (PKU) type I
   e. Hyperammoniaemia and tricarboxylic acid cycle defect

6. Which of the following is recommended concerning tests for inborn errors of amino acid catabolism instituted by Guthrie?
   a. Carrying out the assay for the offending amino acid in blood rather than for a metabolite of the amino acid in urine
   b. Ensuring that blood samples (dried spots of blood) are withdrawn after the child has had several protein-containing meals
   c. Carrying out the test when the child reaches 5 years of age
   d. Both a and b are recommended
   e. a, b and c are all recommended

True/false questions

Are the following statements true or false?
1. The mutation that results in the formation of HbS (sickle cell haemoglobin) rather than HbA is a single base change in the DNA coding for beta chains of haemoglobin.
2. Albinism results from a defect in melanin biosynthesis.
3. PCR stands for polymerase chain reductase.
4. Familial hypercholesterolaemia is an example of a disease for which the inheritance is autosomal recessive.
5. Restriction enzymes recognise sequences in DNA that are often palindromic.
6. Differential clinical symptoms may result from different mutations in a given gene.

7. Prenatal diagnosis of an inherited disease requires that the biochemical nature of the defect is understood.

8. Linked polymorphisms (RFLPs) are of greater value in disease diagnosis than mapping conventional genes.

9. DNA probes can be used to identify the chromosomal location of genes.

10. Recombinant methods always employ bacteria as the host cell for producing proteins to be subsequently used in therapy.

11. Southern blotting cannot be carried out at the North Pole.

12. A cDNA library prepared from a tissue such as liver would be much smaller than a genomic library prepared from liver.

Short essay question

Contrast the testing procedures used in the diagnosis of phenylketonuria (PKU) with those used in Tay–Sachs disease (TSD).

Self-assessment: answers

Single best answer MCQ answers

1. a. **False**. Inheritance is horizontal in AR disorders.
   b. **True**. The affected individual inherits a defective gene from both parents.
   c. **False**. Both sexes are equally affected.
   d. **False**. Both sexes are equally affected.
   e. **False**. The mutant gene is on one of the 22 autosomes.

2. a. **False**. Inheritance is vertical in AD disorders.
   b. **False**. Only one mutant gene need be inherited.
   c. **False**. Both sexes are equally affected.
   d. **False**. Both sexes are equally affected.
   e. **True**. The subject has one abnormal gene leading to the disorder.

3. a. **False**. The defective enzyme is phenylalanine hydroxylase or dihydropteridine reductase.
   b. **False**. Mature red cells do not have mitochondria where PDC is located.
   c. **False**. Liver glucose-6-phosphatase is the defective enzyme.
   d. **True**. This enzyme is in the catabolic pathway for all three branched-chain amino acids.
   e. **False**. Homogentisic acid oxidase is the defective enzyme.

4. a. **False**. All are autosomal recessive with the exception of Fabry's disease.
   b. **False**. The defects are in catabolic pathways involving lysosomal hydrolases.
   c. **True**. This enzyme removes an N-acetylgalactosamine from ganglioside GM_2.
   d. **False**. The defective enzymes are lysosomal.
   e. **False**. Sphingomyelin accumulating in Niemann–Pick disease is not a glycolipid.

5. a. **True**. G6PD deficiency leads to haemolytic anaemia (favism).
   b. **False**. It is methionine metabolism that is affected.
   c. **False**. Sphingomyelin accumulates, not ganglioside.
   d. **False**. In PKU type I it is phenylalanine hydroxylase that is defective.
   e. **False**. It is the urea cycle that is defective.

6. a. **True**. The sensitivity is greater and potential renal problems avoided.
   b. **True**. False negatives are possible if the child isn't challenged.
   c. **False**. In PKU a 1-month delay can severely affect mental ability.
   d. Obviously, this is the single best answer.
   e. **False**. Since c is incorrect.

True/false answers

1. **True**. Codon 6 of the beta chain changes from GAG in HbA to GUG in HbS. Valine substitutes for glutamate.
2. **True**. Tyrosinase is defective and this enzyme is required for melanin synthesis.
3. **False**. It stands for polymerase chain reaction.
4. **False**. Inheritance is autosomal dominant.
5. **True**. The palindromic sequence occurs in four to eight base pairs of DNA.
6. **True**.
7. **False**. Duchenne's muscular dystrophy is an example of a disorder for which prenatal diagnosis was available before dystrophin was identified as the affected protein.
8. **True**. It is the linkage that is critical in terms of their utility in disease diagnosis.
9. **True**. The DNA probes contain radioactive or fluorescent markers.
10. **False**. Bacteria cannot deal with introns nor can they carry out post-translational modifications of the required protein.
11. **False**. Southern was the name of the scientist who developed the technique.
12. **True**. It corresponds to the exons, whereas the genomic library would include exons and introns.

Short essay answer

Both disorders are autosomal recessive. However, a key difference between them is that at this time there is no treatment for TSD, whereas for PKU adoption of a strict dietary regimen prevents the development of the major symptom, mental retardation. TSD homozygotes die within 3 years of birth after a life that features blindness and mental retardation.

In TSD, the important testing that has been introduced is to find heterozygotes in the population. This is done by measuring the defective enzyme, hexosaminidase A, in blood samples from susceptible populations. Heterozygotes have half the normal amount of the enzyme. Heterozygotes who are married and wish to have children are offered amniocentesis carried out around week 13 during any pregnancy. Amniocytes are cultured and hexosaminidase A measured. The absence of activity indicates that the fetus is a homozygote for the disorder. Heterozygotes will have half normal activity but that ensures them a normal life.

In PKU, it is the newborn baby that is evaluated. The baby's phenylalanine hydroxylase activity is determined by measuring their blood phenylalanine. PKU infants will have highly elevated blood phenylalanine levels, which appear after the baby has had several meals containing protein. The finding of elevated phenylalanine in a dried spot of blood leads to a follow-up test for confirmation of the finding. Since PKU babies are normal (because their mother prevented phenylalanine accumulating), the testing (Guthrie test) is carried out on all newborn babies. Since PKU can also be caused by defects in the biopterin coenzyme for phenylalanine hydroxylase, dihydropteridine reductase is measured in babies who have hyperphenylalaninaemia since the therapy for this form of PKU is more complicated.

Index

Notes: Page numbers in **bold** indicate the importance of the text, those followed by "f" and "t" refer to figures and tables/boxed material respectively. Question and Answer sections are indicated in the form 15Q/17A.

F-1-P aldolase, 102f
Fabry's disease, 138
Facilitated diffusion, 50, 76, 76f, 79, 79t
FAD, 170Q/172A, 264, 265, 272A
  enzyme prosthetic group, 28, 272A
  synthesis, 169
FADH$_2$, reducing power in metabolism, 71, 72, 72f, 88
Familial hypercholesterolaemia (FH), 134t, 140Q/142A, 141Q/143A, 288
Familial mitochondrial encephalomyopathy, 288t
Farnesyl pyrophosphate, 133, 133f
Fasted state, 106Q/108–109A, **147–149,** 158Q/160A, 159Q/161A, 162t, 225
  ACC regulation, 128
  adipose tissue, 151–152, 153f
  amino acid metabolism, 226
  brain metabolism, 99, **149–150,** 150f
  counter-regulatory hormones, 149, 159Q/161A
  glucagon, 148, 148t
  glucose metabolism, 100–102, 101f, 148
  glycogen metabolism, 98f, 99
  lipid metabolism, 226
  liver metabolism, 150–151, 152f
  muscle metabolism, 152, 155f
Fast-twitch muscle cells, mitochondria, 156
Fat(s), **260–261**
  coronary heart disease and, 261, 261t
  dietary, 77–78, 260, 261, 269Q/271A
  digestion and absorption, 77, 78
  energy stored in, 260
  metabolism, 71–95
    see also Fatty acid oxidation
  mobilisation, 84f, 157
  see also Fatty acid(s); Lipid(s); specific fats
Fat-soluble vitamins, 270Q/272A, 272t
Fat tissue see Adipose tissue
Fatty acid(s), 77f, 91–92Q/94A
  calcium absorption and, 267
  cell membranes; 48, 49, 49f
  chylomicrons, 130, 131f, 132, 132t, 225
  essential, 261
  glucogenicity, 106Q/108A, 127, 128f
  metabolism, 72, 73f, 91–92Q/93–95A, 131f, 159Q/161A
    adipose tissue, 151, 152, 153f
    brain, 149–150
    kidney, 155
    liver, 150, 151, 151f, 152f, 225–226
    muscle, 152, 154–155, 155f, 157
    vitamin requirements, 270Q/272A
    see also Fatty acid oxidation
  mobilisation, 83, 84f, 148, 151–152, 157
  oxidation see Fatty acid oxidation
  structure, 6Q/8A, 77, 77f
  synthesis, **127–129,** 128f, 129f, 140Q/142A, 151f
    oxidation vs., 144t
Fatty acid desaturases, 129
Fatty acid oxidation, 73f, 83–86, 84f, 92Q/94–95A, 157
  ATP yield, 90
  fasted vs. fed state, 150, 152f, 155f, 158Q/160A
  synthesis vs., 144t
Fatty acid synthase (FAS) multiple enzyme protein, 127, 128, 128f, 141Q/143A
Fatty acyl-CoA, 130, 130f, 136f
Fatty acyl-CoA dehydrogenase, 265
Fatty liver, 225, 226, 231Q/232A

Favism see Glucose-6-phosphate dehydrogenase (G6PDH), deficiency
Fed state, **145–147,** 145t, 225
  adipose tissue, 151, 153f
  brain metabolism, **149–150,** 150f
  glucose metabolism, 100–102, 101f
  glycogen metabolism, 98f, 99, 159Q/161A, 162t
  insulin actions, **146–147,** 146f, 147f, 147t, 148f, 159Q/161A
  liver metabolism, 150, 151f
  muscle metabolism, 152, 154f
Ferric iron, 60, 65, 268
Ferrochelatase, 121, 121f, 124Q/126A
Ferrous iron, 60, 61, 112, 121f, 268
Fetal haemoglobin, oxygen affinity, 62, 63f, 66Q/68A
FH$_4$ see Tetrahydrofolate (FH$_4$)
fibre formation, 17, 209f, 210
fibrin, clot formation, 276–277, 282Q/284A
fibrinogen, 276, 277t, 283Q/284A
fibrinolysis, 276, 279–280
fibrin transamidase, 277
fish oils, 261
Flavin adenine dinucleotide see FAD
Flavoprotein enzymes, 264
Fleming, A., lysozyme discovery, 37t
Fluoride, nutrition, **268**
5-Fluoro-orotate, 168t
5-Fluorouracil (5-FU), 168t, 173A
Fluorouridylate (F-dUMP), anti-cancer drugs, 168t
FMN, 264, 265, 272A
Folate (folic acid), 118, 264, 266, 266t, 267
  pregnancy and, 266, 266t, 270Q/272A
  synthesis, 266, 270Q/271–272A
  'trapping,' 123Q/125A, 267
Folding, polypeptide chains, 20, 20f
Follicle-stimulating hormone (FSH), 239, 240t, 242, 242f, 243, 253Q/255A
'Food Guide Pyramid,' Department of Agriculture, US, 259
Formaldehyde, tetrahydrofolate (FH$_4$) metabolism, 120f
Formic acid (formate), 120f, 165f
Formylmethionyl-tRNA^{Met}, 205, 205f, 212Q/215A
Free energy change (ΔG), in metabolic pathways, 73, 91Q/93A
Fructokinase, 102f, 291t
Fructose, 74, 75f, 92Q/94A, 106Q/108A
  absorption, 76, 76f
  glucose production from, 100f, 102, 102f
  intolerance, hereditary, 291t
  liver metabolism, 225
Fructose 1,6-biphosphatase (F-1,6-BPase), 100f, 101, 101f, 105Q/107A
Fructose 1,6-bisphosphate (F-1,6-BP), 100f, 101, 101f, 102, 102f, 280f
Fructose 1-phosphate, 102f
Fructose 1-phosphate aldolase, defects, 291t
Fructose 2,6-bisphosphatase (F-2,6-BPase) activity, of BFE, 101
Fructose 2,6-bisphosphate (F-2,6-BP), 101, 101f, 102, 105Q/107A
Fructose 6-phosphate, 100f, 101, 101f, 103, 104f, 280f
Fructose 6-phosphate/fructose 1,6-bisphosphate substrate cycle, 101, 105Q/107A, 109A
Fructose membrane carrier (GLUT5), 76

Fructosuria, 74t
Fruit fly, genome size, 176t
Fumarate, 34f, 114f, 115, 164
Fumarylacetoacetate hydrolase, defects, 289t

G1 phase, cell cycle, 183
G2 phase, cell cycle, 183
Gal-1-P uridyltransferase, 102f
Galactocerebroside, 137f, 138
Galactokinase, 102f, 291t
Galactosaemia, 103t, 291t
Galactose, 74, 75f, 92Q/94A, 103t, 106Q/108A, 291t
  absorption, 76, 76f
  glucose production from, 100, 100f, 102, 102f
  liver metabolism, 225
  transport, 76, 77f
Galactose 1-phosphate, 102f
Galactose-1-phosphate uridyltransferase, defects, 103t, 291t
Galactosuria, 74t
γ-Carboxyglutamate, 278–279, 279f
γ-Linolenic acid, essential fatty acid, 129
Gangliosides, 137, 137f, 138t, 141Q/143A
  see also Tay-Sachs disease (TSD)
Gap phases, cell cycle, 183
Garrod, inborn errors of metabolism, 287
Gas transport, by blood, 59–69, 66–67Q/68–69A
Gastric secretory mucoprotein, 266
Gastrin, 78
Gastrointestinal activity, endocrine regulation, 236t
Gastrointestinal hormones, role in digestion, 78
Gaucher's disease, 138
G cells, gastrin production, 78
GDP, allosteric activator of glutamate dehydrogenase, 115
Gelatin, from collagen denaturation, 24Q/26A
Gene(s), 287
  analysis, 294
  control of protein synthesis, **175**
  disease-causing changes, 288t
    see also Genetic disorders; Mutation(s)
  eukaryotic, 197, 197f
  expression, 22, 148f, 248, 253Q/255A, 256A, 288, 295
  Human Genome project, 295
  inheritance, 287–288, 296Q/298A
  prokaryotic, 198Q/200A
  shuffling, immunoglobulins, 276, 283Q/284A
  viruses as model systems, 217, 224A
    see also DNA; Genome(s); Protein synthesis; Transcription; Translation
Gene therapy, 224A, 292
Genetic code, **177,** 198Q/200A, 202, 211–212Q/214A, 213Q/215A
  see also Codons
Genetic disorders, **287–299**
  diagnosis, 292–294
  Human Genome project, 295
  metabolic disorders see Inborn errors of metabolism
  mutations causing, 288t
  patterns of inheritance, 287–288, 296Q/298A

GnRH (gonadotrophin-releasing hormone), 240t
Goitre, 244, 268
Golgi apparatus, 47, 47f, 48t, 53, 141Q/143A, 208, 210
Gonad(s), hypothalamic–pituitary–gonadal axis, 242, 242f, 243
Gonadotrophin-releasing hormone (GnRH, LHRH), 240t, 242, 242f
Gout, 169, 170Q/172A, 171Q/173A
G proteins, 53f, 247, 247t, 248, 248f, 250f, 253Q/255A
Granulosa cell, 242f, 243
Graves disease, **244**, 252Q/254A
Growth, endocrine regulation, 236t
Growth factors, signal transduction system, 249
Growth hormone (hGH), 147, 148, 149, 159Q/161A, 239, **239**, 295
Growth hormone-inhibiting hormone (somatostatin), 239, 240t, 247
Growth hormone-releasing hormone (GHRH, GRF), 239, 240t
GTP (guanosine triphosphate)
    binding to G proteins, 247, 248f, 250f
    protein synthesis, 205
    RNA synthesis, 191
    synthesis, 164, 165f, 166
GTPase activity, of G proteins, 247, 248f
Guanidinoacetate, creatine synthesis, 123Q/125A
Guanine, 164t, 177, 178f, 185Q/187A, 204
    base-pairing, 179, 180f
    catabolism, 169, 169f
    Lesch-Nyhan syndrome, 166t
    synthesis, 166, 166f, 166t
Guanosine, 164t, 169f
    see also specific nucleotides
Guanylate *see* GMP (guanosine monophosphate)
Guanylate cyclase, activation by NO, 251
Guthrie test, 290t, 296Q/298A

HaeIII, cleavage site, 294f
Haem, 12, 28, 61, 66Q/68A, 121f
    bilirubin synthesis in spleen, **227–228**, 228f
    in haemoglobin *see* Haemoglobin
    iron, 12, 60, 61, 65, 66Q/68A, 268
    synthesis, **120–122**, 121f, 122t, 124Q/126A, 126A
Haem–haem interactions, 61
Haemoglobin, **60–65**, 66–67Q/68–69A, 228, 229, 268
    allosteric effects, 61–62, 61f, 62f, 63f, 63t, 64, 66–67Q/68A
    "as enzyme," 67Q/69A
    Bohr effect, 62, 62f
    carbon dioxide binding/transport, 64, 65f, 66Q/68A, 67Q/68–69A, 67Q/68A
    carbon monoxide binding, 62, 63, 63t, 66Q/68A
    haptoglobulin–haemoglobin complex, 274
    mRNA splicing, 197
    oxygen binding/affinity, 11, 12, 60f, 61–63, 61f, 62f, 66Q/68A, 67Q/68A
    physicochemical properties, 66Q/68A
    structure, 16, 60–61, 60f, 66Q/68A
        alpha helical segments, 26A
        haem-prosthetic group, 28, 60, 61, 66Q/68A, 227

histidine residues, 60f, 61
    quaternary, 21
    subunits, 24Q/26A, 60, 60f
    tertiary, 20
    synthesis, iron requirement, 268
    see also specific types
Haemoglobin A (HbA), 65
Haemoglobin M (HbM), 65
Haemoglobinopathies, 64, 65, 65t, 202
    sickle cell anaemia *see* Sickle cell disease
    thalassaemias, 197t, 288t
Haemoglobin S (HbS sickle cell haemoglobin), 64, 65, 65t, 67Q/69A, 296Q/298A
Haemolysis, 229, 263
Haemolytic anaemia, 291t
    G6PDH deficiency, 105Q/107–108A, 105Q/107A, 281t, 282Q/284A, 291t, 296Q/298A
    pyruvate kinase deficiency, 281t, 282Q/284A
Haemophilia A, 278t, 288, 295
Haemophilia B (Christmas disease), 278t, 288
Haemoproteins, biliverdin production, 228
Haemorrhagic disease of the newborn, 264
Haem oxygenase, 228, 228f, 268
Hageman factor, 277t
Half-chair conformation, monosaccharide, 37, 37f
Haptocorrin, vitamin B12 absorption, 266
Haptoglobulin, 274, 274t, 282Q/284A
HDL (high-density lipoproteins), 130, 131t
Heart disease *see* Coronary heart disease (CHD)
Heat, denaturation of proteins, 16
Heavy H chains, immunoglobulin G, 21, 275, 275f, 276
Helical grooves, in DNA double helix, 179
Helicases, 184
Helices
    alpha helix, 17, 18f
    DNA double helix, 177, 177f, 179, 179f, 185Q/187A
    triple helix, 17
Heparin, anticoagulation, 279, 282Q/284A
Hepatitis, liver function tests, 231Q/232A
Hepatocytes, 228f, 230
Hereditary fructose intolerance, 291t
Hereditary non-polyposis colon cancer, 288t
Herpes, 218t
Heterotrophs, 72
Heterotropic allosteric effects, haemoglobin, 61, 61f, 62, 62f, 64
Heterozygosity, 67Q/69A, 138t, 287, 288
HETEs (hydroeicosatetranoic acids), 138
Hexokinase, 29, 35t, 92Q/94A
    ATP hydrolysis prevention, 36
    enzyme specificity, 27, 28, 28f
    glucokinase isozyme, 33, 33f
    glycogen metabolism, 98f
    kinetics, 33, 33f
Hexosaminidase A, Tay-Sachs disease (TSD), 138t, 140Q/142A, 292
High-density lipoproteins *see* HDL (high-density lipoproteins)

'High energy' bonds, in ATP, 71
High molecular weight kininogen (HMWK), 278
High speed centrifugation, ribosome isolation, 203
Histamine, 117, 138
Histidine, 14f, 20, 23Q/25A, 117
    in haemoglobin, 16, 60f, 61, 63, 64, 65
    in serine proteases, 38, 38f
    tetrahydrofolate (FH4) metabolism, 120f
Histones, 12, 176, 183, 184, 184f, 198Q/200A
HIV/AIDS, 218t
    chemotherapy targets, 34t, 220t
    host infection, 219, 222Q/223A
    replication, 220
HMG-CoA, cholesterol synthesis, 132, 133f
HMG-CoA reductase (HMGCoAR), 133, 133f, 134f, 140Q/142A
    inhibitors, 133, 133t
Holoenzyme, 43Q/45A
Homocysteine, 120f, 266t, 289t
Homocysteine-N5-methyl-FH4 transferase (methionine synthase), 119, 123Q/125A, 267
Homocysteinuria, 289t
Homogentisic acid, alkaptonuria, 287
Homogentisic acid oxidase, defects, 289t
Homotropic allosteric effects, haemoglobin, 61–62, 61f, 62f
Homozygosity, 287, 288
Hormone(s), 12, 39, 98f, 99, 235, 252–253Q/254–257A, 274t
    adrenal, **245–246**
    counter-regulatory, 147, 149, 151, 153f, 159Q/161A
    DNA-binding, 199Q/200A
    hypothalamus, **239–240**, 240t
    inactivation in liver, 227
    lipid-soluble, **249–250**, 251f
    mechanisms of action, **246–251**
    physiochemical properties, **238–239**, 239t, 252Q/254A
    pituitary, **239–240**, 240t
    receptors, 53, 53f, 54Q/56A, 249, 250, 251f, 252Q/254A
    structures, 236f, 237f, 238f
    synthesis, **236–238**, 237f, 252Q/254A
    water-soluble, **246–249**, 247f, 247t, 248f, 250f
    see also specific hormones
Hormone-response element (HRE), 250, 251f, 253Q/256A
Hormone-sensitive lipase (HSL), 141Q/143A, 151, 153f, 157, 158Q/160–161A
    adipose tissue, 148, 149
Host–parasite relationship, viruses as model systems, **217–218**
HPETEs (hydroperoxyeicosatetraenoic acids), 138, 139f
Human chorionic gonadotrophin (hCG), 243
Human genome, 176t, 287, 295
Human Genome project, 295
Human immunodeficiency virus *see* HIV/AIDS
Hunger, starch consumption, 260
Huntington's disease, inheritance, 288
Hydration, 4, 6Q/8A
Hydrochloric acid, protein denaturation, 111

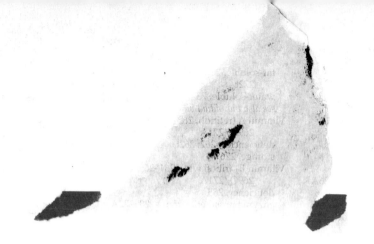